Clinical Investigation
of Respiratory Disease

Clinical Investigation
of
Respiratory Disease

EDITED BY

T. J. H. Clark
MD, BSc, FRCP

Consultant Physician
Guy's Hospital and Brompton Hospital

Professor of Thoracic Medicine
Guy's Hospital Medical School

LONDON
CHAPMAN AND HALL

First published 1981
by Chapman and Hall Ltd
11 New Fetter Lane, London EC4P 4EE

© 1981 Chapman and Hall

Phototypeset in Linotron 202 Times by
Western Printing Services Limited, Bristol
Printed in Great Britain
at the University Press, Cambridge

British Library Cataloguing in Publication Data

Clinical investigation of respiratory
disease.
  1. Respiratory organs – Diseases
  I. Clark, T. J. H.
  616.2   RC731

  ISBN 0 412 15780 2

Contents

Contributors

P. Borum, Assistant Professor, Otopathological Laboratory, University Department of ENT-Diseases, Rigshospitalet, Denmark.

Sherwood Burge, Consultant Physician, East Birmingham and Solihull Hospitals, Department of Thoracic Medicine, East Birmingham Hospital, Birmingham, UK.

T. J. H. Clark, Consultant Physician, Guy's and Brompton Hospitals, Professor of Thoracic Medicine, Guy's Hospital Medical School, London, UK.

G. M. Cochrane, Consultant Physician, Department of Thoracic Medicine, Guy's Health District, London, UK.

Peter Cole, Senior Lecturer in Medicine (Thoracic), Host Defence Unit, Cardiothoracic Institute and Hon. Consultant Physician to Brompton Hospital, London, UK.

John V. Collins, Consultant Physician, Brompton Hospital and St Stephen's Hospital, London, UK.

P. D. B. Davies, Consultant Physician, Whittington and University College Hospitals, London, UK.

D. M. Denison, Director, Lung Function Unit, Brompton Hospital, London, UK.

F. Fazio, Director, Laboratory of Nuclear Medicine, Ospedale S. Raffaele, University of Milano, Italy; formerly Consultant Physician, MRC Cyclotron Unit, Hammersmith Hospital, London, UK.

D. M. Geddes, Consultant Physician, Brompton and London Chest Hospitals, London, UK.

John M. Grange, Reader in Microbiology, Cardiothoracic Institute, Brompton Hospital, London, UK.

Patricia L. Haslam, Non-clinical Senior Lecturer, Department of Thoracic Medicine, Cardiothoracic Institute, London, UK.

Norman L. Jones, Professor of Medicine and Director, Ambrose Cardiorespiratory Unit, McMaster University Health Sciences Centre, Hamilton, Ontario, Canada.

Ian H. Kerr, Consultant Radiologist, Brompton Hospital, London, UK.

N. Mygind, Senior Lecturer, Otopathological Laboratory, University ENT Department, Rigshospitalet, Copenhagen, Denmark.

A. R. Nath, Consultant Physician, Harefield Hospital, Harefield, Middlesex, UK.

A. J. Newman Taylor, Consultant Physician, Brompton and London Chest Hospitals, London and Honorary Senior Lecturer, Department of Clinical Immunology, Cardiothoracic Institute, London, UK.

M. C. F. Pain, Director of Thoracic Medicine, Royal Melbourne Hospital, Professorial Associate, University of Melbourne, Australia.

M. Pedersen, Senior Registrar, Department of Paediatric Lung Disease TG and Danish Cystic Fibrosis Center, Rigshospitalet, Copenhagen, Denmark.

Margaret Turner-Warwick, Professor of Medicine (Thoracic Medicine), Cardiothoracic Institute, Brompton Hospital, London, UK.

Donald C. Zavala, Professor of Medicine, Director of the Pulmonary Diagnostic Laboratories, University of Iowa Hospitals and Clinics, Iowa City, Iowa, USA.

Preface

There have been many advances in the investigation of lung disease over the past decade. These have arisen in part as the result of new techniques, such as fibreoptic endoscopy but also because of our greater understanding of the basic pathogenesis of pulmonary disease. Thus, increased knowledge has led to new ideas about investigation which in turn has stimulated the development of novel diagnostic methods.

Most of these recent advances are now in everyday use and I think it is time for us to take stock of them. It is for this reason that I have persuaded a number of my colleagues to review our present state of knowledge and I am most grateful to them for their willing collaboration in this venture. There is inevitably some overlap between chapters and the occasional conflict of views but the subject fairly easily divides into a number of headings which have provided me with the basis for the organization of this book.

The authors inevitably have employed different approaches to their chapters as most investigations can be reviewed in a variety of ways. Thus, Dr Zavala has concentrated on providing details of how to carry out a bronchoscopy and this practical approach is used in other chapters. Dr Kerr has mainly concentrated on radiological techniques because a diagnostic approach would have required a much more substantial contribution and has been covered fully in other books on the subject. Dr Denison has used a more fundamental approach and has discussed the practical aspects of testing lung function in the context of an appreciation of the physiological basis for employing the tests. Other chapters have a more clinical flavour as they relate the investigations to diseases and I have tried in the introductory chapter to make clear the essential need to relate investigations to clinical requirements. Clinical skills provide the initial and primary items of information upon which the need for further investigation is critically chosen and planned.

Paradoxically, we now are in a position where we have very powerful diagnostic aides at our disposal which can obscure diagnosis by data overload which means that an important skill of the clinician is to be selective and critical in his choice of investigations. One of the main purposes of this book is to help clinicians make that choice wisely. The book is therefore written for all those who see patients with lung disease which will, therefore, include most practising physicians and general practitioners. As the authors have provided the scientific and clinical basis for investigations of lung disease, I hope the book will also be of value to medical students and those who have an interest in the pathogenesis of disease.

I asked authors to provide a readable account of their subject and we have not aimed to supply an exhaustive review full of references. I am aware, however, that readers like a reasonable bibliography both for further reading and to amplify the text and I hope a sensible compromise has been achieved. The size and scope of the bibliography depends on its need and varies from chapter to chapter and I am fully responsible for any miscalculations on this score.

This book would not have been possible without the collaboration of my colleagues but I am also indebted to all the secretaries who have helped to make this book possible; special thanks are due to Joanna Brazier and Alex McVinnie. I am especially grateful to Dr John Rees, whose advice was always of value. Finally, I must thank my wife and children who have given me their full support and encouragement in the preparation of this book.

June 1981   T. J. H. Clark

CHAPTER ONE

Introduction

T. J. H. Clark

Looking after patients depends on information and this applies as much to respiratory diseases as to any other system. This book sets out to review how laboratories and diagnostic departments can provide useful information and help clinicians in its interpretation and application. All information can be valuable in the management of patients and much of it is obtained in the clinic or by the bedside. This clinical information may be just as important as data obtained from the investigations reviewed throughout the rest of this book as the importance of information depends not so much upon its source or apparent scientific veracity but upon its marginal value with respect to the problem posed by the patient. The marginal value of a symptom can often exceed the most exacting laboratory investigation.

This becomes particularly important as investigations become more complex, more invasive and more dependent on an increased knowledge about abnormal structure and function. By tradition, the clinical process starts with the history and passes through physical examination to investigations to reach a diagnosis; this historic approach has helped to create the idea that investigations provide the important marginal data upon which a final diagnosis can be made and management determined. In reality, the diagnostic process is bi-directional with clinical information both cueing and helping with the interpretation of investigations and providing the practical bedrock upon which additional intervention can be judged.

The clinician, therefore, assembles all pieces of information from whatever source and, although they are basically equivalent, weights them according to his judgement about their discriminant function. Thus, a cough in isolation may mean little to the clinician but associated with an abnormal chest radiograph indicates the need for further investigation, particularly if the abnormality on radiograph is of recent origin and the cough persistent. On the other hand, a normal radiograph does not mean that a clinician can ignore a cough if it is associated with another piece of information, such as wheezing and sputum production. This collection of symptoms assumes even greater importance if the patient is a non-smoker and wakes up at night short of breath, as this suggests bronchial asthma. If a patient is known to have bronchial asthma and has a normal radiograph, no further action may be required which may also be appropriate if a radiological abnormality consists of a known complication of asthma such as broncho-pulmonary aspergillosis. Thus, the interpretation of these various items of information, depends largely upon their relationship with each other and upon the likely consequences of that association; this is well known to those interested in diagnostic decision theory and devising computer assistance for diagnosis. The weighting of information has no absolute value but depends upon the clinical context; a cough may be an important piece of clinical information in one context and trivial in another.

The clinician collects pieces of information as soon as the patient walks through the door. When considering respiratory disease, perceptive clinicians will note the exercise capacity of patients during interview and examination. Signs such as cyanosis and clubbing will also be quickly sought as will any obvious deformity of the chest wall. These items of information will be added to those culled by history taking, which usually takes the form of directing questions to confirm or refute clinical hypotheses entertained as soon as the history unfolds. If the patient complains of nocturnal dyspnoea with wheeze, clinicians usually work on the assumption that the likely diagnosis is either bronchial or cardiac asthma or some other conditions which may resemble them; subsequent questions are usually directed towards resolving this diagnostic dilemma. The patient will be asked about other cardiac symptoms and further respiratory symptoms of asthma.

The clinician therefore finds all information of value and in the context of this book, it is important to remember that history taking still remains pre-eminent. Information has to be obtained from fellow human beings and some communication with patients is required before more complex investigations can be instituted although computer interrogation has an increasing role in selection. In the process of making human contact, a good history can be obtained which often makes the need for further investigations unnecessary. A detailed history may enable complex and expensive investigations to be avoided or can provide the clinician with the necessary information to justify further investigations and to judge their value to both patient and physician. Furthermore, a good clinical rapport itself helps the investigator and facilitates a successful investigation by gaining co-operation and goodwill.

The constant aim of a clinician should be to acquire sufficient knowledge about the results of investigations to sharpen his ability to do without them or ask for them more critically. Thus, clinicians should try to relate clinical features to information provided by non-clinical means and, by doing so, identify the value of signs and symptoms in relation to the results of investigations. Computer-aided diagnosis demands such an appraisal. In respiratory disease, for example, studies have shown that physical signs are poor predictors of airways obstruction but symptoms can provide useful information both about lung function and its trends. It is a useful and sobering exercise to predict *in writing* what the investigation will reveal when asking for it. This policy need not be taken to excess but can enable clinicians to look at investigations critically and to know why they are being done. Such a critical approach will also enable clinicians to know the weakness of items of clinical information; the clinician who looks after asthmatic patients without measuring peak flow is materially handicapped as peak flow or another assessment of lung function provides such valuable additional information as to improve significantly clinical management. At the same time regular peak flow measurements improve the ability of patients to identify clinical progress and co-operate with treatment. Where the test can be simply obtained without much cost to patient or physician, it is churlish not to take advantage of the additional information provided. On the other hand, clinicians must avoid investigating patients for every possible contingency in every conceivable way to rule out disease as a substitute for taking a good history and carrying out an orderly examination. A combination of critically applied bedside skills can thus eliminate many investigations and much cost of hardship to patients.

1.1 Practical aspects

By the very nature of the traditional clinical process, most information comes sequentially and clinicians often take advantage of the enforced delay introduced by the time required to deploy investigations. This judicious use of time (also known as constructive delay) is based upon knowledge about the natural history of respiratory diseases as many are self-limiting and require no detailed investigation or are untreatable. Thus, a patient who presents with an acute febrile illness with cough, sputum and pleurisy, is usually not investigated substantially even if his chest radiograph is abnormal, because the majority of these patients have a short-lived illness which recovers spontaneously. Even if the chest radiograph remains abnormal most clinicians would not begin further investigations until some weeks have elapsed and the febrile episode has entirely cleared. Similarly, investigation for asthma is not employed as soon as children have an attack of wheezy bronchitis; the child has to earn further investigations by having repeated attacks which, in turn, makes the diagnosis of asthma more likely and may indicate the need for further investigations to confirm this diagnosis and lead to appropriate treatment being started.

As patients need to have symptoms to seek medical attention, history and physical examination are usually the first pieces of information obtained and can usually provide a diagnosis. There are times, however, when the sequence is reversed, as patients are increasingly being screened for disease and this having been identified, the patient is then interviewed and asked about symptoms and subsequently examined (see Chapter 5). This emphasizes the iterative nature of information and investigation and that clinical data can be used in the same marginal manner as other more conventional investigations. It is important to appreciate that clinical data such as symptom enquiry are as much an investigation as the most complex technological investigation employed by clinicians.

1.2 Cost benefit approach

Clinicians ask for investigations based upon their calculations of the need for them but this, in turn, is conditioned by the cost of those investigations and the benefits produced by them. Cost is assessed in terms of patient inconvenience and time spent on the test, as well as the actual financial cost of carrying it out. In general, tests which are costly and do not provide useful marginal information are less readily done than those tests which are simple and highly discriminant. This involves making a judgement as to the likely benefit of the results of an investigation and as, by definition, the results are not known in advance, it means that there is a temptation to do an investigation on the off-chance that it might reveal useful information. This view needs to be resisted strongly, particularly for those tests which are potentially harmful to patients and costly to perform.

1.3 Procedural constraints

The deployment of investigations is also affected by the likelihood of certain diagnoses or the need for specific action. When a patient presents with cough, haemoptysis, radiological shadowing and a history of heavy cigarette consumption, the clinician may go straight to diagnostic bronchoscopy and miss out tomography and other less direct tests, particularly if the patient is young with good lung function and has other information suggesting operative treatment if the lesion happens to be a bronchial squamous carcinoma. The timing and organization of investigations may also be influenced by immediate practical needs. Thus, if the patient is very ill and clearly requires admission to hospital, out-patient investigations will be dispensed with and will be carried out in hospital, often bunched together in a less orderly manner than those carried out in sequence as an out-patient.

Other constraints are more obvious and less rational but on the other hand assume greater importance. These include the availability of such diagnostic agents as 81m krypton (see Chapter 7) or a computerized tomography (CT) whole body scanner (see Chapter 6). If these are not available, clearly the tests cannot be carried out or the patient will have to be transferred to a centre where they are available. In locations where such facilities are not available, or no one is trained to carry out diagnostic bronchoscopy, patient care will be dictated by such deficiencies and the clinician's role will be to select those patients who require further investigations. This places an even greater premium upon critical use of history, physical examination and simple radiological procedures. Such a selective system requires close co-operation between the referring clinicians and specialist centres so that both are clear as to criteria for selection and the need for further communication if unexpected problems emerge. These criteria depend on the local organization of health care and prevalence of disease; for example, what may be appropriate for London may not apply to New York or Cairo and may be quite wrong for African rural areas.

1.4 Use of information

Once a clinician has begun to assemble items of information, be they clinical or laboratory based, such data are sorted in such a way as to provide for diagnosis, an assessment of severity of the abnormality, prognosis and the provision of information suitable for judging the response to any treatment given. Thus, the uses to which information is put depend upon these different needs, which can be briefly discussed in turn.

1.4.1 Diagnosis

The initial thrust of information gathering is towards reaching a diagnosis but it is not essential to have a diagnosis before treatment and further investigations can proceed. Failure to reach a diagnosis by preliminary investigations, usually requires further information to be sought and clinicians need to think ahead to decide on the likely cut-off point where further investigations are likely to be unrewarding and some treatment may be required without a diagnosis being reached.

Diagnosis is not always required solely for the management of an immediate clinical problem. Thus an abnormal shadow in a chest radiograph of an asymptomatic man of 80 years is investigated both to exclude treatable disease, i.e. tuberculosis, and also to diagnose disease such as cancer. Although no action may be required, knowledge of the diagnosis is often useful later if other disease or social disintegration supervenes.

1.4.2 Assessment of severity

If abnormality is detected by an item of information, it is often useful for clinicians to use this information to assess the severity of the abnormality detected. This assessment can apply to clinical items of information as well as to more easily quantified data such as lung function tests and helps determine treatment requirement, as well as the need for further investigations. Thus, severe pneumonia will demand a more forceful and resourceful application of microbiological tests to identify the causal agent than a trivial acute febrile respiratory illness for which most investigations are unnecessary. In another context, severe asthma will require more intensive treatment which may include corticosteroids as opposed to mild asthma which can often be controlled by inhaled bronchodilators alone taken on an occasional symptomatic basis. Thus, the severity of abnormality as determined by data of a clinical or laboratory nature is of considerable clinical importance even in the absence of a final diagnosis.

A comprehensive assessment of severity from time to time in chronic disease, e.g. sarcoidosis or cystic fibrosis, is also useful in identifying trends which may be missed if only strictly relevant tests are carried out *ad hoc*. Thus periodic assessment may help with prognosis (see below) and a better understanding of the natural history of disease.

1.4.3 Prognosis

The importance of information for diagnosis and assessment of severity lies in the ability it provides clinicians to make an accurate prognosis, although this can be done even in the absence of precision about a diagnosis. For example, patients with chronic airways obstruction are known to have a worse prognosis if the obstruction is severe and they have CO_2 retention; this does not require the clinician being able to define accurately the relative contributions of intrinsic airways disease or emphysema to the airways obstruction and prognosis. Prognosis also does not hinge exclusively on information from laboratory sources and this is exemplified by the prognostic information provided by smoking habit in those patients found to have a deficiency of α_1 anti-trypsin , or by information about working habit in those patients whose illness may be related to asbestos exposure. Thus, symptom enquiry about cigarette smoking and work are as useful prognostically as apparently more subtle tests of lung function or biochemistry.

1.4.4 Response to treatment

All items of information may also be used to enable clinicians and patients to assess response or monitor adverse effects of treatment. Success of asthmatic treatment may, therefore, be monitored by a questionnaire enquiring about dyspnoea, nocturnal episodes of wheezing and consumption of bronchodilator aerosol as well as recording peak flow measurements. This realization that clinical data could be as important as laboratory information led to the emergence of diary cards for monitoring asthmatic treatment but this can also be employed in the context of other diseases and it is a basic reason why most doctors simply ask patients if they feel any better as their preliminary assessment of response to treatment. This crude initial judgement is followed by an opinion as to whether the patient looks any better and it is only after these very general assessments are made that more specific measurements are employed and interpreted in the light of this broad clinical judgement.

1.4.5 Future use

Occasionally investigations can be justified when information is being systematically garnered to learn more about a disease even if it is of little immediate practical value. This should only be carried in circumstances when such information is likely to be put to such use and cannot be justified otherwise, especially if the information is costly to acquire and the investigation is significantly more hazardous than the disease.

1.5 This book

In this Introduction I have, at some length and with some repetition, attempted to try to introduce the subject by discussing how items of in-concentrate largely on laboratory-based methods for investigating respiratory disease. These techniques are of great value and have helped enormously in the ability of clinicians to manage patients but they have to be kept in perspective. The purpose of these introductory comments is to try to achieve a proper balance by emphasizing how important is a good history and examination, as such information may enable a more critical and useful application of the various procedures referred to in subsequent chapters of this book.

Most clinicians approach investigations strictly from the viewpoint of the problem immediately posed by each patient and, as such, a book explaining investigations from the point of view of the investigator rather than the problem may lose some of its clinical relevance. A more clinical approach would be to produce a book based upon the varieties of respiratory problems seen in clinical practice but such an approach does not allow a systematic review of the many methods of investigation now available to clinicians. For this reason, I felt it best to ask the authors to write about their own method of investigation in a way which will enable clinicians to judge their place in the management of any individual problem. In this chapter, I have attempted to try to introduce the subject by discussing how items of information can be used in concert to help in the management of patients and I have stressed the central importance of bedside skills. Without them, detailed investigations become monsters out of the control of patients and doctors. Only by having a detailed, clinical appreciation of the problem, can investigations be used in a thoughtful, critical manner to the best value for the individual patient. Only by acquiring a detailed history and a deep understanding of the individual patient in relation to his problem, can a clinician control the powerful technology at his disposal. Our problem is not so much identifying appropriate investigations but being strictly selective in choosing which ones are useful in individual circumstances. Thus the clinician is faced more often with the problem of deciding what *not* to do rather than the decision of what to do. Critical selection demands a higher level of education about the scientific basis of investigations, their strengths and weaknesses and above all their clinical usefulness. One investigation done unnecessarily is as much a fault as one too few. The purpose of this book is to aid clinicians in the critical choice of investigation so avoiding both faults.

Further reading

Campbell, E. J. M. (1976), Basic science, science and medical education. *Lancet*, **1**, 134–6.

Campbell, E. J. M., Scadding, J. G. and Roberts, R. S. (1979), The concept of disease. *Br. med. J.* **2**, 757–62.

Card, W. I. (1973), The computing approach to clinical diagnosis. *Proc. R. Soc.* B, **184**, 421–32.

de Dombal, F. T. (1973), Surgical diagnosis assisted by computer. *Proc. R. Soc.* B, **184**, 433–40.

Editorial (1979), The value of diagnostic tests. *Lancet*, **1**, 809–10.

Hampton, J. R. *et al.* (1975), Relative contributions of history-taking, physical examination and laboratory investigations to diagnosis and management of medical outpatients. *Br. med. J.*, **2**, 486–9.

Horrocks, J. C. and de Dombal, F. T. (1978), Clinical presentation of patients with 'dyspepsia'. Detailed symptomatic study of 360 patients. *Gut*, **19**, 19–26.

Lillington, G. A. and Jamplis, R. W. (1977), *A Diagnostic Approach to Chest Disease; Differential Diagnosis based on Roentgenographic Patterns*. 2nd edn, Williams and Wilkins.

Lucas, R. W. *et al.* (1976) Computer interrogation of patients. *Br. med. J.*, **2**, 623–5.

Sandler, G. (1979), Costs of unnecessary tests. *Br. med. J.*, **2**, 21–24.

Shim, M. D. and Williams, M. H. (1980), Evaluation of the severity of asthma: patients versus physicians. *Am. J. Med.*, **68**, 11–13.

CHAPTER TWO

Lung Sounds

A. R. Nath

Laennec distinguished breath sounds and their variations in health and disease from added sounds. He correlated what he heard at the bedside with what he found at postmortem. Our traditional interpretation of lung sounds is based on morphological changes in the lung. The advances in lung physiology and the improved methods of sound recording has made it possible to link lung sounds simultaneously with the dynamic events of breathing. The functional approach to lung sounds, as with the heart sounds, has improved our understanding of the underlying mechanism of sound production and enhanced their clinical significance. Auscultation of the lung should no longer be a ritual performance but a deliberate attempt at eliciting the functional and the structural abnormality in the lung.

2.1 Breath sounds

Breath sounds are continuous sounds of no definite pitch (Fig. 2.1). They contain a wide range of oscillations of random amplitude and frequency with approximately even distribution of sound energy. By analogy with white light, they are referred to as a respiratory white noise. The noise is produced by rapid fluctuations of gas pressure associated with random collisions of the gas molecules in the airways during air flow.

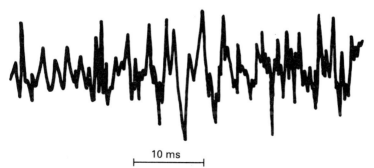

10 ms

Fig. 2.1 Breath sounds showing random variations in amplitude.

The source and generation of breath sounds is closely related to the pattern of gas flow in the airways. In the upper airways, trachea and the main bronchi, the gas flow is turbulent at physiological rates of breathing. As the bronchi divide and subdivide, the velocity of gas flow progressively diminishes towards the periphery. The transition from turbulent to laminar gas flow, however, does not occur until the gas stream reaches the most peripheral airways. The gas flow in the intermediate airways, which extend to about the fifteenth generation bronchi, remains non-laminar because its smooth passage is disturbed at the branching sites [1, 2]. Here the gas stream splits into layers, moving at different velocities with the formation of vortices which are carried downstream by the flow of gas. Since the flow velocity decreases at each bronchial division, the rate of formation of vortices and the velocity at which they are carried downstream falls. In the airways beyond the fifteenth generation of bronchi, the gas stream moves at a very slow velocity and the pattern approximates true laminar flow.

Breath sounds are likely to be generated only within those airways where the flow conditions are appropriate for oscillations to occur. The random movements of gas molecules in regions of turbulent airflow particularly favour sound production. An additional source of sound may be expected in the intermediate airways where abrupt changes in the direction of airflow at the branching sites result in the formation of turbulent eddies. However, the slow flow velocities at physiological rates of breathing in the peripheral airways and the alveoli are incompatible with sound production in a gas phase.

2.1.1 Breath sounds at the mouth

Auscultation of the lung is usually limited to listening with a stethoscope at various points on the chest wall. Noisy breathing at the mouth, however, is common in diffuse airway obstruction. Laennec described the loud breathing of an asthmatic patient which he could hear twenty paces away [3]. He believed that the noisy breathing originated in the pharynx since the breath sounds on the chest wall were not correspondingly loud. An alternative explanation was suggested in a study where the intensity of breath sounds at the mouth of healthy subjects was compared with the breath sounds of patients with asthma, chronic bronchitis, primary emphysema and of the patients with tracheal and bronchial stenosis [4]. For technical reasons, the measurements were confined to the inspiratory component of the breath sounds. The inspiratory sound intensity in asthma and chronic bronchitis was found to be greater than normal at similar inspiratory flow rates. In asthma and chronic bronchitis, the inspiratory sound intensity correlated significantly with the various indices of airways obstruction. The louder the inspiratory breath sounds, the lower the forced expiratory volume in the first second (FEV_1) and the peak expiratory flow rate. Isoprenaline inhalation reduced the inspiratory sound intensity and increased the FEV_1 while in exercise asthma, prior inhalation of isoprenaline prevented a rise in sound intensity. An exception to the rule were the patients with primary emphysema and the patients with bronchial and tracheal stenosis. The inspiratory sound intensity in primary emphysema was normal in the face of a very low FEV_1 while in bronchial and tracheal stenosis, the breath sounds were disproportionately loud when the FEV_1 was not greatly reduced (Fig. 2.2).

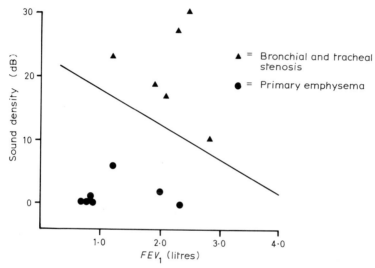

Fig. 2.2 The inspiratory sound intensity at the mouth in relation to FEV_1 in primary emphysema and in bronchial and tracheal stenosis. Regression line of sound intensity and FEV_1 is obtained from patients with chronic bronchitis.

Noisy breathing in patients with asthma and chronic bronchitis may originate exclusively in the upper respiratory tract as Laennec believed. Adduction of the vocal cords in response to changes in intrathoracic airway resistance has been shown in animals [5]. Such a reflex capable of varying the width of glotic aperture in parallel with calibre changes of the intrathoracic airways may also exist in man. The most plausible explanation, however, is that the loud breathing in asthma and bronchitis results from turbulence intensified in the narrowed proximal intrathoracic airways from the high velocity of gas flow. The limits of turbulent zone in diffuse airway obstruction is not defined but it is likely to extend beyond the main bronchi due to acceleration of gas flow in the narrowed airways. An inverse correlation between the inspiratory sound intensity and the FEV_1 suggests that the intermediate airways contribute to loud breathing in asthma and chronic bronchitis. The low FEV_1 in this situation may be explained by a sharp drop in the intrabronchial pressure as a result of high flow resistance in airways between the alveoli and the main bronchi. In primary emphysema, the inspiratory sound intensity is normal because the inspiratory calibre of the proximal bronchi is normal while the loss of elastic recoil and premature dynamic compression of the bronchi contribute to severe reduction in the expiratory flow. Inspiratory loud breath sounds in bronchial and tracheal stenosis result from turbulence intensified by the acceleration of gas flow at the site of narrowing.

2.1.2 Breath sounds through the chest wall

Breath sounds, it was suggested, originate in the upper airways, trachea and the main bronchi by turbulent gas flow and in the intermediate airways from disturbance to gas flow at the branching sites. The sound waves travel well in wide tubes and so the transmission of breath sounds to the mouth from the upper airways, trachea and the proximal bronchi is accompanied by a relatively small loss of frequency or sound energy. Breath sounds to the chest are transmitted through the lobar and segmental bronchi and across the lung and the chest wall. During their transmission the higher frequencies are selectively filtered out with the loss of sound energy. The spectrum of breath sounds at the mouth contain a range of frequencies from 200–2000 Hz; breath sounds at the upper chest contain frequencies from 200–800 Hz while at the lower chest the frequency band narrows from 200–400 Hz. Thus the lung and the chest wall act as a low pass filter with the greatest attenuation of frequencies at the lung bases.

Breath sounds over the trachea are harsh, loud and audible in both phases of respiration while the breath sounds at the lung bases are quieter, confined to inspiration with a short early expiratory component. The clinical distinction between the two varieties led Laennec to believe that the 'vesicular' breath sounds originated peripherally by the friction of air on the terminal bronchioles and the alveoli. In the 19th century a good deal of controversy followed between those who believed in the peripheral origin of breath sounds [6, 7] and those who questioned this view and suggested transmission of the breath sounds from a proximal source [8, 9]. More recent observations favour the transmission of breath sounds from the proximal bronchi.

The flow conditions known to prevail in the intrathoracic airways make it improbable that breath sounds can be produced by laminar flow in the terminal airways and the alveoli. Further evidence in support of this view comes from two sources. If the turbulent flow in the larger airways and the disturbed flow conditions in the intermediate airways generate breath sounds, the sound intensity should change when the density of the inspired gas is altered. However, if breath sounds are produced by laminar flow in the terminal airways and the alveoli, the sound intensity should not alter with the changes in gas density. The experimental observations [10, 11] confirm that the intensity of breath sounds recorded on the chest wall is reduced when a low density gas (helium) is inspired and increased in a high density gas (SF_6). The inference is therefore, that breath sounds are produced in the larger airways.

The heart beat is known to alter the flow conditions in different regions of the lung [12]. The effect of ventricular systole on the lung is two-fold. It is accompanied by a transient fall in intrathoracic pressure [13] and there is a sudden linear displacement of the heart away from the left lower lobe with consequent abrupt expansion of the adjoining pulmonary alveoli [14, 15]. The result is that during inspiration, volume flow rate is augmented in the left lobar bronchus synchronously with the cardiac systole. The magnitude of the volume rate of gas flow in the lobar and segmental bronchi caused by the heart beat can be large and may reach up to a third of the inspiratory volume flow rate. The pulsatile gas flow continues during breath holding when a large proportion of gas moving into the left lower lobe is directed to abruptly expanded alveoli in the vicinity of the heart.

Comparison of the velocity of gas flow in the terminal airways and the alveoli during inspiration and breath holding in subjects with marked cardiac pulsation is of interest. In inspiration the mean velocity of gas flow becomes progressively slower towards the periphery because of increase in the total cross-sectional area of the smaller airways. Thus at an inspiratory flow rate of 50 l/min, the velocity of gas flow in the terminal airways and the alveoli is quite small and is of the order of 5 mm/s. The velocity of gas flow in the peripheral airways of the left lower lobe during breath holding is not known. However, since the volume rate of cardiogenic gas flow in the lobar and segmental bronchi is large and mainly directed to the region of the left lower lobe adjoining the heart, it is probable that the velocity of gas flow in the abruptly distended alveoli adjacent to the heart is at least of the same order of magnitude as that during inspiration. If the breath sounds were generated by the slow rate of inspiratory flow into the peripheral airways and the alveoli, they should also be audible during breath holding in the region of the apex of the heart. The breath sounds are in fact absent during breath holding even in subjects with forceful cardiac pulsations.

Breath sounds on the chest wall evidently originate in the principal underlying lobar and segmental bronchi with a limited contribution from the upper airways. The contribution to breath sounds from airways beyond the segmental bronchi is uncertain but it is likely to be of diminishing importance as the flow rate progressively falls towards the periphery. The intensity of breath sounds in healthy subjects correlates with the regional differences in the flow rate [16]. At the lung apex, in the upright position, the peak intensity of the breath sounds parallels the highest flow rate at the beginning of inspiration. At the lung base, the peak intensity is reached at mid-vital capacity corresponding with the peak flow rate. In a study of patients with diffuse airway obstruction, the loudness of breath sounds on the chest wall was compared with the regional ventilation measured with xenon-133 [17]. A broad correlation was obtained between the loudness of the breath sounds and the corresponding regional ventilation. The correlation between the sound intensity and the regional flow rate is further improved if the transmitting properties of the lung and the chest wall is taken into account [18]. The intrathoracic source of breath sounds can also be inferred from subjects with cogwheel breathing in whom the inspiratory flow rate to the left lower lobe bronchus is augmented, synchronous with the heart beat. The rise in inspiratory flow rate intensifies turbulence in the lobar and the segmental bronchi and the inspiratory breath sounds become louder in systole.

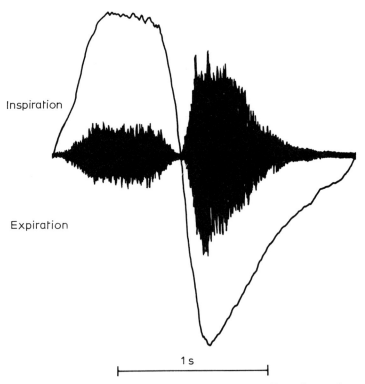

Inspiration

Expiration

1 s

Fig. 2.3 Variations in sound amplitude with the flow rate of breath sounds recorded at the mouth. The maximum amplitude of sound in early expiration and approximate even distribution in inspiration can be seen.

The observed difference in the duration of breath sounds over the trachea and the chest wall can be related to the threshold of hearing. The sound intensity in both phases of respiration parallels the flow rate (Fig. 2.3.) and over the trachea it remains above the hearing threshold throughout the respiratory cycle. The breath sounds on the chest wall are attenuated and contain low frequencies to which the ear is less sensitive. With reference to Fig. 2.4, it can be seen that the sound intensity is below the threshold of audibility in the later part of expiration because the sound intensity falls in parallel with the diminishing flow rate. The shorter duration of the expiratory sound may also be explained by different distribution of turbulence in inspiration and expiration. The turbulent eddies decay further towards the periphery in inspiration and the breath sounds are more readily transmitted to the chest wall. In expiration, the combined effect of the falling expiratory flow rate and decay of the turbulent eddies away from the listening point may account for the absent breath sounds in the later part of expiration.

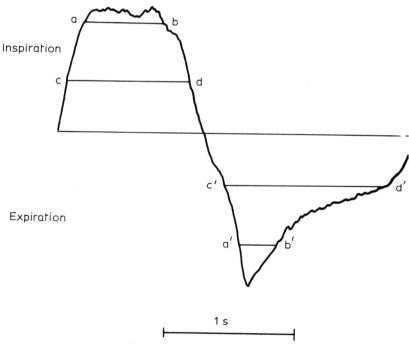

Fig. 2.4 Duration of breath sounds related to the threshold of audibility. Breath sounds on the chest wall are audible at flow rates arbitrarily set by lines *ab*, *a'b'*. Breath sounds at the mouth or trachea are audible at lower flow rates indicated by the line *cd*, *c'd'*.

2.1.3 Clinical application

The loudness of breath sounds at the mouth can provide a useful index of the calibre changes of the proximal bronchi. The value of the clinical sign is enhanced when it is correlated with the simpler expiratory tests of airway obstruction.

Breathing of a healthy person at rest is barely audible with the ear close by. Breath sounds of patients with asthma and chronic bronchitis breathing at rest are frequently loud. The skill in appreciating the loudness of breath sounds in relation to the rate and the depth of breathing is readily acquired. As a rule, the louder the breath sounds, the more severe the airways obstruction. Loud breath sounds in the absence of airways obstruction, suggest stenosis of the larynx, trachea or the main bronchus. In pure emphysema, breath sounds at the mouth are normal because the sound intensity at source is normal while the FEV_1 and the peak expiratory flow rate are often very low. Hence the loudness of breath sounds related to the forced expiratory tests can help to distinguish chronic bronchitis from pure emphysema and stenosis of the larger airways.

The loudness of breath sounds at a particular listening point on the chest wall reflects flow variations in the underlying lobar and segmental bronchi and the transmitting properties of the lung and the chest wall. The transmitted sounds are attenuated and contain the lower frequencies to which the ear is less sensitive. An airless lower lobe due to consolidation, fibrosis or collapse will transmit the higher frequencies resulting in bronchial breathing provided the lobar bronchus is patent. When the bronchus is occluded there is no direct path of transmission of sound from the trachea and the breath sounds are absent. The consolidated upper lobe, however, can transmit the higher frequencies with or without bronchial obstruction because its mediastinal surface is in contact with the trachea. Breath sounds are typically absent over a pneumothorax or a pleural effusion. In these conditions, the sound attenuation occurs at the pleural surface. In widespread airflow obstruction due to chronic bronchitis and emphysema, faint breath sounds result from regional variations in the flow rate and from attenuation of the sound at the pleural surface which separates the distended lung and the chest wall with widely differing acoustic properties. The loudness of breath sounds is therefore not synonymous with 'air entry' and should take into account the filtering effect of the lung and the chest wall.

2.2 Wheezes

Wheezes are continuous musical sounds with a definite pitch (Fig. 2.5). A parallel has naturally been drawn between the musical quality of wheezes and the sound produced by musical instruments. Forgacs [19] pointed out that

Lower pitched wheeze

Higher pitched wheeze

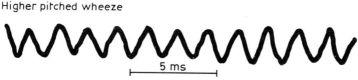

5 ms

Fig. 2.5 Inspiratory monophonic wheeze recorded from a patient with bronchial stenosis. The pitch of the note rises when the inspiratory flow rate is increased.

while the analogy with the wind instrument was obviously correct, the choice of the right model was important in explaining the mechanism of wheeze production.

Wind instruments are of three kinds. An example of the first group is a recorder or an organ pipe. A hiss is generated by the impact of air on a sharp edge which is changed to a musical note when the gas in the body of the instrument is set in resonant oscillations. The pitch of the musical note depends upon the length of the pipe and the velocity of sound. The longer the pipe, the lower the note and the pitch of the note can be raised by blowing helium because the sound waves travel faster in a low density gas. The second variety is represented by the clarinet and the oboe which have in common a single or a double reed. The musical note is produced as the reed opens and closes with air flow which sets into resonant oscillation the gas column within the body of the instrument. As with the recorder and the organ pipe, the pitch of the note is determined by the length of the pipe and the density of the gas. Blowing with a low density gas raises the pitch of the note. The third type of wind instrument is the simple toy trumpet. When air is blown the reed is set in oscillation and a musical note is produced. The attachment to the trumpet is entirely ornamental and serves no acoustic function so that the same note is produced with or without the attachment. The important difference from the orchestral reed instruments is that there is no acoustic coupling between the note produced by the reed and the column of gas. Hence the pitch of the note of a toy trumpet is independent of the density of gas and is determined entirely by the mass and the elasticity of the reed.

It is generally assumed that wheezes are produced by an acoustic mechanism similar to that of an organ pipe. It is believed that the impact of gas streams on the cartilaginous spur or viscid mucus at the bifurcation of the bronchi generate a noise which sets the gas column in the adjoining airway in resonant oscillation, thus generating the musical sound of a wheeze. Clinical and experimental observations do not support this view. The pitch of a wheeze which can be generated in the chest varies from 60 to 2000 Hz. If the analogy with the organ pipe was correct, an instrument of the size of a bassoon would have to be imagined to produce a very low pitched wheeze in the human chest. Theoretically, the lowest note that can be produced by a length of pipe extending from the mouth to the pleura is 500 Hz whereas the pitch of a wheeze is often much lower. In an excised bronchus a musical note cannot be produced in a narrowed bronchus until it is compressed to the point of closure so that the opposite walls are in apposition like a reed. A wheeze is generated when the walls lightly touching at the site of stenosis are set in oscillation by a jet of air. The pitch of the note is unchanged whether a high or a low density gas is blown. Furthermore, a wheeze of a wide range of frequencies can be produced independent of the size of the airway by simply increasing or diminishing the velocity of airflow at the point of stenosis. The experimental findings are confirmed when a wheezy patient is made to breathe alternately air and a helium–oxygen mixture. The pitch of the wheeze remains constant. These observations show that wheezes are produced by a reed mechanism when the bronchial walls are in apposition and their pitch is independent of the density of the gas. Of the reed instruments, the toy trumpet most closely resembles the mechanism of wheeze production [19, 20].

The physical conditions required to produce a wheeze are unstable. The bronchus should not only be narrowed but closed to the point when the walls lightly touch like a reed. The walls are set in oscillation by a gas stream flowing at a critical velocity. A bronchus already narrowed by spasm, oedema, mucus or a tumour mass may be further narrowed to the point of closure by physiological factors. In expiration, the flow is initiated by the pressure gradient between the alveoli and the mouth. As the flow begins, intraluminal pressure drops progressively with increasing distance from the alveoli because energy is expended in overcoming the frictional resistance. At a certain point in the airway, usually at a lobar or segmental level, the pressure outside the airway exceeds intraluminal pressure and dynamic compression of the airway occurs. The compression of the larger airways is augmented by a venturi effect as the flow accelerates from the periphery to the larger bronchi. The narrowing of the cartilaginous supported larger airways is brought about by invagination of the posterior membranous wall forming a slit like orifice [21].

2.2.1 Expiratory polyphonic wheezes

In chronic bronchitis and asthma several musical notes in expiration may be heard either at tidal breathing or on modest expiratory effort. The wheezes are audible at the mouth in the background of loud noisy breathing. When listened to on the chest wall, the higher frequencies of the breath sounds are filtered out and the wheezes dominate. A cluster of wheezes so heard contain harmonically, unrelated sounds called polyphonic wheezes which contrast with the single note of a monophonic wheeze.

Polyphonic expiratory wheezes are common and well recognized in widespread airflow obstruction. Their significance is better appreciated when attention is paid to the underlying physiological events. Normal subjects can generate polyphonic wheezes on forced expiration but their timing and sequence differs from wheezing in diffuse airways obstruction. The airways resistance and the lung compliance are evenly distributed in a healthy lung and during forced expiration the dynamic compression of the bronchi occur simultaneously. When the forced expiratory effort is mild or moderate, only the loud noise of breathing is heard. As the forced expiratory effort is brought to maximum the wheezes appear synchronously and continue to the end of expiration. The wheezes are loud but few in number because dynamic compression occurs at the level of the larger bronchi. By contrast, there are regional variations of the airways resistance and the lung compliance in widespread airflow obstruction and so the dynamic compression of the bronchi tends to be sequential and occur at submaximal expiratory effort. When polyphonic wheezes are already present at tidal breathing, it is a reliable sign of severe widespread airflow obstruction. They may be absent at tidal breathing but become obvious as the expiratory effort is gradually increased. The wheezes appear in sequence; initially only one or two wheezes are heard; the number increases with increasing expiratory effort until the full component of polyphonic wheezes is reached. Hence the interpretation and the significance of expiratory wheezes should be related to the expiratory effort and to the mechanical properties of the lung.

2.2.2 Fixed monophonic wheezes

When the bronchus is narrowed by cicatricial stenosis or an intrabronchial tumour, a low pitched monophonic wheeze may be heard, often in inspiration in association with noisy breathing. The low note of the wheeze is related to the mass of the tumour which is set in slow oscillation by the high velocity of gas flow. The pitch can be varied within a narrow range by altering the velocity of gas flow (Fig. 2.5). The wheeze, however, does not appear until the tumour mass is in contact with the opposite wall of the bronchus. When the bronchus is narrowed by the tumour, the breathing is noisy. In this situation, the wheeze can be elicited by a rapid inspiratory effort when the venturi effect comes into play and the bronchus, already stenosed, is further narrowed to the point of closure.

2.2.3 Random monophonic wheezes

A particular variety of wheezes distinct from the polyphonic expiratory wheezes may be heard in widespread airflow obstruction. These are random monophonic wheezes which arise from individual airways brought to the point of closure by spasm or mucosal oedema. The wheezes may be high or low pitched; they vary in duration and overlap each other, creating an illusion of many wheezes when heard on the chest wall. The timing of the wheeze makes it evident that only a few wheezes are in fact present. It is usually not possible to indicate the source of an individual wheeze but a proximal site may be inferred if the wheeze is transmitted to the mouth.

2.2.4 Stridor

Stridor should be distinguished from noisy breathing commonly present in widespread airflow obstruction. The noisy breathing of stridor is accompanied by a high pitched inspiratory wheeze audible at a distance. Inspiratory stridor in whooping cough is associated with laryngeal spasm, adduction of vocal cords and swelling of the mucosa. It is exaggerated in inspiration by the venturi effect as the lateral pressure falls with accelerating flow while the atmospheric pressure outside remains the same. In tracheal stridor a similar mechanism operates. The noisy breathing in bronchial stenosis accompanied by a fixed monophonic wheeze is essentially a form of inspiratory stridor.

2.2.5 Paradoxical absence of wheezing

The absence of wheezing is compatible with severe widespread airflow obstruction. The production of a wheeze requires an airway on the point of closure and an optimum velocity of gas flow at the site of stenosis to set the bronchial walls in oscillation. In patients with severe ventilatory failure, wheezing may be absent because the flow rate is too slow to oscillate the airways on the point of closure. Asthmatic patients on the other hand are markedly wheezy during an acute attack. Further deterioration may make the chest silent creating a false clinical impression of improvement although the peak expiratory flow rate remains low or even unrecordable. These patients are known to have high peripheral resistance and mucous plugging which displaces the site of dynamic compression further towards the periphery. The gas flow in the peripheral airways is too slow to set the bronchial wall in oscillation which accounts for the silent chest. In emphysema, the additional effect of low elastic recoil contributes to the low flow rate in the peripheral airways.

2.2.6 Sequential inspiratory wheezes

In patients with lung restriction due to pulmonary fibrosis, oedema or infiltration, a brief high pitched wheeze can frequently be heard late in inspiration in association with the inspiratory crackles. The musical note may repeat from breath to breath, disappear and reappear at different times. A number of wheezes may be heard in sequence in a single inspiration. The airways in the basal territories of the lung close early in expiration. They open late in inspiration when the critical opening pressure is reached. The opening of the airway is usually sudden. The walls of some airways, however, may remain momentarily in light contact and oscillate before they open and produce a short high-pitched wheeze [20].

2.3 Lung crackles

The present-day classification of added sounds is unsatisfactory. Laennec's original classification may have served us well if the meaning of the words he chose did not get distorted with the passage of time [22].

Non-musical explosive sounds are variously called rales, crepitations, dry and moist sounds. There is no clear distinction between them; crepitations are usually more profuse and higher pitched than rales. The association between crepitations and pulmonary oedema has come to mean that they are produced by bubbling in oedema fluid in the peripheral airways. As will be discussed later, such an explanation is inconsistent with similar sounds heard in a wide range of lung disorders where secretions play no part in their production. The distinction between dry and moist sounds is essentially subjective and prejudges the mode of sound production. In an attempt to avoid a particular connotation with regard to the mechanism of sound production, it has been suggested that all non-musical explosive sounds are named crackles which may be further distinguished by a more objective criteria.

Lung crackles may be heard in either phase of the respiratory cycle. The commonest variety of lung crackles, however, are confined to inspiration. Attention to their timing in inspiration, distribution and transmission has helped to identify distinct patterns common to certain groups of lung disorder and have suggested possible clues as to how they may be produced.

2.3.1 Late inspiratory crackles

Late inspiratory crackles are so named because they continue to the end of inspiration but may begin at any point in the inspiratory cycle [23] (Fig. 2.6). They are heard in a wide range of restrictive lung disorders characterized by diffuse pulmonary infiltration, fibrosis or oedema. They may also be heard over consolidated and contracted lobes and during the first breath after recumbency. In the upright posture, they are more profuse at the lung bases with an upper horizontal level. A striking clinical feature of the late inspiratory crackles is that they can be silenced or made less abundant on bending forwards when the lung bases are no longer dependent [19, 24].

The lungs in widely varied pathological conditions like fibrosing alveolitis, asbestosis and pulmonary oedema share a common functional abnormality. They tend to be small and stiff reflected in the measurement of a low lung compliance and reduced functional residual capacity. Lung deflation predisposes to the closure of peripheral airways and the distribution of airway closure is gravity dependent [25, 26]. When a subject inspires from residual volume, the gas is preferentially directed to the upper zones in early inspiration. Thereafter, the gas reaches the upper and lower zones at an equal rate and by the end of inspiration only the lower zones ventilate [28]. The difference in regional ventilation is related to the effect of gravity which results in increasingly more negative (subatmospheric) pleural pressure from the base to the apex of the lung. The effect is most striking in various body positions; whether the subject is erect head up, inverted head down, supine, prone and in a right or left lateral decubitus position, pleural pressure in the uppermost region is always more sub-atmospheric than in the lower dependent region. The pleural pressure gradient parallels recoil ten-

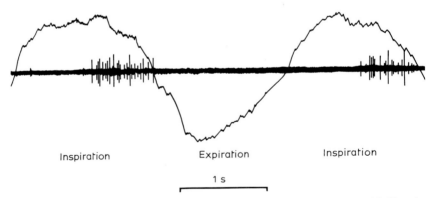

Inspiration   Expiration   Inspiration

1 s

Fig. 2.6 Phonopneumogram of late inspiratory crackles from a patient with fibrosing alveolitis. This is a simultaneous recording of inspiratory crackles and airflow rate. The crackles start in mid-inspiration and continue to the end of inspiration.

sion in the lung which is low at the lung base compared to the apex in the upright position. The peripheral airways are correspondingly narrow in dependent lung regions where the recoil tension is low. They close early in expiration and do not open until the next inspiration is well advanced. The timing of the lung crackles coincides with the late opening of the peripheral airways in the dependent lung regions. An important clue in explaining how the inspiratory crackles may be produced comes from the observation that they do not appear at random but repeat from breath to breath in the same sequence implying that their occurrence is determined by the pressure and volume changes during each breath (Fig. 2.7) [19]. Indeed, the measurements confirm that an individual crackle identified by its timing and amplitude recurs at a similar lung volume and transpulmonary pressure in successive breaths [27].

The genesis of explosive sounds is related to delayed opening of the peripheral airways in deflated lung regions. During inspiration the outward pull on the closed section of the airway by the surrounding lung is opposed by the tension of the airway wall. With the expanding lung, a further rise in radial traction results in abrupt opening of the airway with sudden equalization of gas pressure between the upstream and the downstream section of the closed airway. It is believed that the momentary gas oscillations which follow instantaneous equalization of gas pressure at the moment of airway opening generate the explosive sound of a crackle. The mechanism of crackling in surgical emphysema is similar when air is squeezed from an inflated to the airless compartment of the skin with sudden equalization of pressure.

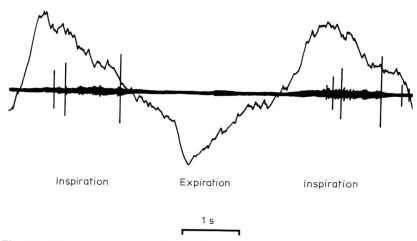

Inspiration   Expiration   Inspiration

1 s

Fig. 2.7 Phonopneumogram of repetitive late inspiratory crackles. The pattern shown here continued for several consecutive breaths.

2.3.2 Eary inspiratory crackles

Early inspiratory crackles are so named because they are confined to the early phase of inspiration and contrast with the late inspiratory crackles which continue to the end of inspiration (Fig. 2.8). Early inspiratory crackles are a feature of widespread airflow obstruction due to chronic bronchitis, emphysema and to asthma. In a study of patients with diffuse airway obstruction, the presence of early inspiratory crackles was correlated with the severity of airway obstruction [23]. Early inspiratory crackles were present only when the FEV_1/VC ratio was less than 45%. Thus the presence of early inspiratory crackles suggest severe narrowing of the airways.

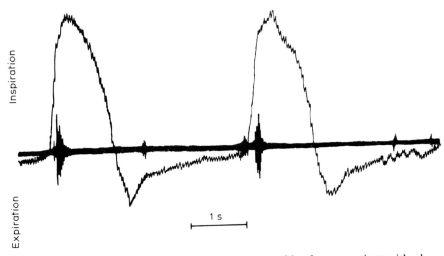

Fig. 2.8 Phonopneumogram of early inspiratory crackles from a patient with obstructive chronic bronchitis. FEV_1/VC ratio was 32%.

The difference in timing between the early crackles of severe airways obstruction and the late crackles of restrictive lung disorder can be related to the site of airway closure. A source in the proximal and larger airways may be inferred for the early inspiratory crackles since they are frequently well transmitted to the mouth and are few in number. The closure of the larger airways at the end of expiration is favoured by high bronchial compliance or if the retractive pressures around the bronchi are low [29]. In the subsequent inspiration, the onset of crackles coincides with the early opening of the closed airways at a low transpulmonary pressure. Late inspiratory crackles, by contrast, originate in the peripheral airways and so they are often profuse and rarely transmitted to the mouth.

2.3.3 Early and mid-inspiratory and expiratory crackles

The presence of coarse inspiratory and expiratory crackles is a well-recog-
nized auscultatory sign of bronchiectasis. Closer attention to their inspiratory timing in bronchiectasis uncomplicated by fibrosis shows a distinct
pattern. The crackles start early in inspiration, continue to mid-phase of
inspiration and fade by the end of inspiration (Fig. 2.9). In this respect the
pattern differs from the early inspiratory crackles of chronic bronchitis and
emphysema and the late inspiratory crackles of fibrosing alveolitis and
related disorders.

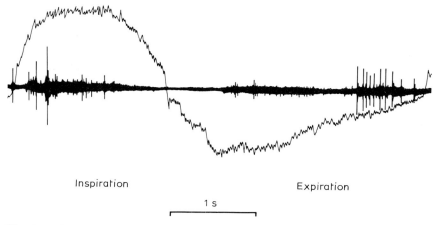

Inspiration   Expiration

1 s

Fig. 2.9 Phonopneumogram of early and mid-inspiratory crackles from a patient
with bronchiectasis. Note the expiratory crackles are also present.

As in chronic bronchitis, the lung crackles in bronchiectasis are transmitted to the mouth suggesting their origin in the proximal airways. This
observation is in keeping with the bronchographic findings which show
abnormalities of the larger and the medium-sized bronchi. It seems likely
that the crackles relate to retained secretions in the damaged and dilated
bronchi. They are typically present in inspiration and expiration and
become less abundant after expectoration. Bubbling in retained secretions,
however, is probably only one of the causes of these crackles. The bronchial
wall compliance is increased in bronchiectasis [30]. A bronchus with a high
compliance lined by mucus will tend to close prematurely in expiration and
will open early in subsequent inspiration at a low transpulmonary pressure.
The airway opening in inspiration may be abrupt or it may remain lightly
closed and open intermittently as a bolus of gas passes when upstream gas
pressure rises above a critical level. Another mechanism which may operate

is suggested by the observation that in bronchiectasis, especially in the varicose and cystic variety, the emptying of dilated sacs is prevented by the collapse of the bronchi downstream (towards the mouth) so that the secretions are retained in them [31]. In this situation, early inspiratory crackles are likely to coincide with the opening of the bronchiectatic airway and their continuation in the middle phase of inspiration result from bubbling in retained secretions as inspiration progresses.

2.3.4 Expiratory crackles

Expiratory crackles usually accompany the inspiratory crackles. Expiratory crackles which occur towards the end of expiration are commonly heard at the mouth in association with the early inspiratory crackles. A characteristic pattern observed is that the crackles are of equal loudness and evenly spaced. At the mouth a series of clicks are heard at regular intervals terminating in a short polyphonic wheeze. The mechanism of sound production is similar to the low-pitched sounds generated when gas passes through the oesophagus or the bowel. As the lung deflates in expiration, the proximal bronchi narrow. A loosely closed bronchus may open intermittently, each click coinciding with the passage of gas. By the end of expiration, the airways are more tightly closed, the walls oscillate like a reed to produce an end-expiratory polyphonic wheeze.

When the larger airways are flooded with secretions, the crackles produced by true bubbling occur in inspiration and expiration. The sequence of crackles is then random and they can be silenced or made less abundant on coughing.

In fibrosing alveolitis and related lung disorders, expiratory crackles are usually present in a more advanced stage of the disease. The likely mechanism is that some of the peripheral airways which close in early expiration, paradoxically reopen with the redistribution of gas flow during expiration.

2.3.5 Pleural crackles

When the pleural membrane is inflamed or infiltrated, the movement of the adjacent surfaces becomes jerky in a manner similar to the bow of a stringed instrument. Pleural crackles so generated are coarse and non-musical but may acquire a musical quality if the chest wall is set in resonant oscillation. They are usually present in both phases of respiration; the crackles appear superficial but may be indistinguishable from the pulmonary crackles.

2.3.6 Crackling sounds in pneumothorax

Clicking sounds may sometimes be heard when there is a shallow pneumothorax on the left side. The sounds are louder when the patient leans over to the left. They are produced either by the impact of the heart on the mediastinal surface of the lung or by sudden displacement of trapped air in the mediastinal pleura by the direct impact of the heart. Clicking sounds disappear either when the lung reinflates or when the pneumothorax deepens.

2.3.7 Clinical application

The interpretation of the lung crackles should be based on their timing, distribution, transmission, the effect of cough and the body position (Table 2.1). Late inspiratory crackles are a feature of restrictive lung disorder due to pulmonary infiltration, fibrosis or to oedema. Spirometrically the FEV_1/ VC ratio is usually normal or high. The inspiratory crackles of fibrosing

Table 2.1 Common features of lung crackles in obstructive chronic bronchitis, bronchiectasis and fibrosing alveolitis

	Obstructive chronic bronchitis	*Bronchiectasis*	*Fibrosing alveolitis*
Timing of inspiratory crackles (typically)	Present early phase inspiration	Present early and mid-phase inspiration	Present end phase inspiration
Number of crackles (typically)	Always few	Usually moderate	Can be profuse
Effect of cough	No change	Temporarily reduced	No change
Effect of position	No change	No change	Modified or abolished
Intensity	Faint	Loud	Moderately loud
Pitch	Low pitched	Low pitched	High pitched
Expiratory crackles	May be present	Typically present	May be present
Transmission at the mouth	Transmitted	Transmitted	Not transmitted

alveolitis and pulmonary oedema from left heart failure share all the important features and are indistinguishable. Lung deflation in both conditions results from either interstitial infiltration or oedema. The flooding of the larger airways in pulmonary oedema is a late feature of the disease when the crackles are produced by true bubbling. They are present in both phases of respiration, they occur at random and are modified by coughing. Although the distribution of late inspiratory crackles is typically basal, the disease process may be generalized. The effect of gravity on lung crackles can be exploited clinically to assess the functional state of the lung. In the early stages of fibrosing alveolitis, for example, the basal crackles in the upright position are silenced on bending forwards. In a more advanced state, bending forwards makes the crackles less abundant while in the most advanced state of the disease, the crackles are present in all body positions indicating more severe lung deflation. The reverse situation applies in the recovery phase. The upper horizontal level of crackles regresses with recovery. The crackles previously present on bending forwards are now silenced and finally they disappear in all body positions as the lung regains normal elasticity and volume.

Early inspiratory crackles are also heard at the lung bases. They are low pitched, faint, few in number and often transmitted to the mouth. They are a feature of severe airways obstruction and reflect premature closure of the larger airways. Spirometrically the FEV_1/VC ratio is well below 45%. In ventilatory failure, early inspiratory crackles are frequently present in the absence of wheeze and their presence may be misinterpreted to indicate pulmonary oedema from left heart failure.

The crackles of uncomplicated bronchiectasis extend from the early to the mid-phase of inspiration and contrast with the early inspiratory timing of crackles in diffuse airway obstruction and the late timing in restrictive lung disorder. Expiratory crackles are usually present and spirometrically the airways obstruction is mild. The pattern of lung crackles when bronchiectasis is complicated by chronic bronchitis or pulmonary fibrosis remains to be evaluated.

2.4 Summary

Auscultation of the chest should be a deliberate attempt at eliciting the functional and pathological state of the lung. Its value is enhanced when correlated with observations made on inspection, palpation and percussion of the chest as well as the chest radiograph and simpler lung function tests. The time for a more manageable classification of lung sounds is ripe. It should take into account the known physiological events of breathing and the acoustic characteristics of lung sounds.

Lung sounds heard in health and disease may be classified into Breath

Sounds, Wheezes and Crackles. Breath sounds result from turbulent airflow in the upper airways, trachea and the proximal bronchi. When the bronchi are narrowed, turbulence is intensified and breath sounds become louder. The loudness of breath sounds is best appreciated by listening at the mouth because the sound transmitted from proximal bronchi is relatively unattenuated. By contrast the breath sounds heard on the chest are attenuated during their transmission through the lung and chest wall as higher frequencies are selectively filtered out and some sound energy is lost. In health, the greatest attenuation occurs at the lung bases which explains the observed difference between breath sounds heard at the upper and lower chest. The transmission of sound is impeded in the presence of a pleural effusion or a pneumothorax and when the lung is distended by air as in emphysema. The consolidated lung favours transmission of higher frequencies resulting in bronchial breathing. The interpretation of breath sounds therefore should take into account the source of sound production as well as the transmitting characteristics of the lung and the chest wall.

Wheezes are musical sounds produced by airways narrowed to the point of closure. The opposing walls of the airway in light contact behave like a reed of a musical instrument and are set in oscillation by gas flowing at an optimum velocity. The pitch of a wheeze depends upon velocity of gas flow and mechanical properties of the vibrating reed. The physical conditions required to produce a wheeze are unstable so that only a few wheezes are usually heard even in widespread airflow obstruction. The polyphonic expiratory wheezes, commonly heard in asthma, result from structural narrowing of larger airways and dynamic compression of bronchi during expiration. In tracheal and bronchial stenosis, noisy breathing may be accompanied by an inspiratory wheeze. It can be elicited by rapid inspiration when the airway is already narrowed and brought to the point of closure by venturi effect. The absence of wheeze is compatible with widespread airflow obstruction. In ventilatory failure, the velocity of gas flow may be too slow to generate a wheeze. A particular variety of inspiratory wheeze associated with the late inspiratory crackles is heard in fibrosing alveolitis and related lung disorder. It is a high-pitched wheeze and of brief duration caused by momentary oscillations of the peripheral airway before it abruptly opens late in inspiration.

Crackles are explosive non-musical sounds. In diffuse lung disorder due to infiltration, fibrosis or oedema, inspiratory crackles result from abrupt opening of the closed peripheral airways in deflated territories of the lung. The inspiratory crackles so produced continue to the end of inspiration but may start in the early, mid or late phase of inspiration. They are often profuse, basal in distribution and modified by a change in body position. The late inspiratory crackles of fibrosing alveolitis and related lung disorders are associated with a 'restrictive' spirometry. By contrast, early inspiratory crackles are a feature of severe widespread airflow obstruction with FEV_1/VC ratio well below 40% and are few in number being confined to the early phase of inspiration. They result from opening of the larger airways prematurely closed in previous expiration and are often heard simultaneously at the mouth and at one or both lung bases. They are unaffected by cough or a change in body position. The inspiratory lung crackles in bronchiectasis uncomplicated by fibrosis occur typically in the early and the mid-phase of inspiration associated with expiratory crackles. They are modified by cough but are independent of body position. As with early inspiratory crackles, they are well transmitted to the mouth while spirometrically the airways obstruction is mild. Lung crackles may also originate by true bubbling when larger airways are flooded with secretions. They occur at random in both phases of respiration and are made less abundant after coughing. The crackles generated by a pleural rub are often coarse, loud and present in both phases of respiration. However, they may be indistinguishable from lung crackles. In this situation the presence or absence of a pleural rub is inferred by associated clinical features and in particular by the presence of pleuritic chest pain.

Closer attention to the various features of lung sounds is of value in the diagnosis of a wide variety of lung disorders and should enhance and revive interest in auscultation of the lung.

References

1. Schroter, R. C. and Sudlow, M. F. (1969), Flow patterns in models of the human bronchial airways. *Resp. Physiol.*, **7**, 341.
2. Jaeger, M. J. and Matthys, H. (1970), The pressure flow characteristics of the human airways. In: *Airway Dynamics*, Charles C. Thomas, Springfield, Illinois, p. 21.
3. Laennec, R. T. H. (1819), Translation of selected passages from *De l'Auscultation Mediate*, 1st edn. With a biography by Sir William Hale-White (1923), John Bale, Son and Danielson, London, No. 183, p. 75.
4. Forgacs, P., Nathoo, A. R., and Richardson, H. D. (1971), Breath sounds. *Thorax*, **26**, 288.
5. Stransky, A., Malgorzata, Szereda-Przestaszewska and Widdicombe, J. G. (1973), The effect of lung reflexes on laryngeal resistance and motoneurone discharge. *J. Physiol.*, **231**, 417.
6. Bullar, J. P. (1884), Experiments to determine the origin of the respiratory sounds. *Proc. R. Soc.*, **37**, 411.
7. Sahli, H. (1892), Ueber die Entstehung des vesciularathmens. *Cor. Bl. Schweiz, Aerzte*, **22**, 265.
8. Gee, S. (1877), *Auscultation and Percussion Together wtih the other Methods of Physical Examination of the Chest*, 2nd ed, Oxford University Press, London, p. 129.

9. Bushnell, G. E. (1921), The mode of production of the so-called vesicular murmurs of respiration. *J. Am. med. Ass.*, **77**, 2104.
10. Nathoo, A. R. (1972), *On Breath Sounds*, M. D. Thesis, University of London.
11. Krumpe, P., Perez, L., Engel, L. and Macklem, P. (1976), The effect of breathing gas mixtures of different densities on breath sounds in normal subjects. 1st Int. Conf. on *Lung Sounds*, Boston, Massachusetts.
12. West, J. B., and Hugh-Jones, P. (1961), Pulsatile gas flow in bronchi caused by the heart beat. *J. appl. Physiol*, **16**, 697.
13. Mills, R. J. (1969), The mechanical effect of the heart beat on the plethysmographic pressure. *Prog. resp. Res.*, **4**, 164.
14. Palmiere, C. C. (1953), Ulteriori raffronti radiochimografici ed elettromanometrici sulla meccancia dei diversi territori polmonari nella piccola respiraxione cardiaca. *Minerva Med.*, **44**, 1655.
15. Palmieri, C. C., Petrucci, D. and Lura, A. (1953), Ricerche comparative radiochimografiche ed elettromanometriche sulla cinematica e sulla dinamica dei diversi territori polmonari. *Minerva Med.*, **44**, 125.
16. Leblanc, P., Macklem, P. T. and Ross, W. R. D. (1970), Breath sounds and distribution of pulmonary ventilation. *Am. Rev. resp. Dis.*, **102**, 10.
17. Nairn, J. R. and Turner-Warwick, M. (1969), Breath sounds in emphysema. *Br. J. Dis. Chest*, **63**, 29.
18. Ploy-Song-Sang, Y. *et al.* (1977), Breath sounds and regional ventilation. *Am. Rev. resp. Dis.*, **116**, 187–99.
19. Forgacs, P. (1967), Crackles and wheezes. *Lancet*, **ii**, 203
20. Forgacs, P. (1978), *Lung Sounds*. Baillière Tindall, London.
21. Pride, N. B. (1971), The assessment of airflow obstruction. *Br. J. Dis. Chest*, **65**, 135.
22. Robertson, J. A. and Coope, R. (1957), Rales, rhonchi and Laennec. *Lancet*, **ii**.
23. Nath, A. R. and Capel L. H. (1974), Inspiratory crackles, early and late. *Thorax*, **29**, 223.
24. Forgacs P. (1969), Lung sounds. *Br. J. Dis. Chest*, **63**, 1.
25. Forgacs, P. (1974), Gravitational stress in lung disease. *Br. J. Dis. Chest*, **68**, 1.
26. Collins, J. V. (1973), Closing volume – a test of small airway function? *Br. J. Dis. Chest*, **67**, 1
27. Nath, A. R. and Capel, L. H. (1974), Inspiratory crackles and mechanical events of breathing. *Thorax*, **29**, 695.
28. Dollfuss, R. E., Milio-Emili, J. and Bates, D. (1967), Regional ventilation of the lung studied with boluses of Xenon-133. *Resp. Physiol.*, **2**, 234.
29. Macklem, P. T., Fraser, R. G. and Brown W. G. (1965), Bronchial pressure measurements in emphysema and bronchitis. *J. clin. Invest.*, **44**, 897.
30. Fraser, R. G., Macklem, P. T. and Brown, W. G. (1965), Airway dynamics in bronchiectasis. *Am. J. Roentg.*, **93**, 821.
31. Bass, H. *et al.* Retional structure and function in bronchiectasis. *Am. Rev. resp. Dis.*, **97**, 598.

CHAPTER THREE

Physiology

D. M. Denison

This chapter discusses the clinical value of making physiological tests on the lung, and takes as its starting points the arguments that:

1. There is little value in making a measurement of any sort unless it is reliable, can be interpreted unequivocally and correctly (two separate conditions!), and potentially leads to some clinically useful action.
2. Before selecting a particular test it is essential to identify the property that the test overtly measures (e.g. airways obstruction), the property that it actually measures (airflow limitation), and the errors introduced by the act of measuring (unnaturally forceful expiration).
3. When the measurement has been made, it has to be assessed. This is usually done at two distinct levels. Firstly, the result is *compared* with values obtained from *real* lungs of normal subjects or people with particular disorders. Secondly, it is *interpreted* using some properties of *imaginary* lungs. Interpretations are obviously no stronger than the mental models that generate them.

At first sight these may seem dry and dull points to make, and you may even hold that view to the end of the chapter, but they have a serious aim since it is surprisingly easy to make unreliable measurements that are difficult to interpret and lead to no useful clinical action. In fact, lung function tests can be of great clinical value, because physiological changes which are characteristic of particular conditions can be used to confirm or modify a diagnosis and to select or follow treatment.

3.1 Finding a suitable mental model of the lung

The choice, conduct and interpretation of tests obviously cannot be considered in a vacuum. The first need is to agree on a clinically adequate model of the lung, but the problem is that the very clear models which are so successful in teaching are too simple for clinical use. The most basic view of the lung (Fig. 3.1) is that it is a 'black box' which produces arterial blood of

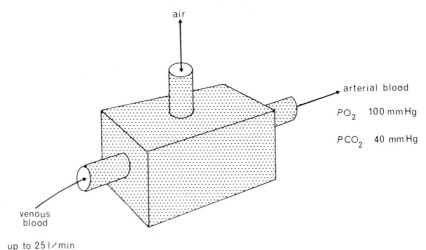

air

arterial blood

PO_2 100 mm Hg

PCO_2 40 mm Hg

venous
blood

up to 25 l/min

Fig. 3.1 A simple 'black-box' model of the lung.

normal gas composition, regardless of the quantity or quality of the mixed venous blood that is offered up to it. It is certainly true that even when healthy people exercise maximally, their lungs continue to provide blood with an arterial oxygen tension (P_aO_2) close to 100 mm Hg and a CO_2 tension (P_aCO_2) that is 40 mm Hg or less. Some determined athletes are able to push themselves hard enough to just beat the equilibrating capacity of the lung, so that their arterial blood desaturates slightly on extreme exertion, but this is very rare. The 'black box' view rightly draws attention to the lungs' primary function of gas exchange, and to the value of testing it under load by measuring arterial gas tensions during maximal exertion. However, it clearly ignores the cost of achieving that function, overlooks all the physiological events that precede a frank breakdown, and fails to draw attention to the many non-respiratory functions of the lung, that are of clinical interest. The latter will not be discussed further here but are described in this book by Geddes, and in monographs [1–3]. The 'testing under load' approach also ignores most people's natural dislike of riding cycles and running on treadmills in laboratories.

3.1.1 Work of ventilation and perfusion

The work of any pump is the product of the pressure it generates and the flow it produces. A rational extension of the 'black box' view would be to measure the cost of lung perfusion (right heart pressure × pulmonary blood flow) and ventilation (pleural pressure × respired gas flow). If we had methods of measuring these variables non-invasively there is no doubt that they would be widely used. At present we do not have them. It is often possible to arrive at the cost of ventilation indirectly, since respired gas flows are readily available and alveolar pressures can be obtained at the same time by whole-body plethysmography. This procedure estimates the work done in forcing gas through the airways but overlooks the cost of stretching alveoli. However, if the latter is suspected to be high, i.e. if the lung is thought to be uncommonly stiff, pleural pressures can be measured with little discomfort or risk, by oesophageal balloon studies. Determining the cost of perfusion is much less satisfactory. Although some measure of pulmonary blood flow can often be obtained from respired gas composition there is, as yet, no reliable method of determining pulmonary arterial pressure non-invasively. Possibly, one may be developed from right heart echocardiography [4]. It is certain that the incidence of pulmonary hypertension in chest disease is underestimated because of this difficulty. It may be that chest physicians should consider right heart catheter studies more frequently than hitherto.

A very valuable 'tube and balloon' view of the lung is shown in Fig. 3.2. This model, which recognizes the existence of an anatomical dead-space (V_D), an alveolar volume (V_A), a pulmonary diffusion characteristic (D_L), pulmonary capillary and anatomical shunt blood flows $(\dot{Q}_p$ and $\dot{Q}_s)$ and the metabolic flows $(\dot{M}O_2$ and $\dot{M}CO_2)$, is essential to any understanding of pulmonary gas exchange. In particular it illustrates two fundamental relationships, the alveolar–ventilation and the alveolar–air equations.

3.1.2 Alveolar ventilation equation

This assumes that the CO_2 diffusing from venous blood to the alveoli behaves as if it were diluted in a stream of CO_2-free gas, the effective alveolar ventilation $(\dot{V}_A)$. Therefore the partial pressure of CO_2 in the alveolar space (P_ACO_2) is proportional to the number of CO_2 molecules diffusing into the stream, divided by its volume:

$$P_ACO_2 = k\,(\dot{M}CO_2/\dot{V}_A). \tag{3.1}$$

It follows that doubling alveolar ventilation will halve alveolar PCO_2 and halving alveolar ventilation will double it. As mentioned earlier, alveolar ventilation is normally adjusted to hold arterial PCO_2 close to 40 mm Hg whatever the level of exertion. In heavy exercise $\dot{M}CO_2$ increases some twenty-fold and $\dot{V}_A$ rises more or less proportionately. *Hyperventilation*, which is ventilation in excess of metabolic need, implies an abnormally low arterial PCO_2, (i.e. <35 mm Hg). People with a normal P_aCO_2 who are ventilating rapidly because their lungs are inefficient or their metabolic rate is high, are hyperpnoeic but not hyperventilating. Similarly, *hypoventilation* implies insufficient ventilation for metabolic needs, $(P_aCO_2 >43$ mm Hg). People

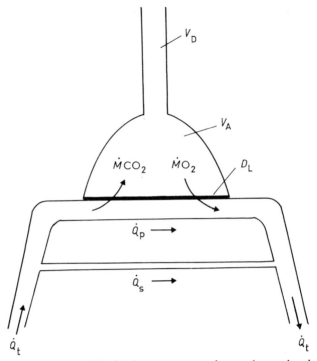

Fig. 3.2 An elementary model of pulmonary gas exchange, in an alveolar compartment V_A ventilated via a dead-space V_D, and linked by a membrane of diffusion conductance D_L to a flow of blood $\dot{Q}_t$, of which a fraction $\dot{Q}_p$ is in contact with the pulmonary membrane and the remainder $\dot{Q}_s$ by-passes it. Molar flows of the exchanging gases are also shown ($\dot{M}O_2$ and $\dot{M}CO_2$).

whose P_aCO_2 is normal but whose ventilation is slight because their metabolic rate is low, are hypopnoeic but not hypoventilating.

3.1.3 Alveolar air equation

This rests on a particular property of molecules in gases, namely that at any given temperature they all move about with the same momentum and therefore exert pressures which are simply proportional to their abundance. It follows that there is a precise relation between the incoming and outgoing oxygen pressures (P_IO_2 and P_AO_2) in the stream of gas ventilating the alveoli. This depends on the 'trading' or respiratory exchange ratio R, ($R = \dot{M}CO_2/\dot{M}O_2$. If there were no volume differences between inspired and expired air the relation would be very straightforward:

$$P_AO_2 = P_IO_2 - P_ACO_2/R. \tag{3.2}$$

As it is, unless $\dot{M}O_2$ and $\dot{M}CO_2$ are identical, small differences in volumes are created and have to be taken into account:

$$P_AO_2 = P_IO_2 - P_ACO_2[F_IO_2 - (1 - F_IO_2)/R] \qquad (3.3)$$

In practice these corrections are very slight and the simple equation is quite suitable for most clinical purposes, but not for studies of gas exchange at high altitudes.

One of the conclusions which can be drawn readily from this equation is that hypoventilation alone is very unlikely to produce sufficient hypoxaemia to cause cyanosis in people at sea level. Even a halving of alveolar ventilation, raising P_ACO_2 to 80 mm Hg, would only drop arterial PO_2 by 40 or 50 mm Hg. This would still leave the blood almost fully saturated.

Fig. 3.2 also provides a basis for calculating the right-to-left blood flow which appears to by-pass ventilated alveoli entirely ($\dot{Q}_s$). The amount of oxygen in systemic arterial blood must be the sum of the contributions from the pulmonary capillary and the by-pass streams:

$$\dot{Q}_tC_aO_2 = \dot{Q}_sC_vO_2 + (\dot{Q}_t - \dot{Q}_s)C_pO_2 \qquad (3.4)$$

Therefore the ratio of shunted to total flow can be calculated from C_aO_2 if C_pO_2 and C_vO_2 are known or can be assumed:

$$\dot{Q}_s/\dot{Q}_t = (C_aO_2 - C_pO_2)/(C_vO_2 - C_pO_2) \qquad (3.5)$$

Measurements of the anatomical shunt fraction ($\dot{Q}_s/\dot{Q}_t$) are usually made from an arterial blood sample alone, taken when the resting patient has been breathing pure oxygen for sufficient time to flush the alveolar space free of nitrogen. Under these circumstances pulmonary capillary blood is assumed to be fully saturated. To calculate the shunt, mixed venous blood is taken to be 75% saturated, alveolar PCO_2 is presumed to equal arterial PCO_2, and an idealized alveolar PO_2 is determined from the alveolar air equation. As a useful 'rule-of-thumb', each 1% of anatomical shunt fraction contributes 20 mm Hg to the apparent $P_{a-A}O_2$ gradient calculated in this way. For accurate studies, as in children with congenital heart disease, it is essential to obtain reliable determinations of C_vO_2 and to take account of the additional oxygen carried in simple solution at high PO_2, ($>$100 mm Hg). It is also important to remember that the shunt flows measured under these circumstances are artificial, since high alveolar oxygen pressures tend to cause pulmonary arteriolar dilatation and so reduce the shunt fraction. These points are discussed again later.

Normally, in resting people, blood takes about one second to traverse the pulmonary capillary, and is fully equilibrated with alveolar gas within the first one-third of this journey. In exercise $\dot{Q}_p$ rises five-fold but, due to recruitment of capillaries that were previously under-perfused, the mean capillary transit time only falls to one-third of a second. This leaves just enough time for complete equilibration. Equilibration is slower when the alveolar membrane is damaged or alveolar PO_2 is low, as at altitude. Although it may still be completed under resting conditions, there is an inevitable widening of the $P_{a-A}O_2$ gradient on exertion. This phenomenon explains why people at high altitude, who are fully conscious at rest, lose consciousness when they exert themselves. It also emphasizes the value of exercise studies in the early stages of conditions such as fibrosing alveolitis and pulmonary sarcoidosis where impairment of diffusion may not be evident at rest. A shortening of capillary transit time may also account for the systemic arterial desaturation that is seen following pulmonary embolization, which forces a normal flow of blood to travel more rapidly through fewer channels.

3.1.4 Bronchial circulation

A major clinical drawback of Fig. 3.2 is its failure to draw attention to the bronchial circulation. The bronchial arteries originate from the thoracic aorta and form an annular plexus around each main bronchus. Several smaller vessels arise from the plexus and radiate out to the extreme tips of the bronchial tree, supplying them and acting as vasa vasorum to the pulmonary arterial tree. Distally, bronchial capillaries can be traced at least to the level of the alveolar ducts.

At birth there are pre-capillary anastomoses between the bronchial and pulmonary circulations, but these are believed to disappear soon after. In healthy adults there are extensive post-capillary connections between the two circulations. Two-thirds of the bronchial flow returns to the left atrium via the pulmonary veins. The remainder goes to the right atrium via the azygos system. Normally the total flow is 1–2% of cardiac output. However, in several diseases, particularly those leading to pulmonary oligaemia, bronchial flow can rise markedly, and often enters the pulmonary circulation at precapillary levels. For example, enlarged bronchial arteries have been found in pulmonary stenosis and atresia, patent ductus arteriosus, transposition of the great vessels and Fallot's tetralogy, and in bronchiectasis, pulmonary embolization and primary lung tumours. It also appears temporarily in consolidation of the lung, persisting for some weeks after. Its existence is thought to explain why less than 10% of pulmonary emboli lead to pulmonary infarction. Similarly, if bronchial arterial blood flow is poor, e.g. in transplanted lungs, it is augmented by blood from the pulmonary circulation.

Increased bronchial blood flow is commonly associated with clubbing and it has been suggested that the abnormal vascular route permits some agent to by-pass the lung and appear in systemic blood in an abnormal state or amount. This attractive theory is contentious and has not been formally proved or disproved.

In pulmonary arterial oligaemia the bronchial flow usually enters the pulmonary circulation at segmental level via the vasa vasorum which break through the media and endothelium of the pulmonary arteries. The bronchial flow then serves respiration but contributes more to CO_2 exchange than to oxygen uptake. Indirect estimates of bronchial blood flow can be obtained from comparisons of right and left lung gas exchange during air and oxygen breathing, and by comparisons of right and left heart outputs derived from dye-dilution studies. A simple non-invasive measure would be of great value but none exists. A detailed account of the bronchial circulation has been given [5].

3.1.5 Maldistribution of air and blood flow

Another clinical drawback of Fig. 3.2 is that it ignores the very important concepts of ventilation/perfusion inequality, parallel dead-space, collateral ventilation and series inhomogeneity. These omissions are overcome in Fig. 3.3.

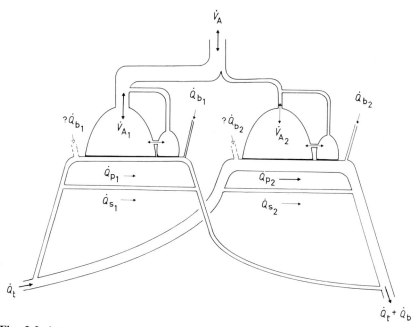

Fig. 3.3 A two-compartment extension of the model in the previous figure, that takes account of normal and pathological flow ($\dot{Q}_b$) in the bronchial circulation, of ventilation/perfusion inequality, and of collateral ventilation.

The nature of *ventilation/perfusion inequality* is simple. If, as in Fig. 3.3, we consider two ventilated and perfused alveoli with perfect equilibration of alveolar gas and end-capillary blood, then the composition of the mixed gases from the two alveoli will be biased by the disproportionate contribution from the compartment which is better ventilated and that of the blood coming from the two chambers will be biased by the disproportionate contribution from the one that is better perfused. This will inevitably generate $P_{a-A}O_2$ and PCO_2 gradients although the alveolar membranes themselves are perfect. It happens that this effect will be more marked for O_2 than CO_2 because of the shapes of their dissociation curves. In an ideal lung there would be perfect matching of ventilation and perfusion, which requires that they are similarly, but not necessarily evenly, distributed. Any departure from this leads to an inefficient lung.

Normally vasomotor and bronchomotor reflexes operate at a subsegmental level, continually matching local ventilation and perfusion. In this respect vasoconstriction in response to hypoxia is more important than bronchodilation in response to hypercapnia. In health, these reflexes keep the contribution of $\dot{V}/\dot{Q}$ inequality to the $P_{a-A}O_2$ gradient to about 5 mm Hg, despite large variations in both variables between the top and the bottom of the lung. Derangements of matching are the commonest clinical cause of arterial hypoxaemia. Some of these, e.g. poor perfusion of the apices or insufficient ventilation of the bases, are reversed by exertion, which then narrows the $P_{a-A}O_2$ gradient. Ventilation/perfusion inequality due to some other causes, e.g. structural defects, may be exaggerated by exertion.

Suppose, for the moment, that one of the compartments in Fig. 3.3 had no perfusion at all but continued to be ventilated normally. Following an inspiration, the composition of the gas entering that compartment would remain unchanged. On expiration, the gas in the anatomic dead-space would emerge first, but that from the unperfused compartment would empty *in parallel* with that from the compartment with a blood flow. It is a simple matter to calculate the contributions of these series and parallel dead-spaces to the total inefficiency of ventilation. The volume of CO_2-free gas appearing at the start of expiration is the series dead-space ventilation. The volume of the series dead-space is rarely affected by disease but its proportionate contribution to ventilation rises as tidal volume falls, from whatever cause. It is, of course, extremely sensitive to the added volumes of any laboratory apparatus and to the use of breathing equipment in anaesthesia, flying, diving, and so on. This is particularly important in patients with low vital capacities. When the breathing equipment consists only of simple fairly rigid tubes the added volume can be measured directly. When the equipment is compliant or its geometry is complex, as in an astronaut's helmet, its effective volume is often less than the actual volume and is strictly defined as the volume common to the inspired and expired streams.

The parallel dead-space ventilation (V_D/V_A) is calculated in a similar way to the anatomical shunt blood flow, i.e. since:

$$\dot{V}_A P_A CO_2 = (\dot{V}_A - \dot{V}_{D'}) P_a CO_2 + (\dot{V}_{D'} \times zero) \qquad (3.6)$$

so:

$$\dot{V}_{D'}/\dot{V}_A = (P_a CO_2 - P_A CO_2)/P_a CO_2 \qquad (3.7)$$

In essence, this fraction expresses the proportion of alveoli in the lung that are ventilated but not perfused, but in fact it also includes an underestimate of those with some blood flow but high $\dot{V}/\dot{Q}$ ratios.

3.1.6 Airflow limitation

If an airway is totally obstructed the alveoli beyond it will collapse due to gas absorbtion. This process takes place in two stages. The first phase, which is rapid, is due to the equilibration of O_2, CO_2 and other soluble gases, such as nitrous oxide. The nett resorption which results, raises the partial pressures of the less soluble residual gases, forcing them into solution until absorption is complete. Pneumothoraces and bubbles of surgical emphysema are resorbed in the same way.

Although airways are commonly obstructed in disease, this form of collapse is uncommon because alveoli and airways below segmental level are interconnected. Total obstruction above that level is needed to produce absorption atelectasis. Although total obstruction in distal airways may not lead to atelectasis, it does impair the efficiency of ventilation, because it lengthens the path incoming air must take to reach affected alveoli. It also leads to series inhomogeneity, i.e. the gas passing through communicating channels has already given up some of its oxygen and gained some CO_2 before it reaches the final alveolus. The vessels in the latter constrict in response to the hypoxia, which diverts blood flow centripetally, creating series, rather than parallel, $\dot{V}/\dot{Q}$ inequality.

All of the models discussed so far have ignored the mechanical aspects of ventilation. These are often tackled, as in Fig. 3.4, by putting a 'tube and balloon' into a bottle. In this model the tube has resistance but no compliance and the balloon is compliant but not resistant. This approach neatly distinguishes the work needed to force gas through the airway from that neccesary to stretch alveoli. It is helpful, for example, because it suggests that in the presence of airway obstruction the total work of ventilation is minimized by slow deep breathing. In the presence of alveolar fibrosis it would be minimized by ventilation that was rapid and shallow. However, it is interesting to see how this model fails to account for the most obvious aspects of a normal forced respiration, let alone the hyperinflation seen in asthma or the compression of alveoli by neighbouring bullae in emphysema.

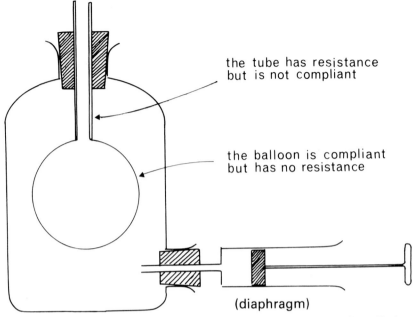

the tube has resistance
but is not compliant

the balloon is compliant
but has no resistance

(diaphragm)

Fig. 3.4 A 'tube and balloon in a bottle' model of the mechanics of ventilation.

The first of these difficulties is illustrated in Fig. 3.5a which plots pleural pressure and ventilatory flow versus lung volume, observed in a normal subject making a maximal flow–volume loop manoeuvre. The subject began with his lung filled to its maximum (i.e. to total lung capacity, *TLC*) and breathed as forcibly as possible into a spirometer until expiration was complete (i.e. to residual volume, *RV*), creating the triangular trace which forms the upper part of the record. He then inspired air from the spirometer as forcibly as possible until inspiration was complete, producing the semi-circular return trace which forms the lower part of the record. The broken line shows the pleural pressures that generated these flows. The graph on the right illustrates superimposed records of three consecutive manoeuvres. Maximal flow-volume loops of this sort are highly reproducible and typical of normal subjects. It is not possible to explain the shapes of these traces using the 'rigid tube and elastic balloon in a bottle' model of Fig. 3.4.

The explanation lies in the construction and geometry of the real airway. The constraints on the design of this structure are very precise. If the branching angles or the ratios of daughter to parent tube diameters were more than slightly different to their actual values, respiration would become impossible, either because the respiratory dead-space would be too large relative to alveolar volume, or because the work of breathing through smaller tubes would be too great. As it is, the total cross-sectional area of the lumina varies with distance along the tree, rising more than a hundred-fold from the trachea to the terminal bronchi, (Fig. 3.6). Incoming air travels speedily and noisily through the trachea and major bronchi but slows abruptly thereafter. Outgoing air leaves the alveoli slowly and quietly but accelerates rapidly as it reaches the lobar and segmental bronchi.

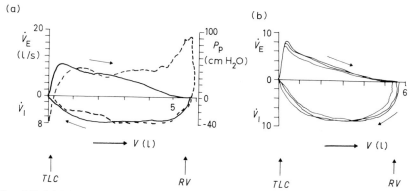

Fig. 3.5 (a) The maximal flow-volume envelope recorded from a normal subject; together with the oesophageal pressure that generated it (broken line). The plot records expiratory and inspiratory flows ($\dot{V}_E$ and $\dot{V}_I$) against respired volume (V). (b) Three consecutive maximal flow-volume loops recorded in another normal subject, in the same manner.

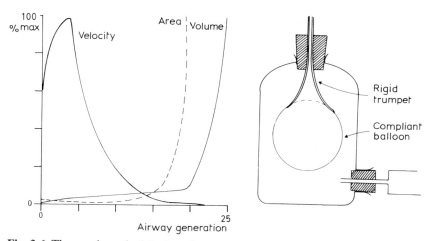

Fig. 3.6 The graph on the left plots the total area of cross-section, the volume of the airway, and the velocity of the air it contains, at each level of the bronchial tree. Variables are plotted as percentages of the maximum value in the tree. Note the steep rise in area of cross-section as the alveoli are approached. The diagram on the right shows the model of Fig. 3.4 amended to take account of this characteristic.

The momentum of the air, and of any particles suspended in it, is proportional to the square of the airstream's linear velocity, (K.E. $= 1/2\ mv^2$), and changes 10 000 to 20 000-fold between the mouth and the alveoli. This means that, on inspiration, inhaled particles tend to travel in straight lines and are caught on carinae and the outer curves of bends in the early rapid part of the journey, and any of the smaller particles which are not trapped in this way fall out of suspension in the later slower part of the journey. Air arriving in the alveoli is generally almost dust-free. During coughing, expired air is moving too slowly to clear the small airways but, because it then accelerates rapidly, is very effective in clearing the major ones. It is not surprising that mucous glands and cough receptors are found in the first few generations of the tree, where the risk of particle deposition and the efficiency of coughing is high, but are not found in the distal parts where deposition is rare and the clearance of secretions is difficult. Equally, it is very understandable that widespread disease can occur in the 'quiet zone' beyond the segmental airways without it being evident to the stethoscope or in measurements of airway resistance. (The effect of airway geometry on lung sounds is described in this book by Nath, and in the monograph by Forgacs [6].)

Although the model on the right of Fig. 3.6 takes account of the variations in cross-sectional area with distance along the bronchial tree, it still fails to explain the shape of the flow-volume loops in Fig. 3.5. These show an expiratory flow that falls to zero when gas is still present in the lung and the pleural pressure remains high. This occurs because the small airways collapse more readily than the alveoli they serve. Premature airway collapse is the commonest cause of respiratory embarrassment in diseased lungs. It might be thought that we would be better off with a bronchial tree made from hypodermic steel tubing, but that view would be wrong because the airway would then provide a rigid skeleton for the lung, preventing it from expanding. This, of course, is the reason why reinforcement is present as divided rings and spirals. Divided reinforcement alone is an unsatisfactory construction which allows the lung to expand but also allows it to buckle and collapse on expiration. In healthy lungs a continuous sheet of longitudinal elastic fibres stretches from the larynx to the alveoli, ensuring orderly retraction of every airway on expiration. With increasing age the elastic fibres in the airways and alveoli degenerate and sag, as they do elsewhere. As a result the lung enlarges and its airways collapse at higher volumes than in youth. In conditions such as progeria, cutis laxa, Marfan's syndrome and $\propto_1$-antitrypsin deficiency this process is accelerated and airway closure is exaggerated.

The trachea and first few divisions of the bronchial tree, which are reinforced with cartilage, are not attached directly to the lung and can move independently of it. The more distal airways, with little or no cartilage, are directly attached to the surrounding lung which can be thought of as a series of guy ropes between the distal airway and the pleura, pulling on each small airway and keeping it patent. This view allows us to think of the whole airway in three parts; an *extrathoracic* element which tends to collapse on inspiration, an *intrathoracic extrapulmonary* part which bellows out on inspiration but is free to collapse as soon as a positive pleural pressure is applied (pressure-dependent expiratory airflow limitation), and an *intrapulmonary* element which collapses progressively as the lung gets smaller (volume-dependent expiratory airflow limitation) (Fig. 3.7).

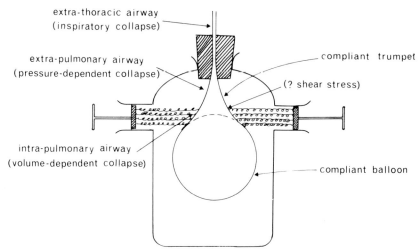

Fig. 3.7 An extension of the previous model to take account of the compliance of the airway. This considers the airway in 3 zones and recognizes the possibility of shear stresses developing at the junction between two zones.

At the start of a maximal flow-volume loop manoeuvre, as the lung is held in full inspiration, pleural pressure is usually 30–50 mm Hg more negative than atmospheric pressure and, since there is no movement of air through the open glottis, pressure within the alveoli is exactly atmospheric. Throughout expiration, alveolar gas pressure (P_A) equals the sum of pleural pressure (P_p) and the elastic recoil pressure of the lung (P_r), but the pressure within the airway must fall continuously, from P_A in the alveoli to atmospheric pressure at the mouth. Somewhere along this course airway pressure must fall below pleural pressure (Fig. 3.8). Upstream of this 'equal-pressure-point' (epp) the airway will be distended. Downstream of this point, if it is within the chest, the remainder of the intrathoracic airway will tend to collapse. The pressure gradient driving gas through the upstream segment will be:

$$P_A - P_p = P_r \qquad (3.8)$$

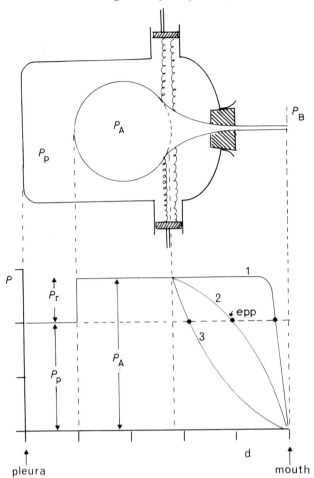

Fig. 3.8 The model of the previous figure used to predict the distribution of lateral air pressures in the airway during expiration; (1) with pursed lips, (2) normally, and (3) in the presence of the extensive small-airway disease. The equal pressure point (epp) is indicated for each case.

that is, when the equal pressure point lies in the chest, maximal expiratory flows are determined by the elastic recoil pressure of the lung and the resistance of the upstream segment, but not by the pressure applied to the surface of the lung. In normal subjects at full inspiration, the epp lies in the trachea or major bronchi. As expiration proceeds, recoil pressure diminishes and the intra-pulmonary airways get smaller, pulling the epp upstream and causing progressive centrifugal airway collapse. It is this phenomenon which explains the shape, remarkable reproducibility and high information content of maximal flow-volume loops. As the epp enters the chest, expiration becomes independent of effort and is determined by physical properties of the lung alone. Pursed lips breathing, and upper airways obstruction, will cause the epp to migrate out of the chest, towards the mouth, opposing premature closure of the small airways. Substantial small airway obstruction, or widespread alveolar destruction, causes the epp to migrate towards the alveoli, favouring early airway closure. Emphysema can be regarded as a process which snips the guy ropes illustrated in Fig. 3.7.

3.1.7 Cough, surgical emphysema and pneumothorax

The model of the lung shown in Fig. 3.7 does account for the shape of maximal flow-volume loops in normal subjects. It also explains another previously puzzling phenomenon which could not be explained by the model of Fig. 3.5, namely that coughing can sometimes lead to surgical emphysema. In this condition air gains access to the sheaths surrounding the intrathoracic extrapulmonary airways and then tracks along the adventitia of central structures escaping from the chest through the neck, and less commonly the oesophageal hiatus of the diaphragm. In the simple model there is no mechanism for rupturing the lung by applying sudden pulses of positive pressure. The model of Fig. 3.8 shows how this could occur, as shearing stresses must develop where airways enter the lung, since the extrapulmonary part is free to collapse the moment that pressure is applied but the intrapulmonary part is held open by the full lung. Holes in airways are often valvular, since the bronchial tree changes shape with the respiratory cycle, usually allowing air to be drawn through the defect when the tree expands on inspiration and obliging it to be pumped along tissue planes as the defect closes on expiration.

Holes on the surface of the lung can behave in the same way. As each pleural cavity is airtight the gas creates an ipsilateral tension pneumothorax. This is aggravated by straining and coughing. When its pressure exceeds 15–20 cm H_2O return of blood to the heart is impeded. This is due to mediastinal shift rather than direct compression of the veins. If the raised intrathoracic pressure is evenly distributed, as in positive pressure ventilation, venous return is less affected. The physiology of coughing has been described recently by Leith [7].

3.1.8 Hyperinflation

Airway obstruction is often *accompanied* by hyperinflation of the lung and it is commonly supposed an increase in lung volume can be a direct consequence of the obstruction, but it is difficult to see how that could be true. The observations to be reconciled are these:

1. Isolated lungs are almost fully distended at a pressure of about 30 cm H_2O and higher inflation pressures produce very little increase in volume (Fig. 3.9a). It is believed that the major part of the pressure-volume curve of the lung reflects extension of its elastic fibres but the limit to expansion is set by the collagen fibres (Fig. 3.9b).

2. At *TLC* the chest is only capable of generating an expansion pressure slightly greater than 30 cm H_2O [8] (Fig. 3.9c). The limit to voluntary chest expansion is muscular rather than skeletal and could be due to loss of mechanical advantage or to active opposition by antagonist muscles [9].

3. In asthma, *TLC* can rise within a minute or two of the onset of airway obstruction and can fall as quickly when the obstruction lapses [10–12].

4. Inhalation of a foreign body can lead to rapid expansion of the part of the lung served by the bronchus it lodges in [13, 14]. The affected part of the lung appears hyperlucent on radiography (see, for example, Figs. 11 and 12 in [15]).

If the chest behaved as a constant pressure ventilator, hyperinflation would only develop if there was a rise in lung compliance *and* a resetting of the upper limit to chest wall expansion. A valvular obstruction to an airway serving normal alveoli would cause them to fill completely but could not cause them to become hyperinflated. If the chest behaved as a constant-

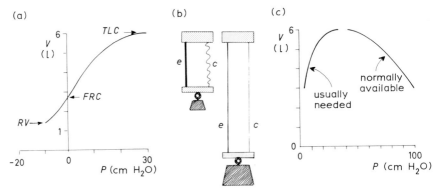

Fig. 3.9 The pressure–volume characteristic of a healthy adult lung. Normally the major part of this curve is determined by the mechanical properties of elastin fibres *e* but its upper limit is set by collagen fibres *c* as indicated in (b). The graph on the right (c) compares the pressures needed to distend the average adult lung in the chest (left-hand curve), with the maximum pressures that the chest wall can normally generate at various lung volumes (drawn form the data of De Troyer and Yernault [8]). This figure shows that at low lung volume the chest wall can develop very large pressures but at high lung volumes it can only just develop sufficient pressures to expand the lung to its maximum capacity.

.volume ventilator, it could never produce a rise in *TLC* but could produce slight hyperinflation of unobstructed elements in the presence of collapse, fibrosis or obstruction elsewhere.

Peress *et al.* [11] believe that there are rapid changes in the compliance of the lung in asthma. These could be due to modifications in the elasticity of alveolar collagen, akin to those in hair as it dampens or dries. Alternatively, it may reflect alterations in surfactant, or in the tone of the contractile fibrils that are known to be present in alveoli. The changes observed after inhalation of a foreign body which behaves as a valve may have a different explanation. On expiration, the unobstructed lung empties and becomes radiographically more opaque, but the obstructed lung cannot empty and remains lucent. In addition, hypoxia distal to the obstruction causes reflex vasoconstriction which increases the radiolucency of the expanded part. It is easy to interpret these changes, seen on a partial expiratory film, as over-inflation of the obstructed lung, when the part may simply be at its total capacity. Trapped gas is rarely found to be under pressure when the obstruction is removed [16]. It is also possible that the compliance of the obstructed part is increased. This could be due to loss of the fire-hose stiffening effect of the circulation or to one of the other mechanisms discussed above. The mediator may be local hypoxia. Generalized hypoxia, as in altitude exposure, is a known cause of hyperinflation of the whole lung. The mechanism is unknown.

3.1.9 Role of bronchial muscle

Another poorly understood aspect of lung function is the physiological role of bronchial muscle. It is usually thought to be primarily a bronchoconstrictor device for matching local ventilation to perfusion. However, in marine mammals, in whom it is particularly well-developed, it appears to act as small airway stiffener, permitting high airflows throughout the respiratory cycle and allowing the lung to empty itself completely on forced expiration [17, 18]. It is interesting that these animals have almost rectangular flow-volume loops [19] as would be expected from the pressure-trace shown in Fig. 3.5a.

None of the models described so far accounts for regional differences in the function of the normal lung. These are thought to be due to the effects of gravity. The lung can be regarded as a lump of isotropic foam, i.e. having identical mechanical properties in all directions (Fig. 3.10a), that has had its surface moistened and has been put in a dome to which it adheres by surface attraction. At rest, in a weightless environment, this would be the only force acting on it. Gravitational forces cause it to hang from the uppermost part of its container, expanding the upper part unevenly, the apical elements bearing most weight and being most expanded, and the basal elements bearing

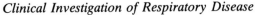

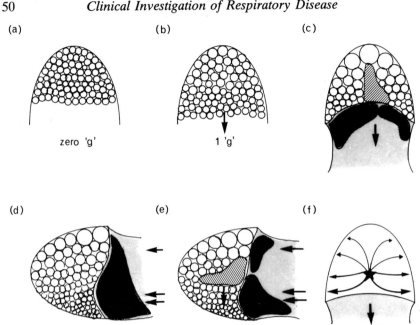

Fig. 3.10 The effects of gravity on the size of alveoli and intrapulmonary airways (a–e) and on the distribution of blood to the lung (f).

least weight and being least expanded (Fig. 3.10b). The weight of the diaphragm, liver and spleen will exaggerate these changes (Fig. 3.10c). With the body lying supine the weights of the lung and abdominal contents are redistributed (Fig. 3.10d). The lung now hangs from its sternal surface and rests on the spine and ribs posteriorly, while the abdominal contents lean on the diaphragm unevenly, compressing posterior lung segments more than those anteriorly. In lateral decubitus, the mediastinum hangs from the upper lung and rests on the lower, and the abdominal contents are redistributed as common sense suggests (Fig. 3.10e). In all of these postures, blood arriving at the lung is normally delivered to the lung at pressures lower than colloid osmotic pressure (to keep the lung dry), reaching the upper parts less readily than those below (Fig. 3.10f).

3.1.10 Summary

Fig. 3.11 attempts to put the various features discussed in this section into a single, and still unsatisfactory, mental model of the lung, mainly as a reminder that simple models can lead to wrong interpretations. It also includes a neurological addition which shows respiration to be controlled by different centres when people are awake and when they are asleep. This

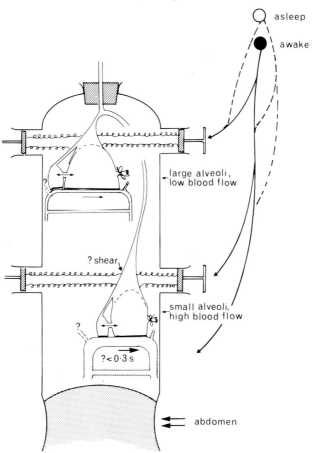

asleep

awake

large alveoli,
low blood flow

? shear

small alveoli,
high blood flow

?< 0·3 s

abdomen

Fig. 3.11 A model lung summarizing the features described in the previous figures. It also indicates the separate control centres regulating breathing in asleep and awake states, and emphasizes the importance of the abdominal wall as a major muscle of expiration.

aspect of breathing has recently been reviewed [20]. Its inclusion is a reminder that some people who have breathing difficulties may appear quite normal when they are awake and should be studied when they are asleep. The model also surreptitiously draws attention to the abdominal wall as a major muscle of expiration. It is often overlooked.

The essential features of the model are reminders that:

1. Airway cross sectional area increases 100–200-fold from the trachea to the terminal airways.
2. Airway calibre varies markedly with lung volume.

3. Although the lung is isotropic the forces acting on it are uneven.
4. As a result, ventilation and perfusion are unevenly distributed.
5. The bronchial circulation can become very important in disease.
6. Alveolar compliance can vary from moment to moment.
7. Blood can flow too quickly through the lung.
8. Shearing stresses may develop at the junction of intra- and extra-pulmonary airways.

3.2 The essential tests of lung function

It is certainly possible to practise chest medicine without access to any tests of pulmonary function at all, just as blind people can be good pianists and others can paint pictures, holding a brush between their toes. From that viewpoint no test of lung function is 'essential'. This chapter is written from a different point of view which asks:

1. What are the minimum of simple, reliable tests needed to provide a clinically helpful, and reasonably complete, functional description of the lung?
2. How should the results of these tests be interpreted?
3. What are the indications that other studies may be helpful?

The Lung Function Unit at the Brompton Hospital sees some 5000 patients with a wide variety of pulmonary disorders, each year. In about two-thirds of these cases, the functional state of the lung appears to be satisfactorily described by results obtained from a fixed battery of four procedures: the maximal flow-volume loop, a measurement of absolute lung volume, the single-breath CO uptake manoeuvre and the spirometric response to an inhaled bronchodilator. In these cases attempts to use fewer manoeuvres have led to errors of interpretation, and the addition of other procedures has added little information. We consider this battery of four as the 'essential' tests of lung function, and apply them to every patient who attends the laboratory, regardless of diagnosis. The conduct and interpretation of these tests will be described first. (We are thinking of adding a soluble-gas estimate of effective pulmonary blood flow and the sampling of arterialized ear-lobe blood as screening tests but cannot comment on their value as routine procedures yet.)

In the remaining patients ear-lobe blood samples, progressive exercise tests, oesophageal and gastric balloon studies, fluoroscopic screening of the diaphragm under load, cardiac catheter measurements and regional tests of lung function at fibreoptic bronchoscopy are the procedures which have most frequently given useful further information. The conduct and interpretation of these tests will be described later.

In almost all lung-function studies the patient wears a nose-clip and breathes through a mouthpiece. It is very easy to forget to check that the clip seals the nose properly, or even to overlook the clip entirely. This can lead to the most bizarre artefacts and creates all sorts of false hares. If any measurement is unexpectedly odd or poorly reproducible, this is the first point to check.

3.2.1 Maximal flow–volume loop manoeuvres

The object of the test is to obtain reproducible records of the flow–volume envelope that limits maximal respiratory manoeuvres. Occasionally the measurements are made with the patient in odd postures in which he has noticed particular dyspnoea, but normally they are conducted with the patient seated upright but comfortably on a firm straight-backed chair. He is told to 'take a deep breath until he cannot get another drop in, then wrap his mouth tightly around a mouthpiece and on a given signal, blow the living daylights out of the machine in front of him until he cannot possibly get another teaspoonful out, and finally suck it all back in again as fast as it will come until he is completely full once more, taking care to keep his back against the chair-back all of the time'. These phrases are given here *verbatim* because the commonest cause of poor reproducibility in this test is poor patient instruction. More delicate indications of what is needed are often ineffective.

The mouthpiece the patient uses is attached to a flow-meter, a spirometer, or both. If a flow-meter (pneumotachograph) alone is used, the flow-signal is integrated to obtain respired volume. If a volume-meter is used by itself, the volume signal is differentiated to obtain respired flow. The flow and volume signals are then plotted on some form of X–Y recorder, providing records of the general style shown in Fig. 3.12. Many indices of respiratory function can be read from this trace. Those derived most commonly are peak expiratory flow ($\dot{V}_{Emax}$), mid-expiratory flow ($\dot{V}_{Emax50}$), late expiratory flow ($\dot{V}_{Emax75}$), peak inspiratory flow ($\dot{V}_{Imax}$), mid-inspiratory flow ($\dot{V}_{Imax50}$), volume expired in the first second (FEV_1), the volume expired in the first three seconds (FEV_3), the volume inspired in the first second (FIV_1) the forced vital capacity (FVC), and the ratio FEV_1/FVC.

A great deal can be learnt by comparing the form of the loop to that which is normally seen, i.e. of a triangle sitting on semicircle, as in Fig. 3.12a. In principle six patterns can be recognized, reflecting various functional disorders. If the intra-thoracic airways collapse immediately expiration begins there is an abrupt early fall from peak flow, i.e. pressure-dependent collapse (Fig. 3.12b). If the airways collapse progressively with expiration, the scooping out of the expiratory limb is more gradual, as in Fig. 3.12c. This is volume-dependent collapse. Conversely, if the lungs are abnormally stiff or springy, airway closure is delayed, as in children and young women, but

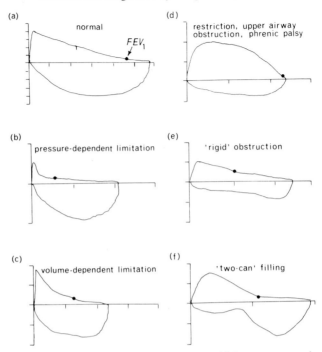

Fig. 3.12 Six types of maximal flow-volume loop which are commonly seen.

inspiration is opposed, producing loops similar to Fig. 3.12d. Flattening of the inspiratory limb is also produced by collapsible obstruction of the upper airway, by pain, and by neuromuscular defects of inspiration. It is a most useful clue to unexpected phrenic palsy. Flattening of both limbs as in Fig. 3.12e, usually reflects rigid airways obstruction. However, very occasionally it can be due to co-existant collapsible obstructions of the upper and lower airways, as in relapsing polychondritis, or to co-existant restrictive and obstructive conditions. Sometimes the two limbs of the loop are flattened in a particular asymmetric way (Fig. 3.12e). This pattern often reflects the lung behaving as if it filled and emptied in two compartments, one fast and the other slow. An example of this, taken from a patient with stenosis of the left main bronchus, is shown in Fig. 3.13.

Many hospitals are not equipped to measure respired flows and volumes in this way. It is still possible to derive a reasonable impression of the flow-volume loop from spirometry alone, by recording separate forced inspiratory and expiratory spirograms and taking tangents at one-eighth, one-quarter, one half and three-quarters of the way through each manoeuvre to derive flows. This is tedious but satisfactory. Fig. 3.14 compares some conventional loops with those constructed in that way.

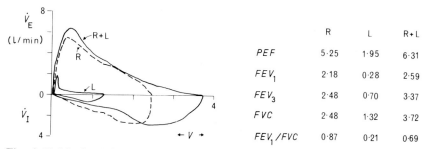

Fig. 3.13 Maximal flow-volume loops recorded at fibreoptic bronchoscopy in a young man with a severely stenosed left main bronchus. (Technique described by Williams *et al.* [26].)

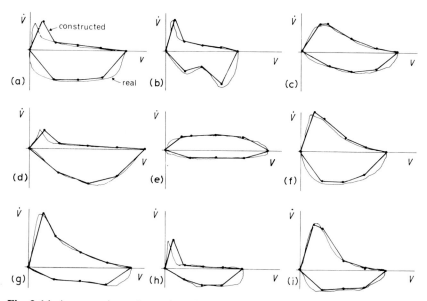

Fig. 3.14 A comparison of actual maximal flow–volume loops with those constructed from conventional spirograms by drawing tangents $\frac{1}{8}$, $\frac{1}{4}$, $\frac{1}{2}$ and $\frac{3}{4}$ of the way through expiration and $\frac{1}{4}$, $\frac{1}{2}$ and $\frac{3}{4}$ of the way through inspiration.

3.2.2 Measurements of lung volume

Absolute lung volumes can be measured in three ways which provide different information. The first of these uses geometrical images of the lung obtained from radiographs and provides an estimate of its displacement volume. The second, employs the body plethysmograph and gives an estimate of the volume of all gas in the thoraco-abdominal cavity, whether or not it is in communication with the mouth. After subtraction of an assumed gut gas volume, this quantity is taken as the lung's compressible gas volume. The third technique calculates the accessible gas volume of the lung, from dilution of an insoluble gas marker. In theory, the differences between the volumes obtained by the first and the second procedure is a measure of the tissue and fluid in the lung, and the difference between the volumes provided by the second and third procedures estimates the trapped gas volume of the lung. The procedures will be described in turn.

(a) Radiographic estimates of lung volume

In this procedure, postero-anterior and lateral films are taken when the patient is at maximum inspiration or expiration. It is essential that the films are not taken until the patient signals that he has actually reached his total lung capacity or residual volume. For the kindest of reasons, radiographers may underestimate how long this takes in people with diseased lungs. The optical geometry of the radiography system must be known or be implicit in the films. The volume of the lung can be calculated from these films in several ways. The method we use, which has an apparent accuracy of $\pm 3\%$, has been described [21]. It supposes that the chest wall, the heart, the spinal mass and the diaphragm are almost, but not quite, elliptical in transverse section, and that the cross-sectional areas of these structure, at any level, can be calculated from the P_A and lateral diameters (Fig. 3.15). These are read repeatedly from the top to the bottom of the lung and the volumes of each structure obtained by summing the volumes present in each thin slice. The procedure lends itself to automation and, at present, takes a few minutes to complete. It has the advantages that it requires very little co-operation from the patient, frequently makes use of radiographs required for other purposes, and is cheaply implemented. Providing their outlines can be seen in both views, it can also be used to calculate the volumes of lobes, segments, cysts, tumours, pneumothoraces, effusions, and the excursions of each hemidiaphragm or costal surface [22].

(b) Whole body plethysmography

In this procedure the subject sits in a gas-tight box, as shown in Fig. 3.16. At first, he warms and wets the air in the box, causing it to expand erratically. Once these initial artefacts have subsided, he is asked to attach himself to a mouthpiece that leads to a pressure sensor and attempt to inspire or expire against it. In doing so he gets bigger or smaller and the manometer senses the alveolar pressure he develops in doing so. A volume or pressure sensor

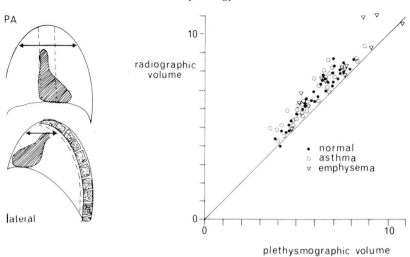

Fig. 3.15 A comparison of radiographic and plethysmographic estimates of total lung capacity in normal subjects and patients with asthma or emphysema. (Method of Pierce *et al*. [21].)

attached to the plethysmograph measures changes in his body volume. Since the changes in body volume and alveolar pressure are known, and body fluids are incompressible, the volume of compressible gas in the thoraco-abdominal cavity can be calculated, using Boyle's Law. It is important to note that this technique measures all of the compressible gas within the cavity, whether or not it is in communication with the mouth. It also measures extrathoracic gas communicating with the mouth, i.e. in the upper airways, including the facial sinuses which do not form part of the conventional dead-space. It does not include or underestimates gas in stiff containers, e.g. obstructed sinuses and thick-walled cysts, or extrathoracic gas, as in surgical emphysema, which does not communicate with the mouth. It will also be in error to the extent to which actual compressing pressures vary from those recorded at the mouth. This can be an important source of error if the volume of gas below the diaphragm is large.

If the patient breathes through an open tube, as in Fig. 3.16b, the resistance of his airways can be calculated, since he still has to change alveolar pressure to push or drag air through the bronchial tree. Instantaneous alveolar pressure can be determined from the apparent change in his body volume, since this reflects the extent to which he is compressing the gas inside him but does not reflect how much he has actually breathed in or out. If actual flow at the mouth is recorded (with a pneumotachograph), plots of alveolar pressure versus respired flow can be obtained. The slope of these curves is airway resistance. Because it is derived from the pressure

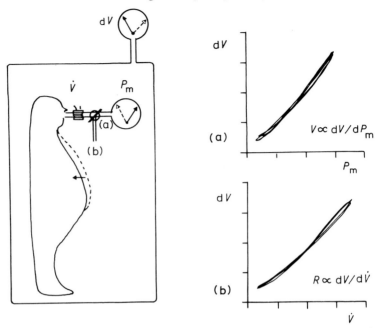

Fig. 3.16 The principle of whole body plethysmography depends on three signals: dV, which reflects the change in volume of the man; Pm, which is the pressure that he develops at the mouth (and in the chest) when breathing through (a); and $\dot{V}$, which is the flow he produces when breathing through (b). The curves on the right show how lung volume and airway resistance are obtained from these measurements.

within the alveolar space rather than that applied to the outer surface of the lung, it is insensitive to changes in pulmonary tissue resistance.

(c) *Gas dilution estimates of lung volume*

In this procedure the patient sits upright, attaches himself to a mouthpiece, and then mixes the gas in his lungs with some air marked with an insoluble gas. An estimate of the volume of his lung at the start of the test is then obtained from the dilution of the insoluble marker. The significance of this volume varies with details of the test.

In the simplest case, the patient expires to residual volume, abruptly inspires a vital capacity (VC) of marked air, holds his breath for a few seconds, and then forcibly exhales to residual volume RV. Some gas from the alveolar part of the expiration is sampled and analysed. It is assumed that this sample is representative of all alveolar gas, and the patient's lung volumes are then calculated as indicated in Fig. 3.17a, i.e.:

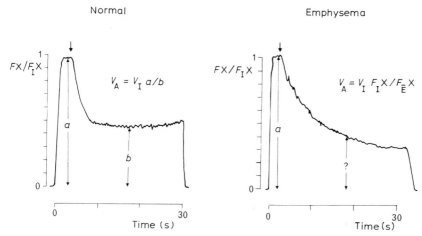

Fig. 3.17 Records of the respired concentration of a marker gas (X) during a sharp inspiration followed by a slow exhalation. Concentrations are expressed as fraction of the inspired value. Equations show how the effective accessible gas volume (V_A) of the lung is calculated in each case. Note it is neccessary to obtain a volume-weighted average of F_EX in patients with unevenly distributed ventilation.

$$TLC = VC \text{ (insp. conc.)/(exp. conc.)} \qquad (3.9)$$

and

$$RV = TLC{-}VC \qquad (3.10)$$

In another simple case, the patient expires to functional residual capacity or residual volume and then rebreathes from a bag filled with a known volume (V_B) of marked gas. Lung volume (V_L) at the moment of entry is calculated as before, i.e.

$$V_L = V_B [\text{(initial conc./final conc.)} -1] \qquad (3.11)$$

In a third simple case, the patient attaches himself to the mouthpiece at a known lung volume and the initial concentration of nitrogen in his alveolar air is noted and he then respires some nitrogen-free gas, usually pure oxygen, for 10–20 minutes. His lung volume, at the onset of breathing the gas, is calculated from the total volume (V_E) and the N_2 concentration of the expired mixture, so:

$$V_L = V_E \text{ (mixed expired } N_2 \text{ conc.)/(initial } N_2 \text{ conc.)} \qquad (3.12)$$

All of these procedures measure that volume of gas in the lung which can be reached by the respired mixture during the time of the test, i.e. they describe an *accessible gas volume* for which a time of access must be specified.

Clinically, it is practical and convenient to use the 10-second single breath volume as the accessible gas volume of the lung, since this period roughly corresponds to the duration of a normal deep inspiration. The difference between it and the plethysmographic volume represents that part of the residual volume, as measured by plethysmography, which cannot be reached by inspired air within 10 seconds. It is a measure of the effective trapped gas volume. It does not imply that the unreached gas is wholly unreachable but does imply that it cannot be reached in the time specified.

The single inhalation technique assumes that the sample of alveolar gas is representative of all the alveolar gas expired, and also of the alveolar gas remaining in the lung at the end of expiration. In diseased lungs neither of these assumptions is justified. Firstly, as in the single-breath trace of Fig. 3.17b recorded from a patient with emphysema, the concentration of marker in expired air may vary continuously throughout expiration. Secondly, even if the alveolar plateau of marker concentration is entirely constant, as in Fig. 3.17a, there can be large differences between the mean expired alveolar and the mean residual alveolar concentrations of marker. Fig. 3.18 illustrates how these can arise. It shows an imaginary emphysematous lung with a *TLC* of 9 litres, divided into 9 compartments of equal capacity but

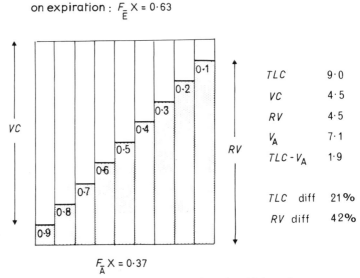

on expiration : $F_{\bar{E}} X = 0.63$

TLC	9·0
VC	4·5
RV	4·5
V_A	7·1
$TLC - V_A$	1·9
TLC diff	21%
RV diff	42%

$F_{\bar{A}} X = 0.37$

Fig. 3.18 A nine-compartment model of the lung in which each compartment has a capacity of 1 l but the residual volumes (shaded) vary from 0.1 to 0.9. As a result, assuming perfect mixing, the concentrations of an inhaled marker vary from compartment to compartment at end-inspiration and differ between mean residual and mean expired alveolar gas at end expiration, as shown.

residual volumes varying from 0.1 to 0.9 litres. Assuming perfect mixing in each compartment, following a vital capacity inspiration of marker, the concentrations of marker in alveolar gas will vary, from 90% to 10% respectively. Mixed expired alveolar air will have a marker concentration of 63%. Mean residual alveolar air will have a marker concentration of 37%. Using the mixed expired concentration will lead to a 21% underestimate of *TLC* and a 42% underestimate of residual volume, whereas a prolonged rebreathing manoeuvre would eventually provide a stable marker concentration of 50%, leading to no error in the estimates of actual *RV* and *TLC*.

At first sight, rebreathing estimates of lung volumes appear to be more accurate, however, rebreathing does not represent real-life respiration, which is a succession of individual breaths. Incoming oxygen and outgoing CO_2 will be treated very similarly to the inhaled marker. The model lung in Fig. 3.18 can properly be said to 'behave as if' it had an accessible gas volume of 7.1 rather than 9.0 litres. The 1.9 litre deficit is a valuable measure of the fraction of residual volume which behaves as if it was not ventilated. Prolonged rebreathing can be used to measure its *actual* accessible volume, but a single inhalation should be used to measure its *effective* accessible gas volume.

Fig. 3.19 compares the 10-s accessible gas volume with the plethysmographic residual volume in 216 people. Of these 56 were normal, 59 had functional emphysema, 43 were asthmatic, 27 were scoliotic, and 31 had

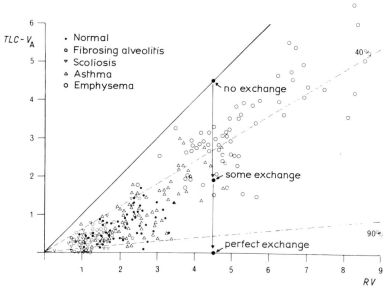

Fig. 3.19 Estimates of the 10-s effective accessible gas volume of the lung, as a fraction of residual volume, in normal people and various patients.

fibrosing alveolitis. We find this plot useful. Any point falling on the abscissa represents a lung in which inspired gas reached all of the residual volume within 10 seconds of a vital capacity inspiration. From the arguments presented in the previous paragraph it would also indicate that there was little unevenness of ventilation. Any point falling on the line of identity represents a lung in which none of the residual volume was reached by inspirate in 10 seconds. Any other point represents a lung which can be treated as if its residual volume were in two parts, of which one was, and the other was not, accessible in this time.

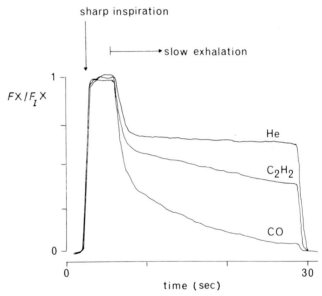

Fig. 3.20 Respired concentrations of helium, acetylene and carbon monoxide seen at the mouth during a sharp inspiration and slow exhalation in a normal subject. Concentrations are presented as a fraction of the inspired value. (Data of Denison *et al.* [27].)

3.2.3 Carbon monoxide transfer

Very similar arguments can be used when thinking of the exchange of *soluble* gases in the lung, during single-breath and rebreathing manoeuvres. Fig. 3.20 shows the concentrations of helium, acetylene and carbon monoxide, that were observed, during an abrupt inhalation and slow exhalation, at the mouth of a normal subject. The initial signals of the three gases have deliberately been scaled to be identical. If acetylene and carbon monoxide were not soluble they would have followed an identical course to that of helium. As it is, acetylene, which is quite soluble in water and fats, dissolves in lung tissue immediately on inspiration, and is carried away by pulmonary and bronchial blood flow thereafter. The initial fall of acetylene relative to helium can be used as a measure of lung tissue volume, and the slope of the subsequent trace relative helium can be used as a measure of *effective pulmonary blood flow*. Exactly as in the previous discussion, it does not measure actual blood flow, but only that part of total lung blood flow which is effective in picking up a soluble gas such as acetylene *or oxygen*.

Carbon monoxide is poorly soluble in water but is extremely soluble in blood; so much so, that its transfer across the alveolar membrane is limited, not by blood flow but by the diffusion resistance between the inspired front and the blood in the pulmonary capillaries. It is also limited by the amount of haemoglobin present at an instant in the pulmonary capillaries. It used to be thought that the behaviour of this gas simply measured the diffusion characteristic of the alveolar membrane. Nowadays it is appreciated that it is most probably reflecting the amount of accessible haemoglobin present at any moment in the effective accessible gas volume. This characteristic of the lung, which is measured from the slope of the carbon monoxide trace relative to that of helium, is the transfer factor of the whole lung ($DLCO$). It can obviously be reduced by two mechanisms; reduction in the effective accessible gas volume (V_A), and reduction in carbon monoxide transfer per litre of effective accessible gas volume ($DLCO/V_A$). The latter is known as the *transfer coefficient* (KCO) of the accessible part of the lung. Clearly it gives no information about the quality of the alveolar membrane, or the quantity of haemoglobin, in the inaccessible part. Neither does it distinguish between haemoglobin in the capillaries and haemoglobin in the airspaces of the lung. Hughes and his colleagues have turned this point to advantage, as an index of cryptic haemoptysis in conditions such as Goodpasture's syndrome [23]. It is also sensitive to variations in whole blood haemoglobin content, both in the anaemias and in polycythaemia.

3.2.4 Spirometric response to inhaled bronchodilator

This test is used to determine whether there is an unsuspected element of reversible airflow limitation in people who are not thought to have asthma, and to document the degree of reversibility at the time of measurement in known asthmatics. It is therefore given to everyone who presents for routine lung-function tests unless there is a clear indication to the contrary. The patient takes two 'puffs' from a salbutamol inhaler, separated by an interval of 30 to 60 seconds. Each 'puff' delivers 100 µg of the bronchodilator. The patient waits 10–20 minutes for it to take effect and then repeats the maximal flow-volume loop manoeuvre. Changes in FEV_1 and FVC are recorded. It is important to note that many people with airflow limitation will show a proportionately bigger increase in *FVC* than FEV_1 (Fig. 3.21), therefore records of peak flows, FEV_1 or the FEV_1/FVC ratio alone may fail to draw attention to responses that are significant.

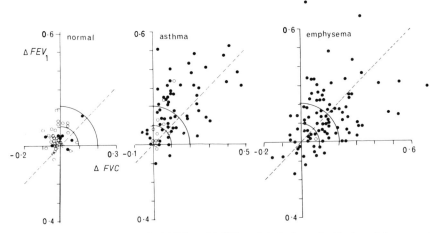

Fig. 3.21 Typical changes in FEV_1 and *FVC* on inhalation of salbutamol in normal subjects, and in patients with asthma or emphysema. All points below the (broken) line of identity represent proportionately greater response in *FVC* than FEV_1. The concentric quadrants confine changes of +10% and +20% respectively.

3.3 Setting up and running a laboratory

Newly appointed chest physicians are often asked to set up or oversee a routine lung-function laboratory. How this is done is, very properly, a personal affair that depends upon the money and space available, the technical skills and equipment that are already there, and the research interests of the physicians. Very few comments apply to every situation but one or two general thoughts may be helpful.

If you have to begin from scratch with little money, firstly discover what local computing facilities are available and whether the new laboratory can be linked to them. Secondly, find out what the hospital machine-shop and electronic laboratory are like. If these are limited, look at the computing, electronic and engineering laboratories in local Universities and Technical Colleges, with the idea of interesting their Sandwich Course and new postgraduate students in joint development projects. Find the best possible technician and then 'shop around' for equipment, with the following priorities:

1. Electrical spirometry (flow and volume), and an *X–Y* plotter.

2. Digital plotting equipment (for radiographic lung volumes).
3. Carbon monoxide transfer analyser.
4. Blood gas electrodes.
5. Pressure transducers for oesophageal 'balloonery'.
6. An ergometer or treadmill for heart and lung stressing.

The more computing and electronic back-up you find, the simpler, cheaper and more flexible these items can be. Any equipment beyond this is a bonus.

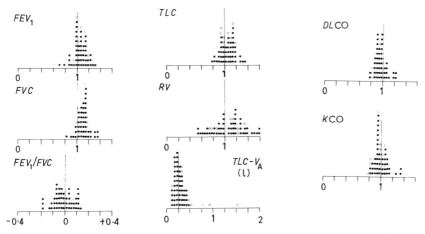

Fig. 3.22 Functional profile of the lungs of 51 'normal' subjects aged 18–72. Solid symbols are people with normal specific conductance, open circles are for those with conductance < 1.3 l/kPa/l.

Supposing the equipment is together and the technicians have been trained, the next step is to offer free lung-function tests to all the normal people you can find. Aim to get the sex, race and age mixture corresponding to that of the population locally. Plot their results, expressed as a percentage of predicted values, as in Fig. 3.22. The predictions we use for white people are those from Cotes [24]. These are reduced by 10% for people from other races, because the evidence available suggests this is a reasonable rule to apply. It should be noted that many of the studies on these people have been conducted in their own countries and may not strictly apply to those living elsewhere. Similarly studies on white people should not be rigidly translated from one part of the country to another. We arbitrarily use Cotes' regression equation to provide us with mean predicted values and set a range of ±15% as a guide to suspicion.

The exercise of looking at 'normal' people has two purposes, firstly to check that results obtained with your techniques are roughly comparable with those of others, and secondly, to establish normal values for your laboratory and the local population. Criteria of normality should not be too exacting. In the study illustrated by Fig. 3.22 the criterion was simply a verbal assurance from the subjects that they had not suffered from major chest disease at any time or experienced minor chest ailments recently. This seems a more appropriate reference population than one narrowed down to a single Swedish housewife and a Marine Commando.

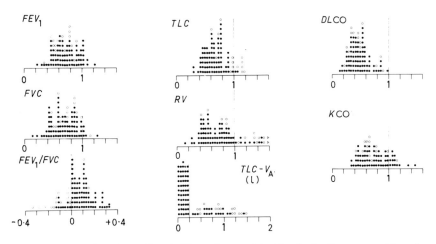

Fig. 3.23 Functional profile of 92 patients with histologically proven fibrosing alveolitis. Symbols as in previous figure.

Once the laboratory is ready to accept patients, insist that they all receive the complete battery of essential tests. This enables you to spot the presence of an unsuspected restrictive element in a primarily obstructive condition, and vice versa. It also allows you to build up functional profiles of various conditions, as in Fig. 3.23, and spot rogue measurements and incomplete diagnoses. This also enables the results to be analysed automatically, to a common standard. A complete set of measurements should be made on at least one member of staff at the start of each day, to check that all the equipment is working correctly, and to identify any slow trends in measurement see (Appendix and Fig. 3.24).

3.4 Interpreting the results of the essential tests

3.4.1 General points

In the Brompton, all routine test results are reported automatically. This 'orang-outang' approach has the advantage that all results are interpreted to

Normal checks : M.L. January–October 1979;   M.L., V.W. and T.S. 1978 and 1979

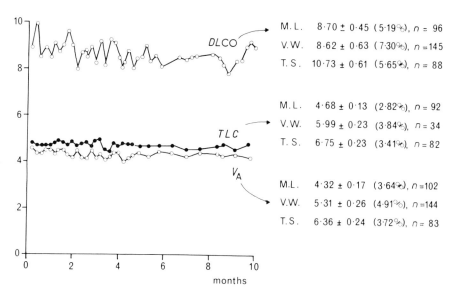

M.L.	8·70 ± 0·45 (5·19%), *n* = 96	
V.W.	8·62 ± 0·63 (7·30%), *n* = 145	
T.S.	10·73 ± 0·61 (5·65%), *n* = 88	

M.L.	4·68 ± 0·13 (2·82%), *n* = 92	
V.W.	5·99 ± 0·23 (3·84%), *n* = 34	
T.S.	6·75 ± 0·23 (3·41%), *n* = 82	

M.L.	4·32 ± 0·17 (3·64%), *n* = 102	
V.W.	5·31 ± 0·26 (4·91%), *n* = 144	
T.S.	6·36 ± 0·24 (3·72%), *n* = 83	

Fig. 3.24 A summary of the normal checks on *DLCO*, *TLC* and V_A, seen in one technician over 10 months, and in three technicians over two years.

a common standard, within minutes of the tests being completed. It also releases the physician for other work. Copies of the programme can be had from this laboratory. The computer is given the age, sex and height of the patient at the time of their first visit and remembers them thereafter. It generates mean predicted values for FEV_1, *FVC*, FEV_1/FVC ratio, *TLC*, *RV*, airway resistance (R_{AW}), specific airway conductance (SG_{AW}), V_A, *DLCO* and *KCO*, and presents these as means ±15%. The upper limit for normal airway resistance is taken as 0.2 kPa/s. Specific airway conductance is a useful measure that checks whether an abnormally high resistance can be attributed simply to the lung being small. If SG_{AW} is between 1.3–3.6 l/s/kPa per litre of lung, then airway resistance is appropriate to lung size. It is obviously particularly important to take it into account when looking at children. V_A is predicted to be 93% of *TLC*. The computer is also given the actual test results for the day and analyses then using the following arguments:

1. If FEV_1 or *FVC* are less than 85% of predicted, there is a ventilatory defect which is classified as mild (70–84%), moderate (40–69%) or severe (<40%).

2. If the FEV_1 and FVC are normal but the ratio is not, it reports 'normal spirometry but note abnormal ratio'.
3. If there is a ventilatory defect, the programme looks for evidence that this is purely obstructive (low FEV_1/FVC ratio, big lungs, high RV, substantial trapping), purely restrictive (normal or high ratio, small lungs, low RV little trapping), or a mixture of the two.
4. If the TLC is outside normal limits it calculates the deviation from the predicted mean and reports this as 'about n litres of hyperinflation or loss of lung volume'.
5. If RV is high when TLC is low, or vice versa, it notes the 'disproportionate' RV/TLC ratio.
6. If inspiratory R_{AW} exceeds the upper limit of normal it reports this as mild (0.2–0.5), moderate (0.5–1.0) or severe (<1.0), stressing that it is an *inspiratory* measurement. (This is important when obstruction is collapsible.)
7. If R_{AW} is high but SG_{AW} is normal it reports that the increase in resistance is appropriate to lung size.
8. If $DLCO$ is above the upper limit of normal it asks 'is there any evidence of pulmonary congestion, polycythaemia or recent haemoptysis?'.
9. If KCO is low it asks for a check on Hb (for anaemia).
10. It notes the state of $DLCO$ and KCO verbally.
11. It compares the pre- and post-bronchodilator spirometry and sums the percentage changes in FEV_1 and FVC. These are reported as normal (<15%), significant (15–30%) or marked (>30%).
12. It notes the shape of the flow volume loop.

Whether or not this is a successful way of interpreting the test data is best seen by studying the case reports that follow. The aims of the analysis are to provide an immediate report for a busy outpatient service, to present the findings in purely functional terms independent of the diagnosis, and to use phrases that will help doctors who are new to chest medicine. All computer reports are checked at the end of each day, and a second copy is then sent out, annotated with any additional comments or suggestions.

3.4.2 Individual cases

The results of essential tests are given in the Appendix, as exercises in interpretation. They are all presented in the same format and can be tackled in the following way. Look first at FEV_1 and FVC and ask if there is a ventilatory defect, then examine the FEV_1/FVC ratio and the flow-volume loop to see whether this defect is likely to be obstructive or restrictive. Then look at the (plethysmographic) TLC and V_T for confirmation or rebuttal. Compare the unforced VC in the plethysmograph with the FVC. Look at the inspiratory R_{AW} to see whether it adequately explains any flattening of the flow-volume loop's inspiratory limb. Move on to the results of the single breath $DLCO$ test, check that the VC in this manoeuvre is similar to the plethysmographic VC and the FVC. If so, compare TLC and V_A. Count any difference beyond 500 ml as 'effective trapping'. Use KCO as a guide to the quality of the alveolar membrane in the accessible part of the lung and consider whether it suggests a check on blood for its haemoglobin content or on sputum for haemoptysis. See whether inhaled bronchodilator (given after the other tests) had any effect. Finally consider whether the results are to be expected from the diagnosis.

3.5 Further tests of lung function

The 'essential' tests of lung function by themselves, fail to give sufficient information in about one-third of the people referred to the laboratory at the Brompton. This is usually in one of six situations.

1. When the essential tests fail to reveal a restrictive lesion which is suspected clinically.
2. When dyspnoea is more severe than the findings suggest.
3. When an unexpected restrictive process is discovered.
4. When a central or upper airway obstruction is found and its site and magnitude need to be determined.
5. When regional lung function studies are required (e.g. in selecting patients for chest surgery, or when a pulmonary embolus is suspected).
6. When pulmonary vascular resistance has to be determined.

The plan of investigation we normally adopt is:

(a) Exercise tests, and arterial PO_2 and PCO_2 measurements in air and oxygen, for 1 and 2.
(b) Oesophageal balloon studies in 2.
(c) Fluoroscopic screening of the diaphragm in 3.
(d) Further measurements of function, during fibreoptic bronchoscopy in situations 4 and 5.
(e) Radio-isotope scans in 5.
(f) Right heart catheterization with Direct Fick studies in air and oxygen for situation 6.

These procedures are described below.

3.5.1 Exercise tests and blood gas studies

These uncomfortable procedures add little information of clinical value to the work-up of most patients whose essential tests are clearly abnormal, but they are invaluable when the essential tests fail to account for the severity of dyspnoea, or fail to reveal a restrictive lesion that is suspected clinically. They are also helpful in disentangling the relative contributions of respiratory and cardiovascular factors in people with both heart and lung disease.

All such patients proceed to blood–gas studies in air and oxygen at rest and in air at the peak of a progressive exercise test. The patient first sits at rest for several minutes, having had a rubifacient cream rubbed on the lobe of his ear some minutes previously. When erythema has developed, a sample of arterialized capillary blood is taken from the lobe, as described by Spiro and Dowdeswell [25]. The patient then breathes oxygen until his end-tidal nitrogen concentration has fallen below 1–2%, and another sample is drawn. After this he breathes air again and runs on a treadmill or pedals a cycle ergometer against a power load which usually rises by steps of 100 kpm/min each minute, until he can do no more. Ventilation and heart rate are measured continuously and a third sample of ear-lobe blood is drawn when the patient signals he is about to stop.

Results are analysed as described by Jones in this book (Chapter 4). A widening of the $P_{a-A}O_2$ gradient on exertion suggests a diffusion defect. A wide $P_{a-A}O_2$ gradient when breathing oxygen at rest suggests than an anatomical shunt is present in the heart or lungs. A rise in alveolar PCO_2 above 43 mm Hg indicates a defect of respiratory control, but it is rare to discover this in someone whose essential tests are only mildly deranged.

3.5.2 Oesophageal balloon studies

Small lungs are usually stiff and large lungs are usually floppy and little is gained clinically by measuring this attribute precisely. However, in some patients there is doubt. For example, 'Are the lungs small because they are stiff or because the expanding mechanism is weak?', or, 'Is there any supporting evidence in favour of centrilobular emphysema in someone with an emphysematous flow-volume loop but normal *TLC* and chest radiograph?', or, 'Is the known phrenic palsy or myaesthenia sufficient to explain the respiratory distress?'.

In cases like these, an oesophageal balloon study can be very helpful. To do this, the patient sits at rest. The more patent of his nostrils is lightly anaesthetized with a gel or spray. A small latex balloon on the end of a fine polythene catheter is threaded through the nose to the oesophagus. Usually, the patient sips water through a straw at this time, to help the balloon on its way. The catheter is attached to a pressure transducer and the balloon advanced until it enters the stomach. (This is recognized by *positive* pressure swings on inspiration.) The catheter is then withdrawn a few centimetres into the mid-oesophagus (where inspiratory pressures are negative), some

40 cm from the external nostril in adults, to a position where cardiac artefacts are least troublesome.

The patient attaches himself to a mouthpiece and makes a series of very rapid, very shallow, respirations, forcing air to move quickly through the airways with very little volume change of the alveoli. Oesophageal pressure and respired flow are then plotted simultaneously on some form of X–Y recorder. Total pulmonary resistance (i.e. that of the lung tissue and airway combined) is measured from the slope of this plot ($dP/d\dot{V}$). Afterwards, the patient makes a single, very slow and relaxed, exhalation from TLC to RV, causing a large change of volume in the alveoli at very low flows through the airways, and oesophageal pressure and expired *volume* are plotted in the same way. Pulmonary compliance is determined from the slope of this plot (dV/dP). Typical graphs of the two measures are shown in Fig. 3.25. Finally, the patient makes maximal inspiratory and expiratory efforts against a closed glottis at TLC, FRC and RV, and these pressures are recorded [8].

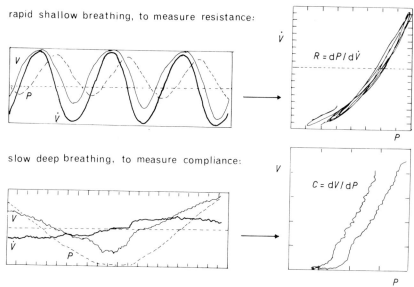

Fig. 3.25 Records of respired volume V and flow $\dot{V}$, and oesophageal pressure P, used to determine pulmonary resistance and compliance; see text for details.

3.5.3 Fluoroscopic screening of the diaphragm

Sometimes, phrenic palsy can pass unnoticed. Whenever the inspiratory limb of the flow-volume loop is unexpectedly flat, or the flattening is unexpectedly severe, it is worth screening the diaphragm. It is best that this is done under load, i.e. with the patient lying supine with a weight on his belly. It is not always appreciated that the diaphragm is often unstressed in the upright position. In this posture, particularly in young patients, very rapid inspiration expands the lower chest smartly, stretching the passive diaphragm like a drumskin, so it appears to move down sharply even though it is weak or paralysed.

3.5.4 Studies of function at fibreoptic bronchoscopy

Regional studies of lung function are clinically necessary in the diagnosis of pulmonary embolus and various developmental defects of the lung and its vascular tree, and in the selection of patients for chest surgery. Functional information can be obtained from chest radiographs, pulmonary and bronchial angiograms, radionuclide scans, and various forms of bronchospirometry. Very few centres have access to all of these techniques, and the procedures used are often determined by availability. The radiographic and scintigraphic techniques are described elsewhere in this book (Chapters 6 and 7). Studies of regional function by means of fibreoptic bronchoscopy are discussed below.

Apart from their value in localizing and determining the size of central and upper airway obstructions, fibreoptic bronchoscopes can be thought of as devices for placing various physical sensors at accurately known sites in the bronchial tree. They open up a wide range of functional investigations that can be conducted in patients who are fully conscious and thus able to perform elaborate breathing manoeuvres on command. Some of the techniques have been described already [22, 26, 27]. Others such as endobronchial pressure measurements are self-explanatory; and others again, such as echobronchography, laser anemometry, endobronchial flow, and regional compliance and resistance measurements, are likely to be developed soon. These techniques have the advantage that they investigate the lung in anatomical terms of interest to the surgeon, using an instrument that is widely available.

Any regional study ought eventually to answer two questions; firstly, what is the present function of this particular region and secondly, would the remainder of the lung be able to support life if this part was removed? The first of these questions is often much easier to answer than the second. It is a relatively simple matter to determine that a cystic or ischaemic part is contributing little to function of the whole, or that a particular lobe or segment *ought* to come out, but it is often impossible to say whether the remainder of the lung is mechanically capable of adapting to the redistribution of tensile stresses and blood flows that follow the resection. We need to develop techniques capable of answering the latter. It is possible to estimate the *immediate* effects of redistribution of blood flow by occluding lobar arteries with a balloon at cardiac catheterization. There is some evidence that this improves the selection of patients for surgery [28]. The problem that persists is that of determining whether the neighbouring lung is capable of expansion, and whether it will rupture if it does.

At present the fibreoptic bronchoscope can be used to study the motion of the bronchial walls on quiet and forced expirations, to isolate one part of the lung from another, to study the composition of gas entering and leaving a particular bronchus, to compare the latter with that contributing to the same breath elsewhere (Fig. 3.26), and to demonstrate the size, shape and position of any lobe or segment (Fig. 3.27). It can also be used to deliver and follow indicators of mucociliary clearance, and to measure pressure-drops across obstructions in the bronchial tree.

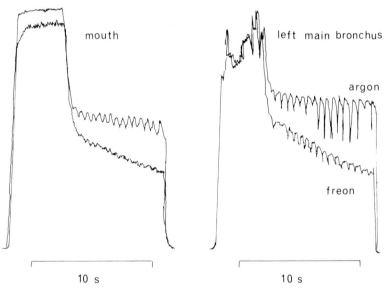

Fig. 3.26 Respired concentrations of argon and Freon 22 recorded in the same breath at the mouth and in the left main bronchus of a subject lying in left lateral decubitus. Note the much higher blood flow apparent in the dependent lung. (Technique of Williams *et al.* [26].)

3.5.5 Cardiac catheter studies

Catheter studies are helpful when patients with chest disease are thought to have a pulmonary embolus, various developmental defects, or pulmonary hypertension. They may also help in the selection of patients for lobectomy

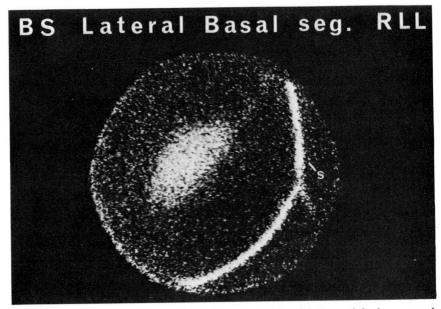

Fig. 3.27 An outline of the lateral basal segment of the right lower lobe in a normal subject, obtained by injecting Krypton 81m down the suction channel of the fibre-optic bronchoscope at the moment of inspiration. (Method of Williams *et al.* [26].)

or pneumonectomy, as mentioned earlier. If pulmonary hypertension is suspected on clinical grounds or because of an unexpectedly low KCO, it is important to determine whether or not it can be reversed by the administration of oxygen or other pulmonary vasodilators. This cannot be done by measurements of pulmonary arterial pressure alone since it is common to see large falls in vascular resistance when these agents are administered, although arterial pressure remains almost unchanged (Fig. 3.28). Measurements of vascular resistance require simultaneous estimation of pulmonary arterial and venous pressures and pulmonary blood flow. Lung Function laboratories can assist here, since they are equipped to measure metabolic gas exchange and blood gas tensions or contents. Steady-state direct Fick estimates of blood flow require adequate proof that a respiratory steady-state exists (e.g. steady end-tidal gas tensions, or little change in the respiratory exchange ratio, R), and simultaneous measurements of VO_2, $P_{\bar{v}}O_2$ and P_aO_2, or CO_2-based equivalents.

Our own practice is to wait until end-tidal gas tensions are steady, then draw simultaneous pulmonary and systemic arterial blood samples slowly over one minute, measuring metabolic gas exchange at the same time. Pulmonary arterial and capillary wedge pressures are measured immedi-

Effects of vasodilators in pulmonary hypertension:

•   oxygen in children
o   diazoxide in adults

all test results ● shown as ratios of control values

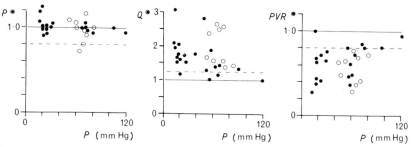

Fig. 3.28 The effects of vasodilators in pulmonary hypertension (*PVR* is the pulmonary vascular resistance) (from data of [30] and [31]).

ately before and after these collections, and the whole procedure is repeated directly to obtain satisfactory measurements in duplicate. The patient is then given oxygen to breath until his end-tidal N_2 concentration falls below 1–2% and further sets of paired samples of blood are taken and gas exchange recorded. If the pulmonary arterial pressure is normal, or only slightly raised, the patient is asked to pedal a cycle ergometer against a light load (100–300 kpm/min) and measurements are repeated once more. The blood samples are labelled very strictly and stored on ice within a minute of sampling. Blood gas contents are calculated from the measured gas *tensions*, using the Tables of Kelman [29], paying particular attention to oxygen in simple solution. Further details are given in [30] and [31].

3.6 Studying respiration in the severely ill

Many patients with chest disease are too ill to come to the laboratory, or to make forced respiratory manoeuvres, and may be unable to respond to commands at all. Certain helpful measurements can be made in these circumstances. It is practical to obtain radiographic estimates of the displacement volume of the lung at functional residual capacity, using a portable machine. The effective accessible gas volume, *DLCO*, *KCO* and effective pulmonary blood flow (at *FRC*) can be measured by rebreathing. It is a simple matter to fill a couple of anaesthetic balloons with appropriate gas mixtures in the laboratory, take them to the bedside, complete a pair of rebreathing manoeuvres, and bring the balloons back to the laboratory for analysis. These measurements are as easy to make on ventilated patients as on those breathing spontaneously. In sick people it is often simpler to obtain a reliable seal with the airway, using an oronasal mask than using a mouth-piece. Pulmonary compliance and resistance can be measured quite easily by oesophageal balloon studies in patients confined to the wards. Often, central venous pressure measurements are available and can be used in lieu. (There is a 1:1 correspondence between swings in oesophageal and central venous pressure with respiration, if cardiac artefacts are ignored.) Serial blood gas measurements are, of course, often quite crucial to the management of the very sick.

Recently, respiratory mass spectrometry has greatly eased studies of respiration in the severely ill. These analysers, which have been used as research tools for many years, have now become simple and reliable clinical aids. They sample gas from any site in the breathing circuit or bronchial tree, at a low continuous rate (2–200 ml/min) and provide accurate estimates of the concentrations of up to eight constituents continuously, or all of its constituents in discrete samples. They have the advantage that they can be used remotely, via long sampling probes (up to 150 ft), and so do not compete for space by the bedside or operating table. Similarly, like computers, they can share time and so serve several sampling sites simultaneously. It is quite practical to measure inspired and end-tidal gas tensions, metabolic gas exchange, minute volume, accessible gas volume, effective pulmonary blood flow and (with some machines) carbon monoxide transfer; and relay these to each bedside individually. Some details of these techniques have been described [32–34]. At present it seems that this type of study will grow.

Further reading

It would be difficult to find simpler or clearer short accounts of the physiology of respiration than those given by West or Murray [35–38], or a better detailed account of present knowledge than the 14-volume series of Lenfant [39], in particular [1, 2, 40–42].

There are valuable sources of information on paediatric aspects which have not been mentioned at all here [43–45]. The reviews by Milner [46] and Janet Stocks [47] are very good starting points in that regard. Harris and Heath [48] and more recently Moser [49] are first ports of call in reading about the pulmonary circulation, and Snashall's [50] brief review is an excellent introduction to the monographs by Staub [51] and Fishman and Renkin [52] on pulmonary oedema. Thurlbeck [53] is essential reading on obstructive lung disease and Cotes [24] and Bates, Macklem and Christie [54] are absolute standbys on the methodology and clinical interpretation of tests of lung function respectively.

Acknowledgements

It is a great pleasure to acknowledge a very obvious debt and thank the Chief Technician (Derek Cramer) and staff of the Lung Function Unit, Brompton Hospital, whose work is reported here.

References

1. Crystal, R. G. (1976), *The Biochemical Basis of Pulmonary Function.* Dekker, Basel.
2. Bakhle, Y. S. and Vane, J. R. (1977), *Metabolic Functions of the Lung.* Dekker, Basel.
3. Robin, E. D. (1978), *Extrapulmonary Manifestations of Respiratory Disease,* Dekker, Basel.
4. Boyd, M. J. *et al.* (1979), Pulmonary hypertension and chronic airway obstruction. *Thorax*, **34**, 697.
5. Cudkowicz, L. (1979), Bronchial artery circulation in man: normal anatomy and responses to disease. In: *Pulmonary Vascular Diseases* (ed. K. M. Moser) Dekker, Basel, pp. 111–232.
6. Forgacs, P. (1978), *Lung Sounds*, Bailliere Tindall, London.
7. Leith, D. (1977), Cough. In: *Respiratory Defense Mechanisms*, (ed. J. D. Brain, D. F. Proctor and L. M. Reid) *II*, Dekker, Basel, pp. 545–92.
8. De Troyer, A. and Yernault, J-C. (1980), Inspiratory muscle force in normal subjects and patients with interstitial lung disease. *Thorax*, **35**, 92–100.
9. Agostoni, E. (1970), Mechanics of the chest wall. In: *The Respiratory Muscles, Mechanics and Neural Control* (ed. E. J. M. Campbell, E. Agostoni and J. Newsom-Davis) Lloyd-Luke, London. pp. 23–114.
10. Freedman, S. Tattersfield, A. E. and Pride, N. B. (1975), Changes in lung mechanics during asthma induced by exercise. *J. Appl. Physiol.*, **38**, 974–82.
11. Peress, L., Sybrecht, G. and Macklem, P. T. (1976), The mechanism of increase in total lung capacity during acute asthma, *Am. J. Med.*, **61**, 165–9.
12. Macklem, P. (1978), Respiratory mechanics. *Ann. Rev. Physiol.*, **40**, 157–84.
13. Chatterji, S. and Chatterji, P. (1972), The management of foreign bodies in air passages. *Anaesthesia*, **27**, 390–5.
14. Aytac, A. *et al.* (1977), Inhalation of foreign bodies in children. *J. thorac. cardiovasc. Surg.* **74**, 145–51.
15. Simon, G. (1971), *Principles of Chest X-ray Diagnosis*, Butterworths, London.
16. Paneth, M. Personal communication.
17. Denison, D. M., Warrell, D. A. and West J. B. (1971), Airway structure and alveolar emptying in the lungs of sea-lions and dogs. *Resp. Physiol.*, **13**, 253–60.
18. Denison, D. M. and Kooyman, G. L. (1973), The structure and function of the small airways in pinniped and sea-otter lungs. *Resp. Physiol.*, **17**, 1–10.
19. Kooyman, G. L. and Sinnett, E. E. (1979), Mechanical properties of the harbour seal lung. *Resp. Physiol.*, **36**, 287–300.
20. Phillipson, E. A. (1978), Respiratory adaptations during sleep. *Ann. Rev. Physiol.*, **40**, 133–56.

21. Pierce, R. J. *et al.* (1979), Estimation of lung volumes from chest radiography using shape information. *Thorax*, **34**, 726–34.
22. Pierce, R. J., Brown, D. J. and Denison, D. M. (1980), Radiographic, scintigraphic and gas-dilution estimates of individual lung and lobar volumes in man. *Thorax*, **35**, 773–80.
23. Ewan, P. W., Jones, H. A., Rhodes, C. G. and Hughes, J. M. B. (1976), Determination of intrapulmonary haemorrhage with CO uptake; applications in Goodpasture's syndrome. *New Engl. J. Med.*, **295**, 1391–6.
24. Cotes, J. E. (1979), *Lung Function*. Blackwell, London.
25. Spiro, S. G. and Dowdeswell, I. R. G. (1976) Arterialized ear lobe blood samples for blood gas tensions. *Br. J. Dis. Chest*, **70**, 263–273.
26. Williams, S. J., Pierce, R. J., Davies, N. J. H. and Denison, D. M. (1979), Methods of studying lobar and segmental function of the lung in man. *Br. J. Dis. Chest*, **73**, 97–112.
27. Denison, D. M. *et al.* (1980), Single exhalation method for the study of lobar and segmental lung function by mass spectrometry in man. *Resp. Physiol.*, **42**, 87–99.
28. Fee, P. W. *et al.* (1978), Role of pulmonary vascular resistance measurements in pre-operative evaluation of candidates for pulmonary resection. *J. Thorac. Cardiovasc. Surg.*, **75**, 519–24.
29. Kelman, G. R. (1966), Digital computer sub-routine for the conversion of oxygen tension to saturation. *J. Appl. Physiol.*, **21**, 1375–6.
30. Davies, N. J. H., Shinebourne, E. A., Scallan, M. J. and Denison, D. M. (1980), A study of pulmonary vascular resistance in children with congenital heart disease. *Br. Heart J.*, (in press).
31. Honey, M., Cotter, L., Davies, N. J. H. and Denison, D. M. (1980), The clinical and haemodynamic effects of diazoxide in pulmonary hypertension. *Thorax*, **35**, 269–76.
32. Davies, N. J. H. and Denison, D. M. (1979a), The measurement of metabolic gas exchange and minute volume by mass spectrometry alone. *Resp. Physiol.*, **36**, 261–7.
33. Davies, N. J. H. and Denison, D. M. (1979b), The uses of long sampling probes in respiratory mass spectrometry. *Resp. Physiol.*, **37**, 335–46.
34. Gothard, J. W. W. *et al.* (1980), Applications of respiratory mass spectrometry to intensive care. *Anaesthesia* **35**, 890–95.
35. West, J. B. (1977a), *Pulmonary Pathophysiology – the Essentials*, Williams and Wilkins, Baltimore.
36. West, J. B. (1977b), *Ventilation, Blood Flow and Gas Exchange*, Blackwell, Oxford.
37. West, J. B. (1979), *Respiratory Physiology – the Essentials*, Blackwell, Oxford.
38. Murray, J. (1976), *The Normal Lung*, Saunders, Philadelphia.
39. Lenfant, C. (ed.) (1976–1980), *Lung Biology in Health and Disease.* **1–16**, Dekker, Basel.
40. West, J. B. (ed.) (1977c), *Bioengineering Aspects of the Lung*, Dekker, Basel.
41. Brain, J. D., Proctor, D. F. and Reid, L. M. (1977), *Respiratory Defense Mechanisms*. Dekker, Basel.

42. Macklem, P. and Permutt, S. (1979), *The Lung in Transition Between Health and Disease*, Dekker, Basel.
43. Scarpelli, E. M., (1975), *Pulmonary Physiology of the Fetus, Newborn and Child*, Lea and Febiger, Philadelphia.
44. Avery, M. E. and Fletcher, B. D. (1974), *The Lung and its Disorders in the Newborn Infant*. W. B. Saunders, Philadelphia.
45. Strang, L. B. (1977), *Neonatal Respiration*, Blackwell, Oxford.
46. Milner, A. D. (1971), Assessment of respiratory function in childhood and infancy, In: *Recent Advances in Paediatrics*' (ed. D. Gairdner and D. Hull), Churchill, London, pp. 217–43.
47. Stocks, J. (1977), The functional growth of the lung during the first year of life. *Early Human Develop.*, **1**, 285–309.
48. Harris, P. and Heath, D. (1977), *The Human Pulmonary Circulation*, Churchill-Livingstone, Edinburgh.
49. Moser, K. M. (1979), *Pulmonary Vascular Diseases*, Dekker, Basel.
50. Snashall, P. (1980), Pulmonary oedema. *Br. J. Dis. Chest*, **74**, 2–22.
51. Staub, N. C. (1978), *Lung Water and Solute Exchange*, Dekker, Basel.
52. Fishman, A. P. and Renkin, E. M. (1979), *Pulmonary Edema*, Am. Physiol. Soc. Bethesda.
53. Thurlbeck, W. M. (1976), *Chronic Airflow Obstruction in Lung Disease*, Saunders, Philadelphia.
54. Bates D. V. Macklem P. T. and Christie R. V. (1971) *Pulmonary Function in Disease*. W. B. Saunders, Philadelphia.
55. Denison, D. M., Bellamy, D. and Pierce, R. J. (1980), Some observations on lung function in scoliosis. In: *Scoliosis 1979*, (ed. P. A. Zorab and D. Siegler) Academic Press, London, pp. 137–47.

An Appendix of case reports follows on p. 80.

APPENDIX OF CASE REPORTS

Case 1   Male   27 yr   1.83 m   smoker
Diagnosis: Normal (smoker)

	pred.	*obsv.*	*(post-bronchodilator)*
FEV$_1$	3.72–5.03	4.57	4.79
FVC	4.52–6.12	5.71	5.70
FEV$_1$/*FVC*	76–88	80	84
TLC	5.92–8.02	7.26	
RV	1.65–2.24	1.76	
VC	4.52–6.12	5.50	
Insp. R_{AW}	<0.2	<0.2	
SG_{AW}	1.30–3.60	<3.6	
DLCO	10.4–14.2	11.4	
V_A	5.51–7.46	6.46	
KCO	1.57–2.13	1.77	
(VC)		5.45	

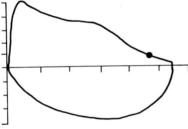

Computer report

Normal *FEV*$_1$, *FVC* and flow–volume loop, with:
   possible obstructive ventilatory defect,
   normal *TLC* and 0.3 l of air-trapping,
   normal inspiratory resistance,
   no response to salbutamol inhaler,
   normal *DLCO* and *KCO*.

Additional comments

This supposedly normal man has an unforced vital capacity which is the same for the plethysmographic study (5.50 l) and the transfer test (5.40 l). Therefore it is legitimate to compare his effective accessible gas volume (6.46 l) and his compressible thoracic gas volume (7.26 l). There is a shortfall of 800 ml, which is slightly greater than normal, (<500 ml). This is probably due to his smoking. However, it is commonly found as an isolated abnormality in trivial lung conditions and in asthmatics in remission. The computer has been programmed to draw attention to it because that is so, hence the phrase 'possible obstructive defect'.

Case 2   Male   34 yr   1.80 m   smoker

Diagnosis: normal (smoker)

	pred.	*obsv.*	*(post-bronchodilator)*
FEV$_1$	3.44–4.65	4.27	4.55
FVC	4.26–5.66	5.59	5.60
FEV$_1$/FVC	73–85	76	81
TLC	5.72–7.75	8.03	
RV	1.68–2.28	2.63	
VC	4.26–5.76	5.40	
Insp. R_{AW}	<0.2	0.22	
SG_{AW}	1.30–3.60	1.00	
DLCO	9.73–13.2	8.86	
V_A	4.83–7.21	6.49	
KCO	1.49–2.02	1.37	
(VC)		5.28	

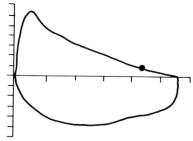

Computer report

Normal *FEV$_1$*, *FVC* with:
    possible obstructive ventilatory defect,
    about 1.3 hyperinflation and 1.0 trapping,
    loop shows mild volume-dependent airflow limitation,
    mild rise in inspiratory resistance,
    no response to inhaled salbutamol,
    low *DLCO* and *KCO*, check Hb.

Additional comments

This 'healthy' smoker shows four obstructive defects (loop shape, hyperinflation, trapping, increased R_{AW}) and low gas transfer per litre of effective accessible gas volume. Blood gases at rest were normal. Although there is clear evidence of airway obstruction, his spirometry is within normal limits, so this is still reported as a 'possible' rather than an actual *ventilatory* defect.

Case 3   Male   65 yr   1.80 m   ex-smoker

Diagnosis: chronic bronchitis

	pred.	*obsv.*	*(post-bronchodilator)*
FEV$_1$	2.71–3.67	1.30	1.55
FVC	3.81–5.15	3.10	3.34
FEV$_1$/*FVC*	62–73	42	46
TLC	5.92–8.02	6.99	
RV	2.20–2.98	4.29	
VC	3.81–5.15	2.70	
Insp. R_{AW}	<0.2	0.50	
SG_{AW}	1.30–3.60	0.42	
DLCO	8.23–11.2	6.48	
V_A	5.51–7.46	4.59	
KCO	1.15–1.56	1.41	
(VC)		2.55	

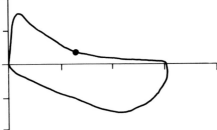

Computer report

Moderate obstructive ventilatory defect with:
   normal *TLC* and 1.9 l of air-trapping,
   contrary/disproportionate change of *RV/TLC*,
   loop shows moderate volume-dependent airflow limitation,
   significant response to salbutamol inhalation,
   low *DLCO* and normal *KCO*.

Additional comments

This finding is typical of chronic obstructive bronchitis, i.e. a clear obstructive spirometry, normal-sized lungs, obvious inspiratory obstruction, modest trapping, low *DLCO* as a consequence, but normal or near-normal *KCO* because the alveolar membrane of the accessible part of the lung is reasonably sound. Note the internal consistency, plethysmographic and transfer test *VC* are similar, so V_A and *TLC* can be compared. *FVC* exceeds the unforced *VC* because airflow limitation is not pressure-dependent. The loop has a slight 'two-can' look about it, that might be worth following up.

Case 4   Male   58 yr   1.80 m   smoker

Diagnosis: asthma

	pred.	*obsv.*	*(post-bronchodilator)*
FEV₁	2.44–3.30	1.81	1.90
FVC	3.28–4.43	3.94	4.26
FEV₁/FVC	65–75	46	45
TLC	4.93–6.67	7.26	
RV	1.76–2.38	3.26	
VC	3.28–4.43	4.00	
Insp. R_{AW}	<0.2	0.41	
SG_{AW}	1.30–3.60	0.53	
DLCO	7.26–9.82	6.91	
V_A	4.58–6.20	5.91	
KCO	1.23–1.66	1.17	
(*VC*)		3.87	

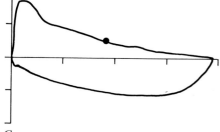

Computer report

Mild/moderate obstructive ventilatory defect with:
>   about 1.5 l hyperinflation and 0.8 l of air-trapping,
>   loop shows inspiratory and expiratory airflow limitation,
>   mild rise in inspiratory airway resistance,
>   no response to salbutamol inhalation,
>   slightly low *DLCO* and normal *KCO*.

Additional comments

Asthma is not diagnosed in the lung function laboratory but at home or in the ward, by serial measurements of peak flow or other spirometry. That point is illustrated by this man who is known to be asthmatic. He shows an almost identical function defect to the previous man (Case 3) who was not asthmatic at any time. Sometimes, though not here, the laboratory can help in the diagnosis of asthma, by showing a marked response to inhaled bronchodilator, or by finding a high *KCO* combined with airflow limitation. However, the latter is also associated with other causes of inspiratory obstruction. On most occasions when testing asthmatics, all the laboratory can do is document the functional state at the time and draw attention to any features that are atypical (e.g. low *KCO*, low *RV*, deep inspiratory limb to the flow-volume loop).

Case 5   Male   47 yr   1.82 m   ex-smoker

Diagnosis: emphysema

	pred.	*obsv.*	*(post-bronchodilator)*
FEV$_1$	3.16–4.27	0.64	0.67
FVC	4.10–5.55	2.82	2.71
FEV$_1$/*FVC*	69–80	23	25
TLC	5.86–7.93	12.1	
RV	1.92–2.60	8.24	
VC	4.10–5.55	3.85	
Insp. R_{AW}	<0.2	0.29	
SG_{AW}	1.30–3.60	0.34	
DLCO	9.18–12.4	0.29	
V_A	5.45–7.37	5.45	
KCO	1.35–1.83	0.37	
(*VC*)		2.75	

Computer report

Severe obstructive ventilatory defect with:
   about 5.2 l hyperinflation and 6.1 l of air-trapping,
   flow–volume loop shows severe pressure-dependent airflow limitation,
   slight rise in inspiratory airway resistance,
   no response to salbutamol inhalation,
   low *DLCO* and low *KCO*, check Hb.

Additional comments

Emphysema is strictly a condition that can only be diagnosed histologically but, as here, it is very likely to be present if the ratio of mid-expiratory to mid-inspiratory flow exceeds 10:1 and the *KCO* is low. This case is a striking example of expiratory flow limitation due to airway collapse. The inspiratory resistance is quite low as would be expected from the deep inspiratory limb of the flow-volume loop. The rise in *RV* and the high trapped-gas volume reflect substantial small airway involvement (compare with Case 7).

Case 6 Male 74 yr 1.72 m ex-smoker

Diagnosis: asthma/?emphysema

	pred.	obsv.	(post-bronchodilator)
FEV₁	2.14–2.90	0.95	1.19
FVC	3.15–4.27	2.04	2.48
FEV₁/FVC	59–69	47	48
TLC	5.19–7.03	6.57	
RV	2.08–2.81	4.07	
VC	3.15–4.27	2.49	
Insp. R_{AW}	<0.2	1.16	
SG_{AW}	1.30–3.60	0.20	
DLCO	6.71–9.08	7.88	
V_A	4.83–6.54	4.14	
KCO	1.05–1.42	1.90	
(VC)		2.60	

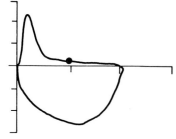

Computer report

Severe obstructive ventilatory defect with:
 normal *TLC* and 1.9 l of air-trapping,
 contrary/disproportionate change of *RV/TLC*,
 flow–volume loop shows severe (delayed) pressure-dependent limitation
 significant response to salbutamol inhalation,
 normal *DLCO* and high *KCO*,
 check for polycythaemia, haemoptysis and lung congestion.

Additional comments

This man has severe pressure-dependent airflow limitation, which probably explains why his *FVC* is so much less than his unforced *VC*. The loop is typical of emphysema but not asthma, while the high *KCO* is seen in asthma but not emphysema. He should be studied in remission to determine the extent of his co-existant emphysema.

Case 7   Male   49 yr   1.82 m   ex-smoker

Diagnosis: relapsing polychondritis

	pred.	*obsv.*	*(post-bronchodilator)*
FEV$_1$	2.77–3.75	1.10	1.35
FVC	3.56–4.84	4.40	4.00
FEV$_1$/*FVC*	69–80	25	34
TLC	5.13–6.94	5.85	
RV	1.69–2.29	1.23	
VC	3.58–4.84	4.62	
Insp. R_{AW}	<0.2	0.48	
SG_{AW}	1.30–3.60	0.73	
DLCO	8.05–10.9	8.52	
V_A	4.77–6.46	5.57	
KCO	1.33–1.80	1.53	
(VC)		4.18	

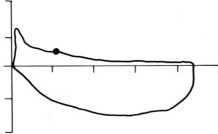

Computer report

Severe mixed ventilatory defect with:
    normal *TLC*,
    contrary/disproportionate change of *RV/TLC*,
    loop shows severe pressure-dependent flow limitation,
    slight rise in inspiratory resistance,
    no response to salbutamol inhalation,
    normal *DLCO* and normal *KCO*.

Additional comments

This man's expiratory spirometry suggests that he has severe emphysema, but several functional findings contradict this. The inspiratory limb of the loop is rather shallow, his *TLC* is normal, his *RV* is low, there is no gas-trapping and gas transfer is normal. He is a good example of collapsible *central* airway obstruction. This does not produce 'trapping', since gas enters all parts of the lung easily on inspiration, as the small airways are patent, the combination of slight trapping with obvious airflow limitation should always suggest central airway obstruction. If this was not obvious on forced expiratory radiographs or tomograms we would proceed to fibreoptic bronchoscopy on the basis of these findings alone.

Case 8 Male 61 yr 1.74 m smoker

Diagnosis: fibrosing alveolitis (smoker)

	pred.	obsv.	(post-bronchodilator)
FEV_1	2.54–3.44	2.25	2.17
FVC	3.49–4.72	2.60	2.17
FEV_1/FVC	64–74	87	83
TLC	5.33–7.21	3.40	
RV	1.94–2.62	1.40	
VC	3.49–4.72	2.00	
Insp. R_{AW}	<0.2	zero	
SG_{AW}	1.30–3.60	>3.6	
$DLCO$	7.64–10.3	1.58	
V_A	4.95–6.71	3.34	
KCO	1.20–1.62	0.47	
(VC)		2.30	

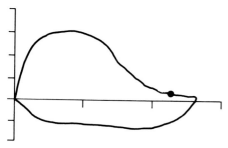

Computer report

Mild/moderate restrictive ventilatory defect, with:
  about 2.9 l loss of lung capacity,
  flow–volume loop shows a restriction, upper obstr. or phrenic palsy,
  low inspiratory resistance,
  no response to salbutamol inhalation,
  low $DLCO$ and low KCO, check Hb.

Additional comments

(At rest, P_aO_2 = 55 mm Hg, P_aCO_2 = 32 mm Hg.) All findings are typical of a moderately severe, purely restrictive, process. Note high FEV_1/FVC ratio, the shape of the flow–volume loop, the absence of trapping, low airway resistance and low lung capacity. The reduction in residual volume is particularly important because optimistic compensation-seekers cannot mimic this. Note also that this gentleman's arterial blood is desaturated at rest, as would be expected from the severe gas transfer defect. This is obviously another change that cannot be produced at will.

Case 9   Male   42 yr   1.73 m   smoker

Diagnosis: pulmonary sarcoidosis (smoker)

	pred.	*obsv.*	*(post-bronchodilator)*
FEV$_1$	2.71–3.67	2.30	2.41
FVC	3.42–4.62	3.55	3.66
FEV$_1$/FVC	63–74	65	66
TLC	4.73–6.41	5.03	
RV	1.48–2.00	1.63	
VC	3.42–4.62	3.43	
Insp. R_{AW}	<0.2	0.11	
SG$_{AW}$	1.30–3.60	2.92	
DLCO	7.77–10.5	3.23	
V$_A$	4.40–5.96	4.29	
KCO	1.27–1.71	0.75	
(VC)		3.41	

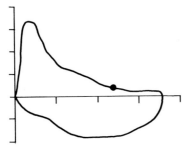

Computer report

Slight mixed ventilatory defect with:
    normal *TLC* and 0.2 l of air-trapping,
    flow-volume loop shows marked restriction and some obstruction,
    normal inspiratory resistance compatible with lung volume,
    no response to salbutamol inhalation,
    low *DLCO* and low *KCO*, check Hb.

Additional comments

This gentleman has a fairly severe restrictive defect which is not all obvious on simple spirometry but is evident from the flow-volume loop. It emphasizes the importance of looking at the inspiratory limb. Note although *FVC>VC* and inspiratory airways resistance is within normal limits, the shape of the expiratory limb of the loop and the presence of 0.2 l of air-trapping indicates some airway involvement (which may simply be due to smoking). The normal inspiratory resistance rules out upper airway obstruction, and the low *KCO* excludes pure extrapulmonary constriction as causes of the flattening of the inspiratory limb of the loop.

Case 10   Female   50 yr   1.52 m   non-smoker

Diagnosis: pulmonary sarcoidosis

	pred.	*obsv.*	*(post-bronchodilator)*
FEV_1	1.84–2.49	0.79	0.89
FVC	2.24–3.04	1.46	1.57
FEV_1/FVC	73–85	54	57
TLC	3.50–4.73	3.37	
RV	1.20–1.62	1.82	
VC	2.24–3.04	1.55	
Insp. R_{AW}	<0.2	0.67	
SG_{AW}	1.30–3.60	0.63	
DLCO	6.12–8.28	1.65	
V_A	3.26–4.41	2.05	
KCO	1.46–1.98	0.80	
(VC)		1.38	

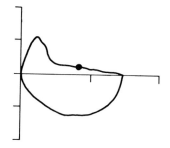

Computer report

Severe, predominantly obstructive, defect, with:
   about 0.7 l loss of lung capacity and 0.8 l of trapping,
   contrary or disproportionate change of *RV/TLC*,
   flow–volume loop shows moderate volume-dependent flow limitation,
   moderate rise in inspiratory resistance,
   slight response to salbutamol inhalation,
   low *DLCO* and low *KCO*, check Hb.

Additional comments

(Hb = 14.6 g%.) These findings, which are commonly seen in pulmonary sarcoidosis
with substantial airway involvement, are due to a mixture of obstructive and restrictive changes, i.e. small lungs but raised *RV*, trapping and high R_{AW} obstructive
spirometry and *VC>FVC*.

Case 11   Male   59 yr   1.72 m   non-smoker

Diagnosis: ? fibrosing alveolitis

	pred.	obsv. 1 22-11-77	obsv. 2 20-2-80
FEV_1	2.53–3.43	2.14 (2.11)	1.34 (1.34)
FVC	3.43–4.65	3.54 (3.58)	3.75 (3.86)
FEV_1/FVC	65–75	60 (59)	35 (34)
TLC	5.19–7.03	5.08	6.55
RV	1.86–2.52	1.58	2.50
VC	3.43–4.65	3.50	4.05
Insp. R_{AW}	<0.2	zero	0.08
SG_{AW}	1.30–3.60	>3.6	2.98
$DLCO$	7.57–10.2	2.75	2.96
V_A	4.83–6.54	4.74	5.71
KCO	1.22–1.65	0.58	0.51
(VC)		3.22	4.84

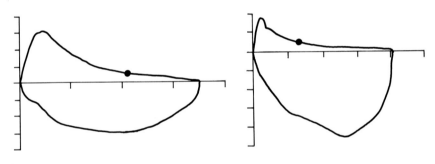

Additional comments

This patient shows a recent, severely obstructive defect, superimposed on an almost purely restrictive process of longer standing. Note that in 1977 he had restrictive spirometry and some flattening of the inspiratory limb of the flow–volume loop, small lungs, low *RV* no trapping and *FVC>VC*. In February 1980 he had obstructive spirometry, an emphysematous flow–volume loop, large lungs, some trapping, measurable airway resistance and *VC>FVC*. The changes were associated with the development of pneumonia and a series of severe airway infections. The findings illustrate how obstructive and restrictive processes work in opposite directions.

Case 12   Female   27 yr   1.56 m   non-smoker

Diagnosis: scoliosis

	pred.	*obsv.*	*(post-bronchodilator)*
*FEV*₁	2.46–3.33	1.68	1.68
FVC	2.77–3.75	1.89	1.86
*FEV*₁*/FVC*	79–91	89	90
TLC	3.92–5.31	2.52	
RV	1.13–1.53	0.77	
VC	2.77–3.75	1.75	
Insp. R_{AW}	<0.2	zero	
SG_{AW}	1.30–3.60	>3.6	
DLCO	7.42–10.0	4.87	
V_A	3.65–4.95	2.25	
KCO	1.60–2.16	2.15	
(VC)		1.72	

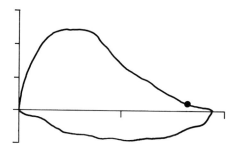

Computer report

Moderate restrictive ventilatory defect, with:
   about 2.1 l loss of lung capacity,
   flow–volume loop shows restriction, upper obstr. or phrenic palsy,
   low inspiratory resistance,
   no response to salbutamol inhalation,
   low *DLCO* but normal *KCO*.

Additional comments

This lady shows the findings typical of a pulmonary fibrosis *but* her *KCO* is at the upper limit of normal, while airway resistance is low. That combination always suggests that the excursion of the lung is limited by external rather than internal factors. Quite often in scoliosis, *DLCO* is low but *KCO* is substantially raised. This occurs because compression of the lung squeezes out more air than blood. Usually airway resistance is increased to an extent compatible with the fall in lung volume, and so specific conductance remains in the normal range. Gas-trapping is uncommon. Other functional aspects of scoliosis have recently been discussed elsewhere [55].

Case 13   Male   24 yr   1.90 m   non-smoker

Diagnosis: teratoma, before and after chemotherapy

	pred.	*obsv. 1*	*obsv. 2*
FEV_1	4.01–5.43	4.83 (4.85)	5.05 (5.05)
FVC	4.88–6.61	5.40 (5.30)	5.87 (5.89)
FEV_1/FVC	77–89	89 (92)	86 (86)
TLC	6.39–8.64	6.56	6.89
RV	1.77–2.40	1.66	1.29
VC	4.88–6.61	4.90	5.60
Insp. R_{AW}	<0.2	zero	zero
SG_{AW}	1.30–3.60	>3.6	>3.6
DLCO	11.2–15.2	10.3	8.76
V_A	5.94–8.04	6.14	6.31
KCO	1.60–2.17	1.68	1.39
(VC)		5.15	5.39

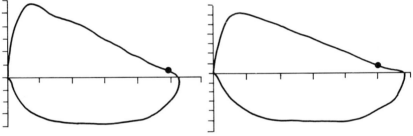

Additional comments

Several cytotoxic drugs produce a restrictive defect, as does radiotherapy. Serial lung function tests can be used to follow its course and alert the therapist before it becomes too severe. In this case, which is typical of satisfactory treatment, improvements in spirometry, *TLC* and V_A, probably associated with greater 'well-being', should be discounted. The significant warnings are the falls in *RV*, *DLCO* and *KCO*. Note also *FVC>VC*.

Case 14   Male   36 yr   1.73 m   ex-smoker

Diagnosis: teratoma, prior to chemotherapy

	pred.	*obsv.*	*(post-bronchodilator)*
FEV$_1$	3.17–4.29	2.22	2.33
FVC	3.91–5.29	2.58	2.54
FEV$_1$/*FVC*	72–84	86	92
TLC	5.26–7.12	3.59	
RV	1.55–2.10	1.49	
VC	3.91–5.29	2.10	
Insp. *R*$_{AW}$	<0.2	zero	
SG$_{AW}$	1.30–3.60	>3.6	
DLCO	8.97–12.1	6.81	
V$_A$	4.89–6.62	3.06	
KCO	1.47–1.99	2.23	
(*VC*)		2.10	

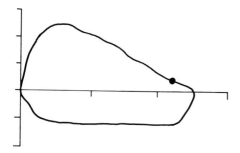

Computer report

Moderate restrictive ventilatory defect, with:
   about 2.6 l loss of lung capacity,
   flow–volume loop shows restriction, upper obstr. or phrenic palsy,
   low inspiratory resistance,
   no response to inhaled salbutamol,
   low *DLCO* but high *KCO*,
   check polycythaemia, haemoptysis, lung congestion.

Additional comments

This man had chemotherapy immediately following an orchidectomy 4 years ago. He was referred for routine studies again immediately before chemotherapy was to start again for a recrudescence. Almost all the functional changes seen here could be attributed to a severe restrictive defect following previous chemotherapy, but this would be a wrong interpretation in view of the high KCO which suggests that he has an upper airway obstruction, phrenic palsy or some more complex inspiratory muscle weakness. In fact, he has a tumour on the right side of his neck. This has certainly involved his right recurrant laryngeal nerve (he has a paralysed R vocal cord). However, the low inspiratory resistance, the low TLC and the high KCO suggest it is also involving his phrenic nerve. The findings suggest that he should have his diaphragm screened under load. (This showed he had an unsuspected right phrenic palsy. His high right hemidiaphragm had previously been attributed to collapse of the right lower lobe. The patient died, from acute ventilatory failure, shortly after these tests were made.)

CHAPTER FOUR

Exercise Tests

N. L. Jones

'The condition of exercise is not a mere variant of the condition of rest, it is the essence of the machine' [1].

The central concept of exercise testing is its use to measure the adaptive potential of the heart, lungs and circulation in responding to the demands for increased oxygen delivery and carbon dioxide removal. The quotation from Sir Joseph Barcroft indicates that this concept has been recognized for many years – and in the last two decades exercise testing has become a routine in many pulmonary and cardiac laboratories. The techniques employed are straightforward and the clinical usefulness of the information well established. However, it needs to be emphasized that the information is physiological, rather than diagnostic in the narrow sense, and must always be interpreted in the light of clinical information. This chapter will review briefly the application of exercise testing to clinical investigation, the normal responses to exercise, some patterns of response in disease, and some applications of the various tests now available.

Bearing in mind that exercise tests seek to measure the responses of a variety of systems to the increased demands for O_2 supply and CO_2 removal, a number of clinical applications may be listed:

1. To obtain a physiological explanation and quantification of effort-related symptoms, such as dyspnoea and chest pain.
2. To assess the severity of an established diagnosis, for example in a patient with diffuse alveolitis.
3. To exclude a functionally important diagnosis, by obtaining a normal response in a patient with suspected cardiac or pulmonary disease.
4. To establish the diagnosis in those conditions having a specific exercise response, e.g. exercise-induced bronchoconstriction.
5. To unmask a disorder complicating another, diagnosed, condition; an exercise response consistent with poor myocardial function in a patient with airway obstruction, for example.
6. To obtain objective assessment of the capacity for work, e.g. in industrial compensation cases.

7. To measure the effects of therapy, such as steroids in diffuse alveolitis.
8. To provide indications for further investigation of pulmonary or cardiac function.

4.1 Types of exercise

Some forms of exercise depend almost entirely on muscle size and strength, either because the power developed is very high but of extremely short duration (the 'explosive power' required to lift heavy weights), or because the muscle contraction is maintained constant for some time ('isometric exercise'). In both these examples oxygen delivery is not much involved, in the first because the time is too short to change O_2 delivery mechanisms, and in the second because the maintained tension virtually prevents any local muscle blood flow. Although playing an important part in everyday life and occupation, these types of exercise will not be considered further in this chapter.

4.1.1 Dynamic exercise

Dynamic exercise employing large muscle groups (as in walking, running and cycling) may be divided into two categories. In 'sprint' activity (high power output and short duration), oxygen demands cannot be met quickly enough and the adenosine triphosphate (ATP) required for muscle contraction is regenerated in part through anaerobic metabolism, with associated lactic acid production. Many activities in everyday life, such as climbing a flight of stairs, involve this type of activity. By contrast, the term 'endurance' exercise refers to situations in which oxygen demands are fully met, and exercise may be continued for a long time. In this form of exercise a steady state of oxygen uptake and the related oxygen delivery mechanisms is achieved. Both types of dynamic exercise may be used in clinical exercise testing. Although strictly 'sprint' activity is seldom used in clinical testing, patients are often gradually taken up to a maximum power output, usually to obtain information regarding limiting factors to exercise. 'Steady state' exercise is used particularly when estimations are made of variables requiring several measurements, such as cardiac output by the Fick principle, which need to be maintained constant for the measurements to be valid.

4.2 Oxygen consumption and delivery

Muscle contraction is associated with the breakdown of ATP to adenosine diphosphate (ADP). Muscle ATP has to be continuously replenished if exercise is to continue because the concentration of ATP in muscle is small. Although the ATP may be reformed from creatine phosphate (CP + ADP

→ C + ATP) and also from the condensation of ADP (2 ADP → ATP + AMP), most is linked to the oxydation of fuels. From the point of view of metabolic economy this regeneration of ATP is best linked to the aerobic breakdown of glycogen, glucose and fats. *Glycogen* is stored in muscle and *glucose* is delivered from the liver by the blood stream: their breakdown is summarized in the following equation:

$$(\text{glycogen–glucose}) \; C_6 H_{12} O_6 + 6 \; O_2 \rightarrow 6 \; CO_2 + 6 \; H_2O \qquad (4.1)$$
$$36 \; ADP + 36 \; P_i \rightarrow 36 \; ATP + 36 \; H_2O$$

Thus 1 mole of O_2 is used for 6 moles of ATP regenerated from ADP, and a mole of glucose yields 36 moles of ATP (strictly 38 if the reaction starts at glycogen). Also 1 mole of O_2 leads to 1 mole of CO_2 (the RQ is 1.0). For a representative *free fatty acid*, mobilized by hydrolysis of triglyceride in adipose tissue and delivered to muscle in blood, but also available in fat stores in muscle, the equation is:

$$\text{Palmitic acid} + 23 \; O_2 \rightarrow 16 \; CO_2 + 16 \; H_2O$$
$$129 \; ADP + 129 \; P_i \rightarrow 129 \; ATP + 129 \; H_2O \qquad (4.2)$$

1 mole O_2 is used to regenerate 5.6 moles of ATP (129 ÷ 23) which is associated with the production of 0.7 (16 ÷ 23) mole CO_2: i.e. the RQ is 0.7.

It follows that if energy requirements are met equally from the aerobic oxidation of fats and carbohydrate the RQ will be midway between 0.7 and 1.0, or 0.85. The equivalent ratio at the lungs (CO_2 output ÷ O_2 intake) is known as the respiratory exchange ratio (R) to distinguish it from the 'true' metabolic RQ in tissues, although in a steady state the two are by definition equal. The oxygen demands of exercise (Fig. 4.1), increase from 0.25–0.30 l/min (12 mmoles/min) at rest to about 1.0 l/min (45 mmoles/min) during walking on the level (50 W), and to 2 l/min (90 mmoles/min) during running at about 6 mph (9.6 km/hr); maximal O_2 intake for an average man will be 2.5–3.5 l/min (110–150 mmoles/min) and for an athlete as high as 6–7 l/min (270–310 mmoles/min). These values are for a 75 kg man aged 20–30: normal standards are established according to sex, age and size [2].

Oxygen demands are met through several linked mechanisms, which may be considered in terms of a chain, as follows:

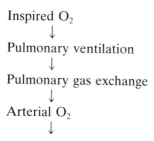

Inspired O_2
↓
Pulmonary ventilation
↓
Pulmonary gas exchange
↓
Arterial O_2
↓

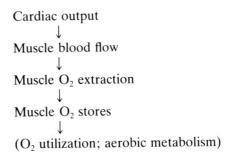

This scheme illustrates that malfunction in one mechanism may be countered, at least in part, by a relative increase in another mechanism further down the chain, acting to maintain oxygen delivery. For example, a fall in arterial O_2 content due to low inspired O_2 (high altitude) or to inadequate pulmonary ventilation or gas exchange, may be countered by an increase in cardiac output. It should also be noted that an 'adaptation' upstream is less effective than one downstream: for example, poor O_2 delivery due to an inadequate cardiac output cannot be countered effectively by an increase in ventilation. The linkage between mechanisms may also be demonstrated for

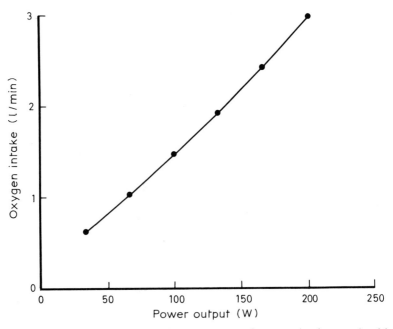

Fig. 4.1 O_2 intake during exercise in a representative untrained normal subject (male, age 30 yr, weight 75 kg) exercising at increasing power outputs, each maintained for 6 min. Maximum power was 200 W and $\dot{V}O_2$ 3.0 l/min.

CO_2 removal, and may be more or less rigorously expressed in terms of a series of equations (see below).

4.3 Carbon dioxide production and excretion

Although adequate O_2 delivery is of prime importance for exercise lasting more than a minute, it should not be forgotten that CO_2 removal is also important, and in some situations may even be more important than O_2 delivery. There are several reasons for this. CO_2 is the end product of aerobic metabolism (as described by the equations above), but in addition CO_2 will be generated through the reaction with bicarbonate of any H^+ ions (protons) produced by metabolic processes. The main source of H^+ ions in exercise is lactic acid, which is the end product of anaerobic glycolysis. Similar equations to those above for aerobic metabolism may be recognized for anaerobic glycolysis:

$$\text{(glycogen} - \text{glucose) } C_6\,H_{12}\,O_6 \rightarrow 2\ CH_3\ CHOHCOO^- + 2H^+$$
$$2\ ADP + 2\ P_i \rightarrow 2\ ATP \tag{4.3}$$

It should be noted that glycolysis of a mole of glucose regenerates only 2 moles of ATP (3 from glycogen), as compared to 36 for aerobic glycolysis. In doing so 2 moles of H^+ are generated, which through their reaction with HCO^-_3 are associated with the production of 2 moles of CO_2; 2 moles of lactate are also produced. As this series of reactions generates CO_2 without using O_2, R increases. Thus CO_2 is generated without the consumption of O_2. Lactate is metabolized aerobically by muscle to CO_2 and incorporated back into glucose in the liver (the Cori cycle); both processes regenerate HCO^-_3 but as energy is required for gluconeogenesis, excess CO_2 is always produced if anaerobic metabolism is occurring, even if the blood lactate is maintained in a steady state. Finally, CO_2 removal from muscle is an important mechanism for the control of muscle pH. If muscle pH falls below a critical level (probably around 6.5), the activities of several rate limiting enzymes are inhibited and ATP regeneration cannot be maintained in spite of adequate oxygen, leading to muscle fatigue.

The mechanisms removing CO_2 from muscle are similar to those which deliver oxygen with some important differences in emphasis: the circulation is pre-eminent in supplying oxygen whereas ventilation is more important in excreting CO_2. As with O_2 a transport 'chain' may be recognized:

(CO_2 production, aerobic and anaerobic metabolism)
Body CO_2 'stores'
$\downarrow$
Venous CO_2 content
$\downarrow$

Local venous flow
↓
Cardiac output (venous return)
↓
Alveolar ventilation
↓
Total ventilation (alveolar ventilation + dead space)

Notice that in the case of CO_2, a low total ventilatory response to exercise will lead to a fall in CO_2 excretion and a rise in venous (and thus tissue PCO_2), which cannot be helped much by increases in cardiac output; as pointed out above, this is the reverse of the situation with regard to O_2 delivery.

4.4 Equations used to describe changes in exercise

The concepts outlined above are described by a series of equations which allow the changes which occur in gas transport mechanisms to be expressed mathematically or graphically, and also may be used to calculate results obtained in exercise tests. The relationships are more fully covered in Chapter 3.

1. Ventilation is the product of tidal volume and breathing frequency:

$$\dot{V}_E = V_T \times f_r \quad \text{(Fig. 4.2)} \tag{4.4}$$

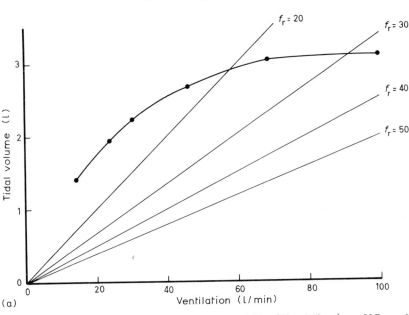

Fig. 4.2(a) Tidal volume in exercise in the same subject (Fig. 4.1), whose *VC* was 6l.

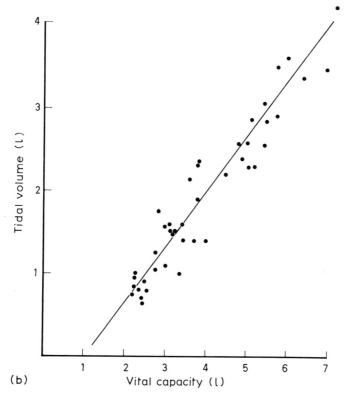

4.2(b) Maximum tidal volume in exercise as a function of *VC* in normal subjects [5].

Also total ventilation is conceptually divided into effective or 'alveolar' and the wasted or 'dead space' components:

$$\dot{V}_E = \dot{V}_A + \dot{V}_D \quad \text{(Fig. 4.3)} \tag{4.5}$$

or

$$\dot{V}_E = \dot{V}_A + V_D/V_T (\dot{V}_E) \tag{4.6}$$

where dead space ventilation is expressed as a proportion of each breath.

2. Alveolar ventilation:

$$\dot{V}_A = \frac{\dot{V}O_2 \times 0.863}{P_IO_2 - P_AO_2} \tag{4.7}$$

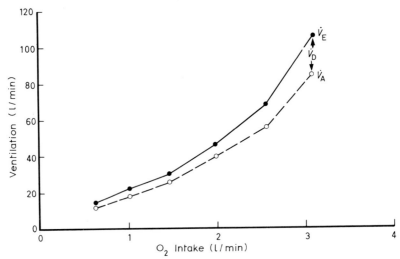

Fig. 4.3 Ventilation during exercise in the same subject shown in Fig. 4.1, related to O_2 intake, showing increase in $\dot{V}_E$ and $\dot{V}_A$ and initial fall in $\dot{V}_D/\dot{V}_E$ (4.6).

Also:

$$\dot{V}_A = \frac{\dot{V}CO_2 \times 0.863}{P_aCO_2 - (P_ICO_2)} \quad \text{(the alveolar ventilation} \atop \text{equation) (Fig. 4.4)} \qquad (4.8)^*$$

3. Cardiac output is the product of stroke volume V_s and cardiac frequency:

$$\dot{Q}_t = V_s \times f_c \text{ (Fig. 4.5)} \qquad (4.9)$$

also:

$$\dot{Q}_t = \frac{\dot{V}O_2}{C_aO_2 - C_{\bar{v}}O_2} \quad \text{(the Fick equation) (Fig. 4.6)} \qquad (4.10)^\dagger$$

and

$$\dot{Q}_t = \frac{\dot{V}CO_2}{C_{\bar{v}}CO_2 - C_aO_2} \qquad (4.11)$$

4. Ventilation–perfusion matching – dead space:

$$\frac{\dot{V}_D}{\dot{V}_E} = \frac{V_D}{V_T} = \frac{P_aCO_2 - P_ECO_2}{P_aCO_2 - (P_ICO_2)} \qquad (4.12)$$

Notionally the V_D/V_T ratio expresses the proportion of each breath

* 1. Equation (4.8) strictly should be written in terms of P_ACO_2 but P_aCO_2 is taken as a reasonable approximation. 2. CO_2 is inspired air (P_ICO_2) is small enough to be ignored.
† Unlike Equations (4.7) and (4.8), which because of a linear relationship between gas concentration and pressure may be written in terms of PO_2 and PCO_2, Equations (4.10) and (4.11) are written in terms of gas concentrations, CO_2 and C_cO_2, as the relationship between concentration and pressure ('dissociation curve') is not linear.

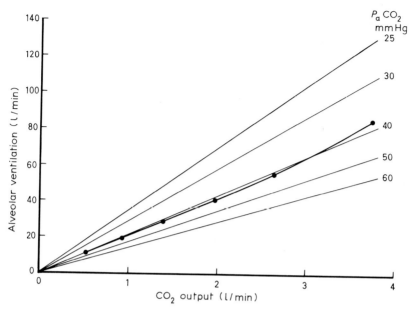

Fig. 4.4 Alveolar ventilation for the same subject (Fig. 4.1) related to $\dot{V}CO_2$; isopleths are P_aCO_2 (4.8), showing constant P_aCO_2 until high levels of exercise are reached, and that the increase in V_A with heavy exercise (Fig. 4.3) is mainly due to a disproportionate increase in $\dot{V}CO_2$ compared to $\dot{V}O_2$.

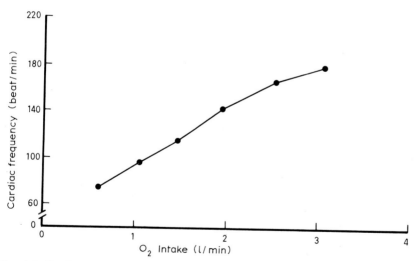

Fig. 4.5 Cardiac frequency response for the same subject (Fig. 4.1) showing a maximum f_c of 180 beats/min.

'wasted' through ventilation of airways ('anatomical dead space') and areas having high or infinite $\dot{V}_A/\dot{Q}_c$ ratio ('alveolar dead space')

5. Ventilation–perfusion matching – venous admixture:

$$\frac{\dot{Q}_{va}}{\dot{Q}_t} = \frac{C_{c'}O_2 - C_aO_2}{C_{c'}O_2 - C_{\bar{v}}CO_2} \qquad (4.13)\ddagger$$

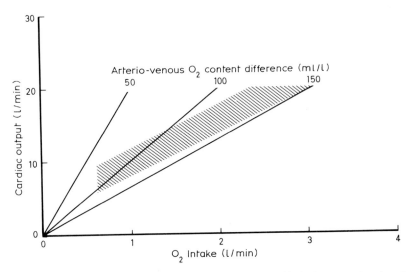

Fig. 4.6 Cardiac output in normal subjects (mean $\pm$ 1 s.d.) during exercise showing increasing arteriovenous O_2 content difference (isopleths) (4.10).

4.5 The normal pattern of responses to exercise

Oxygen intake increases linearly with increasing power output (Fig. 4.1) to a maximum value ($\dot{V}O_2$max), which varies in the normal population with sex, age, size and fitness [2]. For a 70 kg male with a $\dot{V}O_2$max of 3 l/min, the 10–12-fold increase in $\dot{V}O_2$ above resting values is achieved through a four-fold increase in $\dot{Q}_t$ to 20–25 l/min and a three-fold increase in the arteriovenous O_2 difference to 120–160 ml/l (4.10). The increase in $\dot{Q}_t$ with increasing $\dot{V}O_2$ is linear (Fig. 4.6), as is the cardiac frequency, f_c. Stroke volume (V_s) in exercise is related to body size and to fitness but remains relatively constant

‡ 1. The equation is written in terms of concentration as in Equation (4.11). 2. $C_{c'}O_2$ is a function of P_AO_2 Equation (4.7) and $C_{\bar{v}}O_2$ is a function of $\dot{Q}_t$ Equation (4.11). 3. $\dot{Q}_{va}/\dot{Q}_t$ expresses the proportion of a total cardiac output perfusing areas of zero gas exchange – zero $\dot{V}_A/\dot{Q}_c$ ratio and zero $\dot{D}O_2$.

at moderate and heavy exercise [16]. Maximum f_c is related to age (expressed in years) through the expression f_c max $= 210 - (0.65 \times \text{years})$ [3]. Thus maximum $\dot{Q}_t$ is related to size, influencing V_s, and age, influencing f_c max (4.9). In healthy subjects $\dot{V}_E$ in exercise does not reach the ventilatory capacity: values of $80 - 120$ l/min are attained, which compare with ventilatory capacities of $150-200$ l/min for healthy males [4]. $\dot{V}_E$ at low and moderate exercise increases linearly with increasing $\dot{V}O_2$. However, high power outputs (in normal subjects above 60% of $\dot{V}O_2$ max) are associated with lactic acid accumulation and thus 'excess' CO_2 output (see above). This accounts for $\dot{V}_E$ increasing non-linearly with respect to $\dot{V}O_2$ at high power outputs (Fig. 4.2), but maintaining a close relationship to $\dot{V}CO_2$. $\dot{V}_E$ at low power outputs is mainly increased through an increase in V_T, but once V_T has reached about 2/3 of the vital capacity [5], further increases are mainly through increasing f_r. Arterial PCO_2 remains constant, indicating a close coupling between $\dot{V}_A$ and $\dot{V}CO_2$ (4.8; Fig. 4.4); a slight fall in P_aCO_2 during heavy exercise is due to the additional ventilatory stimulus of a fall in pH. As P_ECO_2 tends to rise in normal subjects, the difference between P_aCO_2 and P_ECO_2 narrows, indicating that V_D/V_T has become smaller (4.12); although this is due mainly to the increase in V_T with exercise, a reduction in alveolar dead space also occurs [6, p. 25]. Arterial O_2 content (C_aO_2) remains constant in exercise: as $C_{\bar{v}}O_2$ falls, the denominator in (4.13) increases indicating a fall in $\dot{Q}_{va}/\dot{Q}_t$. The falls in V_D/V_T and $\dot{Q}_{va}/\dot{Q}_t$ in normal subjects may be interpreted as an improvement in ventilation:perfusion relationships with exercise (see Chapter 3).

These normal responses may be contrasted with the patterns of response obtained in patients in whom O_2 and CO_2 transport mechanisms have reduced adaptive capacity.

4.6 Effects of an impaired central cardiovascular response (Fig. 4.7)

Patients with functionally significant cardiac disease show a reduced maximum power output and $\dot{V}O_2$ max, coupled with a reduced $\dot{Q}_t$ at maximum work. If the cardiac response is impaired by low stroke volume, cardiac frequency is usually high at all power outputs (Equations 4.9–11). Sometimes a low cardiac rate response is the primary abnormality and is partly compensated for by an increase in stroke volume. $\dot{V}_E$ is usually normal at low exercise loads but during exercise close to maximum is higher than normal, due to an increase in CO_2 output secondary to lactic acid production. V_T and f_r, when related to $\dot{V}_E$ are usually normal in the absence of pulmonary vascular overload. Arterial O_2 content, V_D/V_T and $\dot{Q}_{va}/\dot{Q}_t$ are normal in the absence of pulmonary complications.

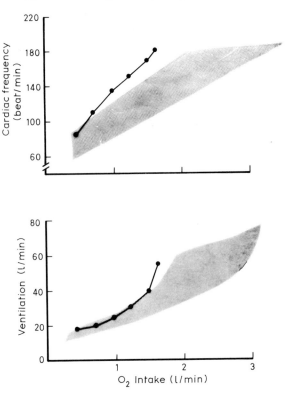

Fig. 4.7 Cardiac frequency and ventilation in exercise ('stage I' test) in a patient with mitral incompetence; contrasted with normal subjects, f_c is high at all $\dot{V}O_2$ and the maximum f_c (180 beats/min) is reached at a low maximum $\dot{V}O_2$ (1.6 l/min). Ventilation shows an increase due to lactic acid production and associated high $\dot{V}CO_2$, but $\dot{V}_E$ at maximum exercise (55 l/min) is well below the ventilatory capacity (*FEV*$_1$ 3 l, *MVV* 100 l/min).

4.7 Impaired ventilatory response due to airways obstruction (Fig. 4.8)

If airway obstruction is mild no impairment of exercise may occur, due to the fact that the ventilatory capacity has to fall below about 70% of normal before it reaches the ventilation normally required in exercise. However, increasing obstruction leads to a progressive encroachment on the ventilatory requirements of exercise. The extent to which this leads to a low exercise performance depends on the interaction between the low ventilatory capacity, and the ventilation required to meet the metabolic demands. Features of the exercise response commonly encountered include a reduced maximum power output and $\dot{V}O_2$ max associated with a ventilation at maximum exercise which is close to the maximum voluntary ventilation (*MVV*). A reasonable approximation of *MVV* is given by the equation.

$$MVV = FEV_1 \times 35 \qquad (4.14)$$

where FEV_1 is in litres and MVV in l/min. $\dot{V}_E$ at submaximum power outputs is variable, and depends on the response of $\dot{V}_A$ and the V_D/V_T ratio (Equation 4.5). A low $\dot{V}_E$ is an indication that $\dot{V}_A$ is also low. However, a 'normal' ventilation response may be a combination of low $\dot{V}_A$ and increased V_D/V_T (Fig. 4.8). The reduced airflow leads to a pattern of breathing of reduced V_T and limited f_r. In patients with severe airway obstruction the expiratory

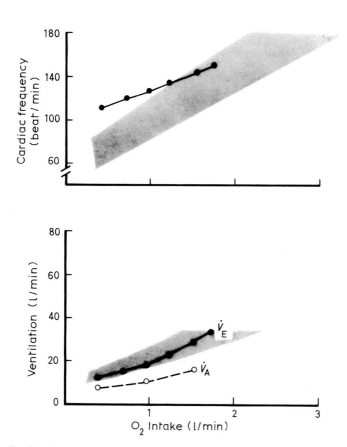

Fig. 4.8 Cardiac frequency and ventilation in a patient with severe chronic bronchitis (FEV_1 1.0 l); because exercise is limited by the reduced ventilatory capacity, the normal f_c max (170 beats/min) is not reached. Although the ventilation is normal, the maximum $\dot{V}_E$ is the same as the ventilatory capacity (34 l/min), and $\dot{V}_A$ is reduced, due to a high V_D/V_T ratio and leading to an increase in P_aCO_2.

airflow is limited by the maximum flow:volume characteristics; their inability to increase expiratory airflow often leads to a situation where an increase in f_r is accompanied by a fall in V_T. This is normally associated with severe dyspnoea. Arterial PCO_2 usually increases with exercise in patients with severe airway obstruction, particularly if a gas exchange disturbance (high V_D/V_T) or an abnormality of respiratory control is present.

4.8 Impaired ventilatory response due to reduced lung volume (Fig. 4.9)

Diffuse alveolitis and other clinical situations associated with reductions in lung volume are associated wtih greater reductions in maximum power output and $\dot{V}O_2$ max than in airway obstruction associated with comparable

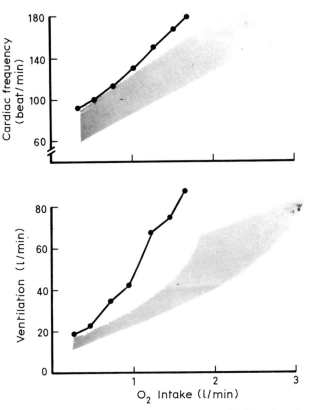

Fig. 4.9 Cardiac frequency and ventilation in a patient with fibrosing alveolitis (bird fancier's lung). There is a gross increase in ventilation, which is accomplished with a low V_T and high f_r. Maximum V_T was only 1100 ml. The hyperventilation was associated with a progressive fall in arterial O_2 saturation to 85% due to a severe gas exchange disturbance.

impairment of ventilatory capacity. This is mainly explained by the finding of a ventilation which is high at all levels of exercise and often reaches the ventilatory capacity. The pattern of breathing is one of low V_T, which is related to the reductions in lung volume, and high f_r which may reach levels of over 60 breaths/min (Fig. 4.9). A gas exchange disturbance is often associated (see below), leading to hypoxaemia; P_aCO_2 is usually low. Lactic acid production may occur at relatively low levels of exercise; although often ascribed to the hypoxaemia in some patients it is circulatory in origin. In such patients an impaired cardiac output response to exercise is found, probably in association with pulmonary vascular disease.

4.9 Impaired pulmonary gas exchange

In normal subjects pulmonary gas exchange improves with exercise, with a fall in V_D/V_T ratio and reduction in venous admixture. Abnormalities in gas exchange are often brought out by exercise, and recognized by high V_D/V_T ratios, increased alveolar-arterial PO_2 differences and venous admixture ratios. A high V_D/V_T ratio may partly be due to low V_T but often is due to areas of high $\dot{V}_A:\dot{Q}_c$ ratio, particularly in patients with thromboembolic pulmonary vascular disease, and in emphysema. Impaired pulmonary oxygen transfer and areas of low $\dot{V}_A:\dot{Q}_c$ cause increases in the alveolar–arterial PO_2 difference and venous admixture, characteristically seen in patients with alveolitis and emphysema. However, some patients with a low P_aO_2 and increased alveolar–arterial PO_2 difference at rest, may improve with exercise. This finding indicates that the gas exchange abnormality is due to areas in the lung with low $\dot{V}_A/\dot{Q}_c$ ratio at rest; the impairment is not fixed and improves with exercise due to the increase in ventilation and associated improvement in $\dot{V}_A/\dot{Q}_c$ distribution. Characteristically patients with chronic bronchitis without emphysema behave in this way [7].

4.10 Impaired respiratory control

Underventilation in exercise, with low $\dot{V}_A$ and high P_aCO_2, is common in patients with chronic airway obstruction, but may also be seen in idiopathic alveolar hypoventilation [8].

4.11 Hyperventilation in exercise

A high $\dot{V}_E$ during exercise may be accounted for by a number of factors acting singly or in combination.

1. An increase in $\dot{V}CO_2$ with appropriate increase in $\dot{V}_A$: this is usually due to lactic acid production.

2. An 'inappropriate' increase in $\dot{V}_A$, leading to low P_aCO_2 (Equation 4.8), may be due to arterial hypoxaemia or acidosis, but sometimes may be accounted for by pulmonary hypertension, by psychogenic factors (Fig. 4.10) or possibly through stimulation of pulmonary stretch receptors (for example in alveolitis).
3. An increase in V_D/V_T due to a low V_T, increases the proportion of $\dot{V}_E$ wasted in dead space (Equation 4.6).
4. An increase in V_D/V_T due to a gas exchange disturbance has a similar effect, and may be associated with poor pulmonary capillary perfusion as in recurrent pulmonary emboli, pulmonary valvular stenosis and emphysema.

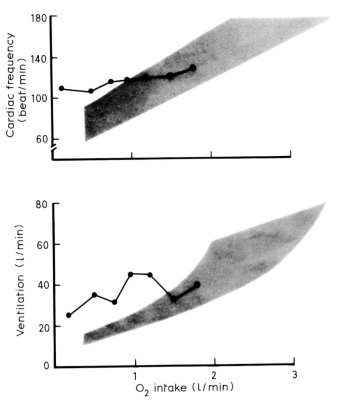

Fig. 4.10 The responses to exercise in a patient investigated for severe breathlessness, with no objective evidence of respiratory disease. Heart rate was high at low power outputs but became normal with increasing work. A similar pattern was seen for ventilation. This response is found in patients with psychogenic hyperventilation, and may be contrasted wth dyspnoea due to organic disorders of the heart or lungs (Figs 4.7 and 4.9).

A high $\dot{V}_E$ during exercise often means that the ventilatory capacity is reached at a lower exercise level than would have occurred, had $\dot{V}_E$ been normal. For this reason it is useful to analyse the symptom of dyspnoea in terms of the ventilatory demand in exercise ($\dot{V}_E$), and the ventilatory capacity (*MVV*). The use of measurements obtained during exercise in this way may often explain the symptom of dyspnoea in a patient who on clinical examination and routine pulmonary function testing does not 'deserve' to be dyspnoeic for purely mechanical reasons.

The patterns of response outlined above together with the related factors influencing exercise performance may often coexist and lead to a relative worsening in exercise. For example, coexisting cardiac malfunction in a patient with lung disease may lead to gross impairment of exercise through a reduction in oxygen delivery, increasing lactic acid production and worsening gas exchange function.

4.12 Exercise tests

Different types of exercise tests will be reviewed briefly, in terms of the relative ease with which information is obtained and the clinical value and indications.

4.12.1 The twelve minute walking test [9]

This is a simple clinical test in which the patient is asked to walk as far as possible within 12 min. The distance is measured, symptoms noted and heart rate recorded. The main application of the test is in the assessment of disabled patients with chronic airway obstruction, and is useful to observe the effects of bronchodilators, O_2 administration and physical training. The test is similar to a stairclimbing test [10], in which the time taken to climb a known height is measured. Both tests have the advantages of simplicity and close resemblance to everyday activities. However, the metabolic load ($\dot{V}O_2$, $\dot{V}CO_2$) is not easy to estimate or measure accurately; for this reason more elaborate measurements usually are not worth the effort.

4.12.2 Standardized, progressive, multistage tests

These tests use a calibrated cycle ergometer or a treadmill; both allow the metabolic load ($\dot{V}O_2$) to be estimated fairly accurately ($\pm$ 15%), or measured ($\pm$ 5%).

In what has been termed the 'stage I exercise test' [6, p. 50], work settings are increased by a small and equal amount every minute, so that most patients are taken to a symptom-limited maximum within 5–15 min. The increments usually amount to 17 W (100 kp m/min) for a cycle ergometer and

2.5% in treadmill grade at a constant speed of 80 m/min, but are modified for elderly patients and children. Ventilation, V_T and f_r are measured continuously by gas meter, Tissot spirometer or pneumotachygraph; the electrocardiograph is recorded to obtain an electrocardiogram and f_c, and blood pressure is also measured periodically. In addition to these basic measurements, others may be added to increase precision or the information obtained from this test. Analysis of expired gas for O_2 and CO_2 using rapid analysers is used to calculate $\dot{V}O_2$ and $\dot{V}CO_2$. Ear oximetry [11] is a useful addition to the assessment of patients with gas exchange abnormalities. All measurements are made during the last $10 - 20$ s of each minute; in this way many points are obtained (Figs 4.7–10). In addition to demonstrating the way in which variables change with increasing exercise up to the patient's maximum exercise capacity, the numerous points in the relationships tend to reduce experimental and biological variation. If exercise-induced bronchoconstricton is suspected the FEV_1 is recorded for the first 15 min of recovery (see below).

The advantage of this type of test is that it is within the expertise of any pulmonary or cardiac laboratory; the power output is standardized; the patient is taken to a maximum exercise capacity, and simple measurements are made from which clinically relevant information is obtained.

The following list is not meant to be exhaustive but will illustrate the clinical use of the progressive test.

1. A normal $\dot{V}O_2$ max, $\dot{V}_E$ and f_c response to exercise virtually excludes serious pathology in the heart or lungs.
2. Limiting values of $\dot{V}_E$ and f_c can be identified.
3. The symptom of dyspnoea may be analysed in terms of the balance between the exercise ventilatory demand and the ventilatory capacity.
4. $\dot{V}O_2$ max and the other measurements may be related to the expected strain of the patient's occupation, or to a prescribed activity régime.
5. Improvement following bronchodilators, steroids, etc. may be measured reliably.
6. Exercise-induced bronchoconstriction may be identified and the effects of treatment observed.
7. The results may provide evidence for further tests: for example, an abnormal cardiac response in a patient with diagnosed psychogenic dyspnoea in origin may be the only clue to obstructive pulmonary hypertension.
8. If a steady state test is needed, appropriate power outputs may be chosen on the basis of the results of the stage I test.

4.12.3 'Steady state' submaximal exercise tests [6, p. 53]

Some measurements and calculations require a steady state of $\dot{V}O_2$ and $\dot{V}CO_2$ for several minutes; these include cardiac output, V_D/V_T ratio and $\dot{Q}_{va}/\dot{Q}_t$. Preferably at least two power outputs are chosen on the basis of a progressive test so that results may be related to the maximum power. In addition to measurement of $\dot{V}_E$, $\dot{V}O_2$ and $\dot{V}CO_2$, arterial or arterialized capillary blood is sampled for measurement of P_aCO_2, P_aO_2, pH and lactate. However, the key measurement in this type of test is the mixed venous PCO_2, measured non-invasively by a rebreathing technique [6, p. 57]. This allows cardiac output to be estimated and all the equations of gas exchange (4.7–13 above) may be solved. The tests are performed on treadmill or cycle, the latter being preferable from a practical point of view.

Although these tests (the 'stage II and III tests') are more complex and thus more difficult to do, the additional physiological information may be clinically important for several reasons.

1. Measurements are obtained to solve all the equations above and so explain in physiological terms substandard exercise performance. As noted above there is no point in going this far if the results of a progressive test are normal, or if they have yielded sufficient information to answer the clinical problem. However, it may be important to know whether a reduced $\dot{V}O_2$ max and high f_c is accompanied by a low $\dot{Q}_t$, or whether a ventilatory abnormality is due to changes in $\dot{V}_A$ or V_D/V_T, for example.
2. Changes in gas exchange variables – V_D/V_T and $\dot{Q}_{va}/\dot{Q}_t$ – are quantified, for example, to follow progress of alveolitis.
3. Mixed problems involving cardiac and pulmonary malfunction may be separated.

Details of the procedures and measurements are given elsewhere [6, pp. 63–112] but it should be emphasized that technically the procedures are not difficult to set up and appropriate equipment is widely available and reliable.

4.13 Tests for exercise-induced bronchoconstriction

Exercise may be used as a potent 'challenge' technique to measure non-specific airway reactivity. Since it was first introduced by Jones *et al.* [12] much research has explored both the best methods for eliciting the response and the mechanisms underlying it, and controversy continues to surround both topics (see [13] for review). The most potent challenge, i.e. the technique required to reveal the least reactive airways response, is treadmill running for 6–8 min, with a heart rate of at least 160, and with the subject breathing cold dry air [14]. A greater degree of reactivity is revealed by a routine 6–8 min treadmill test or the stage I exercise protocol outlined above. The results obtained with these two methods are broadly comparable, and the severity of the broncho-constriction revealed by them is related to the airway reactivity measured by histamine or methacholine [15]. However, subjects who only respond to the inhalation of high doses (over 4 mg/ml) of histamine acid phosphate, generally do not show exercise-induced bronchoconstriction, measurement of FEV_1 or PEF are sufficient, before, immediately after and 1, 2, 5, 10 and 15 min after exercise. Often, there is a transient bronchodilatation immediately following exercise, with an increase in FEV_1 above the pre-exercise value. The most discriminating index is the bronchial lability index of Jones which is calculated as follows:

$$BLI = \frac{\text{Best } FEV_1 - \text{worst } FEV_1}{\text{predicted } FEV_1} \times 100 \qquad (4.14)$$

An index of over 10% is generally taken as significant (see [13] for a fuller discussion).

The realization that asthma may be provoked by airway cooling and that this probably explains the production of asthma by exercise has also led to the development of tests which employ hyperventilation with cold air as a measure of non-specific airway reactivity and such tests may eventually replace exercise as a bronchial challenge. Other ways of assessing non-specific airway reactivity are discussed in Chapter 11.

4.14 Summary

Exercise testing is used to measure the responses of the cardiovascular and respiratory systems to the dual metabolic loads of O_2 intake and CO_2 output. Information is obtained at several levels of exercise to obtain the reserve capacity in the systems and also the extent to which adaptation to malfunction has occurred to maintain the capacity to exercise.

In patients with respiratory disease a number of factors may impair exercise tolerance: reduced ventilatory capacity; the mechanical characteristics of the lungs; pulmonary gas exchange; ventilatory control; cardiac function, and the metabolic processes in exercising muscles. Information regarding these factors may be obtained from exercise studies that are not technically demanding. In addition, the results may be used in a number of clinical applications: to help decide the patient's occupational capacity; the prescription of exercise rehabilitation; the assessment of airway reactivity; the value of ambulatory oxygen, and the response to therapy.

Standardized exercise tests provide information regarding the integrated responses of the total respiratory system to loads and thus usefully complement techniques which measure the individual functions in isolation.

References

1. Barcroft, J. (1934). *Features in the Architecture of Physiological Function.* Cambridge University Press, Cambridge.
2. Shephard, R. J. (1969), *Endurance Fitness.* University of Toronto Press, Toronto.
3. Lange-Anderson, K. *et al.* (1971), *Fundamentals of Exercise Testing,* WHO, Geneva.
4. Freedman, S. (1970), Sustained maximum voluntary ventilation. *Resp. Physiol.,* **8**, 230–44.
5. Jones, N. L. and Rebuck, A. S. (1979), Tidal volume response to exercise. *Bull. Physiopathol. Resp.,* **15**, 321–27.
6. Jones, N. L., Campbell, E. J. M., Edwards, R. H. T. and Robertson, D. G. (1975), *Clinical Exercise Testing.* W. B. Saunders Company, Philadelphia.
7. Jones, N. L. (1966), Pulmonary gas exchange during exercise in patients with chronic airway obstruction. *Clin. Sci.,* **31**, 39–50.
8. Hyland, R. H. *et al.* (1978), Primary alveolar hypoventilation treated with nocturnal electrophrenic respiration, *Am. Rev. Resp. Dis.,* **117**, 165–72.
9. MacGavin, C. R., Gupta, S. P. and McHardy, G. J. R. (1976), Twelve-minute walking test for assessing disability in chronic bronchitis. *Br. Med. J.,* **1**, 822–3.
10. Gupta, S. A., Fletcher, C. M. and Edwards, R. H. T. (1973), Progressive exercise step test. *J. Ass. Physicians India,* **21**, 555–64.
11. Saunders, N. A., Powles, A. C. P. and Rebuck, A. S. (1976), Ear oximetry: accuracy and practicability in the assessment of arterial oxygenation. *Am. Rev. Resp. Dis.,* **113**, 744–9.
12. Jones, R. S., Wharton, M. J. and Buston, M. H. (1963), The place of physical exercise and bronchodilator drugs in the assessment of the asthmatic child. *Arch. Dis. Child.,* **38**, 539–45.
13. Godfrey, S. (1975), Exercise-induced asthma–clinical, physiological and therapeutic implications. *J. Allergy Clin. Immunol.,* **56**, 1–17.
14. Strauss, R. H., McFadden, E. R. Jr., Ingram, R. H. Jr. and Jaeger, J. J. (1977), Enhancement of exercise-induced asthma by cold air. *New Eng. J. Med.,* **297**, 743–6.
15. Anderton, R. C. *et al.* (1979), Bronchial responsiveness to inhaled histamine and exercise. *J. Allergy clin. Immunol.* **63**, 315–20.
16. Wade, O. L. and Bishop, J. M. (1962), *Cardiac Output and Regional Blood Flow.* Blackwell Scientific Publications, F. A. Davis, Co., Philadelphia.

CHAPTER FIVE

Screening

G. M. Cochrane

Population screening for the detection of lung disease has been the subject of much recent debate and controversy. Screening in thoracic medicine is not a recent development as in the early post-war years it was extensively carried out by the mass miniature radiograph service. During these early years this service was cost effective because in conjunction with tuberculin testing and contact tracing, it revealed sufficient sources of active tuberculosis. The prevalence of active tuberculosis was high and the later introduction of chemotherapeutic agents allowed effective treatment. With the reduction in the incidence of tuberculosis (for whatever reason, be it treatment or change in the environment or genetic predisposition of individuals), this screening service to detect patients suffering from active disease is no longer cost effective.

The relative prevalence of pulmonary disease has changed and tuberculosis is no longer the main public health problem. Nowadays, the commonest lung diseases are cancer, chronic obstructive bronchitis and occupational lung disease and these are now the prospective targets for screening in thoracic medicine. Radiology is no longer the best screening method as these diseases are either not detected by radiography or, detected only when diagnosis is likely to be unresponsive to treatment.

5.1 Concept of screening populations

The majority of patients attending hospital clinics routinely undergo recording of blood pressure, urine testing and frequently chest radiographs. These might be regarded as screening procedures as they are carried out irrespective of the presenting complaint, but they are carried out on patients who have specifically sought medical advice. Screening for preclinical lung disease in patients not requesting treatment places the doctor in a different role: he is proffering a service which has not been sought and therefore it obligates the physician to show this service is beneficial. Unfortunately, in both lung cancer and chronic obstructive bronchitis the search for such a screening procedure has not entirely recognized this change in the physician's role, although it has extensively added to our understanding of these disease processes. As a result many of the screening procedures outlined in this chapter are valuable in individuals who have sought advice.

5.2 Assumptions inherent in screening populations for asymptomatic disease

The diseases sought by screening any population should be those which enable presymptomatic detection to be followed by effective treatment. Thus, detection must be at a time when either the disease can be cured or its progression curtailed to such an extent that morbidity is significantly reduced. This goal has yet to be achieved by any form of screening.

Asymptomatic diabetic patients have a reduced life expectancy but controlled trials, in both the UK and the USA, have not shown that early diagnosis and treatment have improved prognosis. The natural history of hypertension can be beneficially altered by the regular administration of antihypertensives and would appear to be a suitable condition for early detection as effective treatment is available. Studies have shown that although control of hypertension is adequate, there is no improvement in morbidity. On the other hand, they have shown that patients, when told that they are at risk of illness because of raised blood pressure, have an increased incidence of headache and a doubling of the incidence of absenteeism, which illustrates the dangers of screening, as health can be converted into disease without benefit [1].

5.3 Criteria for the screening tests

5.3.1 Simple and with no morbidity

The procedures used for screening populations for early detection of disease should not be associated with morbidity. If they are to be effective, they should be simple, requiring minimal training for all socio-economic groups. They should also be able to be carried out quickly as the clinician is persuading a non-symptomatic subject to spend time establishing health. Screening tests are increasingly available at factories, and public gatherings such as exhibitions; unless these criteria are fulfilled, the subjects will not agree to take part because they do not believe they are 'at risk' and therefore lack the motivation to take part in tests of uncertain benefit which may result in discomfort. A factor which may bias results of such surveys is that people who are either mildly unwell but have yet to see their own doctor, or people who know from their exposure to medical educational propaganda that they may be at risk (most smokers and fat people), tend to use the anonymity and convenience of screening 'clinics' to confirm or reject their fears.

5.3.2 Repeatability

The ideal screening procedure must be repeatable (giving the same answer when the subject is re-examined) and valid (measuring the variate it purports to measure in pathophysiological terms). The commonest screening procedure is still the questionnaire. Every clinician when interviewing a patient with a specific illness runs through a 'time-honoured', semi-structured selection of questions to exclude the possibility of other related diseases, and the extension of this technique to screening is useful. Qualitative attributes such as clinical symptoms and signs can be best related by contingency tables. This involves taking the data from questionnaire surveys and comparing observer 1 results to observer 2 results with positive and negative statements, leading to an overall agreement represented by the percentages following in *a* and *d* of Table 5.1.

Table 5.1 Contingency table for determining the accuracy of questionnaire data

	Observer 1	
	Positive	*Negative*
Observer 2		
Positive	*a*	*b*
Negative	*c*	*d*

This measure of repeatability unfortunately reflects the prevalence of the disease, the exactness of the questionnaire and the definition of the disease process, as opposed to the repeatability of the method. The effect of defining the disease can be demonstrated in chronic bronchitis which is defined in terms of quantity and persistence of sputum production, while the disease which may lead to crippling respiratory failure is chronic obstructive bronchitis, rather than simple sputum production. Unfortunately, this obstructive feature is poorly defined until wheezing and dyspnoea are obvious to the patient, albeit too late. As can be seen in Table 5.1, the repeatability for the individual subject based on questionnaire data depends upon the prevalence of borderline cases ($b + c$) and therefore, although questionnaires may be helpful to the epidemiologist concerned with groups rather than individuals, they are often less helpful in screening procedures, where an 'at risk' individual is sought.

Questionnaires are most useful in determining the incidence of certain diseases with populations or subgroups of populations. Questionnaires have shown the increased risk of chronic lung disease in the lower socio-economic groups and in industry have shown the increased incidence of lung disease with certain industrial processes. Advantages of the questionnaire are its ease of administration and simplicity. Analysis of data can be easily handled by computer if the questionnaire is well constructed, so results from a survey are rapidly available. By structuring the questionnaire particular problems, such as nocturnal wheeze following industrial exposure to fumes, may be elucidated whereas respiratory function tests during the day may miss this nocturnal airflow obstruction.

Repeatability in measurements of a numerical variable such as forced expired volume in one second (FEV_1) can be more clearly defined. The repeatability of replicate measurements in the same individuals on separate occasions (intrasubject variation) and in groups of individuals (intersubject variation) can be expressed as standard deviation or as coefficient of variation (standard deviation divided by the mean). These methods can give clear-cut indications as to the probability of any value lying outside the expected limits for that measurement assuming a normal distribution.

5.3.3 Sensitivity and specificity

The sensitivity and specificity of screening has to be defined in relation to a reference test of its validity. Thus screening must be related to a specific diagnostic feature, e.g. a pathological abnormality in the case of lung cancer. By contrast, in screening tests for early chronic obstructive bronchitis where identification of a pathological abnormality is often indirect and, thus morbid anatomical validity is difficult to establish, screening is based on the physiological disturbance of airways obstruction.

A sensitive test is a test with a high percentage of true positives ($a/a+c$), whereas a specific test has a low percentage of false positives ($d/b+d$) (see Table 5.2). The initial problem for any screening procedure is to be specific without losing any sensitivity and to be repeatable.

5.3.4 Prognostic value

Screening procedures may be sensitive and specific but their final performance is also related to the prognostic value of a positive or negative result. The likelihood of a person having a disease can be seen from Table 5.2 as $a/a+b$. If this disease has a low incidence in the group screened the proportion of true negatives ($b+d$) in relation to true positives ($a+c$) is high, and the proportion of false positives (b) will be greater in proportion to true positives (a). The prognostic value therefore will decline in relationship to the prevalence of the disease screened.

Table 5.2 Contingency table classifying subjects as positive or negative first by the screening test, and then by the reference test

	Reference Test		
Screening Test	*Positive*	*Negative*	*Total*
Positive	a	b	$a+b$
Negative	c	d	$c+d$
Totals	$a+c$	$b+d$	

a = true positive identified by screening test
b = false positive identified by screening test
c = false negative identified by screening test
d = true negative identified by screening test

5.4 The identification of individuals within a population who have lung disease

The criteria of sensitivity and specificity outlined above may not be entirely appropriate as implicit in their definition is the idea that there is an abrupt change from health to disease. Unfortunately there is no good evidence for a bimodal distribution of lung function within populations, a continuous distribution is found and a likely explanation of lack of sample size has never been substantiated [2] (Fig. 5.1). This overlap of populations – the well and the ill – makes detection of the individual who is at risk of lung disease at a remedial stage more difficult. However, A. L. Cochrane [2] has proposed the idea of determining the point on the distribution curve at which treatment does more harm than good as a point separating individuals into the two populations. However, although such a technique has been applied to other disease processes it has yet to be used in screening for airways obstruction. Part of the reason for this is the natural history of chronic airways obstruction is so long and that many factors affecting this natural history may change over this period of time.

Screening procedures should in summary be aimed at common treatable diseases, be easy and cheap to perform with no morbidity. They should be repeatable with a low incidence of false positives and false negatives, and have clear cut prognostic value. Finally, even though they are unlikely to be able to separate perfectly between healthy and diseased subjects, a point on their distribution curve for populations can be determined where treatment may do no harm and possibly some good.

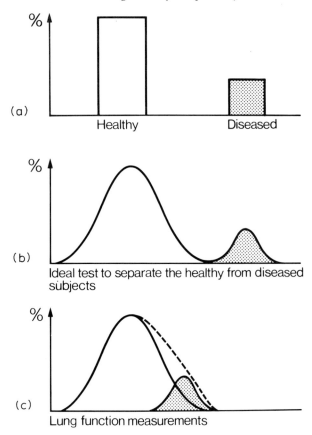

Fig. 5.1 (a) The ideal screening situation where there is an abrupt change between healthy individuals and those with disease; (b) the distribution in performance of the ideal test separating healthy from diseased subjects; (c) the continuous distribution of lung function measurements in subjects classified as healthy or diseased [2].

5.5 Screening for chronic airways obstruction

Chronic airways obstruction whether caused by chronic obstructive bronchitis defined as chronic mucoid sputum production with shortness of breath and wheeze, or emphysema defined in terms of alveolar pathology, or a combination of both, is largely caused by cigarette smoking and is in the terminal stages untreatable. Although a considerable percentage of most populations smoke cigarettes (40–70% depending on the country, sex and age span included of the population), only a small percentage present under 70 years of age with shortness of breath of sufficient severity that the individual is unable to work or care for himself. This suggests an 'at risk' group in the smoking population, and this view combined with the poor results of treatment once symptoms appear, raised the hope that screening for the detection of airflow obstruction at an early stage of the disease might enable the 'at risk' patient to be selected and treated.

Macklem and Mead [3] showed that airways of less than 2 mm in diameter constituted only 10–20% of normal total airways resistance, and that considerable changes in resistance in these airways could occur before there would be significant changes in total airways resistance in man. As early as 1958 McLean in a review of pulmonary emphysema (then a less well-defined term than now) suggested the early changes occurred in the peripheral airways of less than 2 mm in diameter [4]. These observations were supported by Hogg *et al.* [5] who confirmed this pathological site and that pathological changes could be associated with marked ventilation perfusion imbalance while having little effect on the larger airways. Conventional tests such as FEV_1 were postulated to be little altered at this stage and as the patient is asymptomatic, a 'silent zone' of disease could therefore progress without detection until disability appeared rapidly leading to crippling lung disease.

The assumption that airways obstruction silently progresses has never been fully proven. Prieto *et al.* [6] have shown that symptoms occur early in patients most at risk of developing severe irreversible airflow obstruction and significant airflow obstruction is rare in asymptomatic smokers. Thus, symptoms may be more important as an early indication of disease than previously thought, and may be detected by structured questionnaires. Questionnaires for screening working populations have shown their value and this may reflect the more clearly defined populations at risk and nature of pulmonary hazard.

5.6 Screening tests of small airway function

5.6.1 Frequency dependence of compliance

Woolcock *et al.* [7] showed differences in dynamic lung compliance at increasing breathing frequencies in patients with pathological evidence of small airways obstruction compared with patients with no histological evidence of airways obstruction. (Dynamic compliance is determined by measuring the changes in oesophageal pressure and tidal volume during tidal breathing.) These authors suggested that at increasing breathing frequencies, the difference in time constants between obstructed and non-obstructed airways would lead to a fall in dynamic compliance with increasing breathing frequencies. The fall in dynamic compliance at a frequency of 60 breaths/min was found in patients shown to have normal airways resistance but changes in small airways at histology. Unfortunately the repeatability of this test was poor even when the technique was improved. Even knowing the intrasubject variation it always proved too time-consuming, expensive and uncomfortable to be a suitable test for screening, but has often been used as a reference test for other tests of small airway function.

Frequency dependence of compliance has almost completely disappeared as a screening procedure for chronic airways obstruction because of these factors, and also because of its apparent lack of specificity, since it has been reported to be altered in subjects suffering from respiratory viral infections. These studies also showed the reversibility of the decreased dynamic compliance at high breathing frequencies during recovery from such infection. This test of small airway function has been validated by histological evidence of small airway abnormality and the return to normal values of frequency dependence of compliance on cessation of smoking. At a similar time (1968) frequency dependence of flow resistance was also proposed as a screening test but never developed the popularity of dynamic compliance at varying respiratory frequencies.

5.6.2 Arterial blood gases

Further evidence to support the idea that patients with chronic bronchitis (defined in sputum terms) and asthma could have 'relatively normal' routine pulmonary function tests and airways resistance, but abnormal gas exchange came from Levine *et al.* [8]. This study, however, relied on arterial blood gas estimation and was not considered for screening although a number of authors have since suggested measuring arterialized ear lobe oxygen saturation on exercise to determine early abnormalities in gas exchange.

5.6.3 Residual volume

Residual volume determined by the body plethysmograph is raised in many patients with chronic airflow obstruction and it has been suggested as a screening test as it detects overdistention secondary to peripheral airways obstruction. This measurement required expensive equipment (body plethysmograph), a co-operative patient and earlier work has also shown it not to be highly reproducible in poorly trained subjects and thus it has obtained little support as a screening test.

5.6.4 Closing volume

Closing volume is the lung volume at which airways begin to close in dependent portions of the lung. The mechanism for a 'closing volume' test assumes that as a subject exhales towards residual volume, the airways in gravity dependent lung regions close, thus leaving a finite volume of gas peripheral to this point of closure. The tests for detection of closing volume rely on the subject inhaling a small volume of marker gas (e.g. helium, argon or radio-labelled xenon), or a single breath of oxygen, from residual volume. Because of gravity dependent airway closure during the initial part of inspiration, the highest concentration of marker gas will be inhaled into the apices and in the remainder of the lung the concentration of this marker gas will be diluted by air. During controlled slow expiration after clearing the dead space the concentration of the marker gas reaches a plateau as gas is expired from the apices (high marker gas concentration), and mixed with that coming from the bases (low concentration marker gas). As residual volume is approached the gravity dependent airways close, leading to a rise in marker gas concentration because no gas from the bases now dilutes the high apical concentrations (Fig. 5.2). The phases of the closing volume marker gas concentrations are denoted as 1–4: phase 1 reflects dead space,

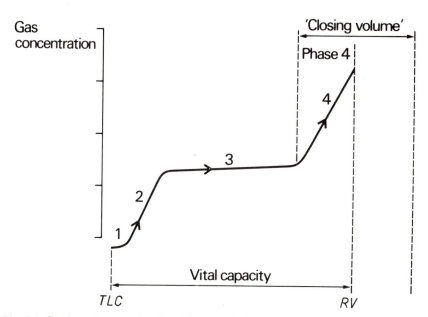

Fig. 5.2 Closing volume estimation. Phase 1, dead space; phase 2, dead space alveolar gas mixing; phase 3, alveolar plateau – mixing of marker gas from all regions of the lung; phase 4, terminal rise of marker gas when emptying ceases from the lower lung zones. Measurements which may be determined from this manoeuvre: Closing capacity (the relationship of phase 4 volume and residual volume over total lung capacity); Phase 4/VC% (percentage ratio of phase 4 volume to the vital capacity); Alveolar plateau estimation (as change in marker gas concentration during phase 3 per litre expired gas).

phase 2 includes the rise in concentration of marker gas as alveolar emptying begins, phase 3 signifies the alveolar plateau with marker gas coming from all regions of the lung, and phase 4 the terminal rise in concentration of marker gas when emptying ceases from the lower zones. Phase 4 volume is sometimes referred to as closing volume and related to vital capacity (VC), but as airway closure occurs above residual volume, phase 4 volume is also added to residual volume and this combined volume is called closing capacity and related to total lung capacity.

Closing volume (expressed as phase 4/$VC\%$) increases with age and this has been considered to be caused by loss of tissue elasticity associated with ageing. Abnormally high phase 4/$VC\%$ measurements have been found in studies of asymptomatic smokers. These changes in closing volume were associated with either loss of external support (a loss of tissue elasticity and thus early emphysema) or intrinsic changes in the structure or properties of the airway itself (early obstructive bronchitis). As airway closure is usually confined to smaller airways, closing volume has been proposed as a suitable test for screening populations.

Early in its career a number of technical problems were found to be associated with the measurement of closing volume; inspiratory and expiratory flow rates needed to be controlled and a high intra-observer variation has been found, and the test has also been shown to be poorly repeatable in individuals when used routinely outside specialist units.

5.6.5 Single breath N_2 test

In normal subjects the phase 3 alveolar plateau either of marker gas or residual N_2 slopes gently upwards, but in patients with lung disease the slope is steeper. Standardization of the measurement of this slope especially when using the single breath oxygen test where the concentration of expired nitrogen is monitored ($\Delta N_2/l$) has suggested that an increase in this slope occurs early in cigarette smokers. Unfortunately, there have been some reported anomalies where subjects have abnormal spirometry yet the alveolar plateau remains normal, and in patients with asthma the response of $\Delta N_2/l$ may vary with bronchodilator therapy despite improvement in spirometry. No accurate tests of specificity are available and the prognostic value is unknown but is likely to be poor, as initial results indicate that the incidence of abnormality thus detected far exceeds the incidence of disabling airways obstruction. The single breath oxygen test measuring $\Delta N_2/l$, is therefore under further investigation to answer these points, but at present appears to be a promising screening test being simple and relatively cheap to perform.

5.7 Tests based on the forced expiratory manoeuvre

The forced expiratory manoeuvre has been described in Chapter 3 and can be measured in terms of volume against time giving a volume expired in one second (FEV_1), total volume (forced vital capacity; FVC) and time taken to insignificant flow (forced expired time; FET). Mean flow measurements can be derived simply from such a trace, producing, for example, a mean flow rate which is usually determined by dividing the time taken expiring forcibly from 25% to 75% of the vital capacity into the volume expired over this time. The other format for measuring the forced expiratory manoeuvre is plotting instantaneous flow rate against vital capacity and determining the flow rates at peak flow rate, 50% of expired vital capacity and 75% expired vital capacity (Chapter 3). The maximal expiratory flow volume curve (MEFVC) can be determined either by measurements obtained at the mouth (with the tendency to exaggerate gas trapping and airflow obstruction), or by volume displacement of the chest wall with a body plethysmograph, the latter method often relating instantaneous flows to total lung capacity rather than vital capacity.

5.7.1 Instantaneous flow rate measurements derived from the terminal portion of the MEFVC

The reason for determining instantaneous flow rates from the MEFVC is that simple spirometric tests such as FEV_1 and FVC are considered to be insensitive to the pathological changes in the smaller airways found in early chronic obstructive bronchitis. The flow rates determined in the terminal portion of the flow volume curve are considered (by the following rationale) to reflect airway changes in the smaller airways. Fry and Hyatt [9] showed from isovolume pressure flow curves that during forced expiration the rate of airflow cannot increase beyond certain maximum values; at large lung volumes these maximum values are effort dependent while at smaller lung volumes maximum flow rate becomes largely independent of the effort applied once it exceeds a certain minimum. Hence, in the lower three-quarters of the vital capacity maximum expiratory flow rates reflect the dimensions of airways between the alveoli and points in the airways where the lateral airway pressure during forced expiration equals pleural pressure. As residual volume is approached these equal pressure points move into the smaller bronchi. In obstructive lung disease the flow limiting segments during the forced expiratory manoeuvre are probably located in small airways at higher lung volumes than in normal people, because of the increase in peripheral airways resistance and loss of lung elastic recoil. Hence, reduction in maximum expiratory flow rates in the lower part of the vital capacity should reflect a reduction in airflow from the smaller peripheral airways. During the early 1970s, many papers were published relating the reduction in flow rate in the terminal portion of the MEFVC to changes in frequency-dependent compliance and closing volume in non-smoking and asymptomatic smoking subjects, thus indicating small airways obstruction. The majority of smokers were shown to have spirometric values of FEV_1, within the normal range but to have significant abnormalities in these tests of small airways function. Available data on normal values for flow rate in the terminal portion of the MEFVC were originally limited and taken from dissimilar populations to the study groups with no repeatability assessment of the variates measured.

Thus, measurements of flow rate in the terminal portion of the MEFVC were thought to be more sensitive than FEV_1 on the premise that they provided a higher percentage of results outside the predicted normal range. This apparent discriminative power of the flow rates of the terminal portion of the MEFVC led to its being considered as a sensitive test of airways function. Repeatability studies in terms of intra-subject variation, diurnal variation and intersubject variation showed later that flow rates in the terminal portions of this curve were less repeatable with higher coefficients of variation than many of the simple tests of forced expiration. These large coefficients of variation are caused in part by variations in normal anatomy. A noticeable feature of a flow volume curve in patients with airflow obstruction is its curvilinearity to the volume axis and this change in shape appears to be reproducible. Unfortunately, despite a number of attempts, a single mathematical description of this curvilinearity has proved difficult to obtain. Of tests derived from the MEFVC, the flow rate after expiring 75% of the vital capacity is probably the most useful.

5.7.2 Flow volume curves using gases of different density

A way of reducing intersubject variation is to use the subject as his own control. Helium (80%) and oxygen (20%) mixtures have been used therapeutically for many years in patients with airflow obstruction of the trachea or larynx. More recently it has been shown that in normal subjects the maximum flow in the first 75% of MEFVC is dependent on gas density: the less dense the gas mixture the greater the increase in flow rates. The nature of the flow of gas at different sites in the airways determines the changes produced with gas mixtures of different densities. Turbulent flow occurs in the larger airways and turbulent flow rates increase with less dense gas. Laminar flow occurs more often in small airways and such flow is independent of gas density. Patients with chronic obstructive bronchitis have no increase in flow rates after helium/oxygen mixtures because the flow-limiting segment is within the smaller airways where laminar flow predominates. Smokers with early changes in small airways function are considered to move the equal pressure point during the forced expiratory manoeuvre into the small airways at high lung volumes. In such subjects a comparison of flow rates at mid-vital capacity when breathing air and helium/oxygen mixtures should show less density dependence of flow rate than non-smokers.

Recent studies have shown a proportion of smokers to have such a reduction in density dependence of flow rates after breathing helium/oxygen mixtures even with normal flow volume curves breathing air, but the repeatability of this test suggests it may not be repeatable enough to provide the necessary discrimination required to detect the earliest changes associated with smoking.

The volume at which flow is the same for air and helium/oxygen mixtures during comparable forced expiratory manoeuvres (volume of isoflow) is a development of this test. The advantage of this measurement is the elimination of the variation inherent with instantaneous flow rate determinations and this test is widely favoured (Fig. 5.3).

5.7.3 Forced expiratory time and mean transit time

Forced expiratory time (FET) has considerable appeal because of its apparent simplicity, but because of the difficulty in determining the end of expiration, both clinically and spirometrically, and its apparent crudeness in merely separating patients with moderately severe airflow obstruction measured in terms of FEV_1 from normal, it has not proved suitable. A recent development of FET has been the introduction of mean transit time analysis of forced expiration. Mean transit time is obtained in a similar manner to that used for cardiac output determination using an injected indicator. Mathematically the mean transit time is determined by integrating the area under a volume time plot of forced expiration, and dividing by the forced vital capacity.

The theoretical advantage of the mean transit time plot is that (assuming an accurate determination of the end of expiration flow can be obtained), it will tend to be increased by a relatively small population of slowly emptying airways while a comparatively large population of rapidly emptying airways will not lead to a marked reduction in transit time. Thus despite measuring the whole of the forced expiratory manoeuvre it will tend to exaggerate changes associated with airflow obstruction in the small airways. Further advantages of the mean transit time estimation are that it is independent of size and can be applied over a full range of age. This test has only recently been promoted as a screening test and is at the stage of initial optimism. Accurate calculation of this measurement requires a microprocesser for speed, but this should provide no significant problem.

5.8 The need for tests of small airway function other than the *FEV*₁

The development of tests of small airway function arose following the finding that the initial pathological process occurred in small airways. These are in the so-called 'silent zone' of the lung as regards routine respiratory function tests. Fletcher and Peto [10] have cast considerable doubt on the assumption that the FEV_1 is insensitive in detecting the middle-aged male smoker who will be seriously incapacitated later in life by chronic obstructive bronchitis or emphysema. Their reasoning is based on a longitudinal survey of male workers whose annual rate of decline of FEV_1 was deter-

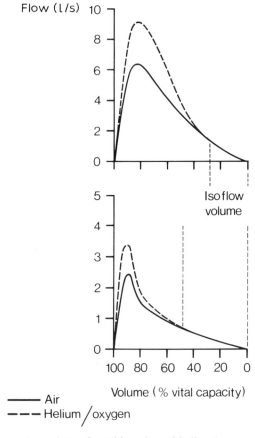

Fig. 5.3 Flow volume loops breathing air and helium/oxygen mixtures in a normal subject (upper) and a patient with moderately severe chronic obstructive bronchitis showing the diminished effect in the patient on flow rates breathing less dense gas mixtures and the increase in isoflow volume.

mined over many years. Severe symptoms associated with airflow obstruction are uncommon in subjects with an FEV_1 of much over one litre. Non-smokers and the majority of smokers were shown to have an annual rate of decline which would maintain an FEV_1 of greater than one litre until over the age of 80. A minority of smokers were shown to have a faster rate of decline in FEV_1. This survey also demonstrated that on stopping smoking cigarettes this faster rate in decline in FEV_1 tended to return to the rate found in non-smokers. Subjects with the faster rate of decline of FEV_1 normally had an FEV_1 well below accepted normal values at the age of 45. Their data support the thesis that screening smoking males in the fifth decade using simple spirometric techniques would detect the individual at risk of developing chronic obstructive bronchitis at an age when stopping cigarette smoking would allow an adequate FEV_1 at the age of 70. Thus more sensitive tests at an early age are unnecessary and may not identify the patients most at risk.

Becklake and Permutt [11], however, have argued that changing the smoking habits in middle age may not be easy, and identifying individuals at risk at an earlier age will lead to a greater success in stopping patients smoking. Although there is little firm data on the age when stopping smoking is most successful, the search for the best test of small airway abnormality continues on the above premise. At present the best of these tests would appear to be flow in the terminal portion of the MEFVC, the volume of isoflow, mean transit time of forced expiration, or the slope of phase 3 of a single breath test ($\Delta N_2/l$). A summary of the tests available is shown in Table 5.3. However, prospective longitudinal trials will be required to elucidate the best test for screening chronic obstructive bronchitis at a reversible stage. Such a trial or series of trials is a considerable undertaking and will require time.

5.9 Genetic predisposition to developing chronic obstructive bronchitis

Physiological screening procedures for the identification of individuals at risk of developing incapacitating airflow obstruction have not been the only approach. Questionnaires and clinical acumen have revealed higher risk in males, lower socio-economic status and first degree relatives of patients with chronic obstructive bronchitis. The apparent relationship between possible genetic predisposition and airways obstruction was given impetus by an association found between severe α_1-antitrypsin deficiency and emphysema (see Chapter 8). It is now recognized that the serum concentration of α_1-globulin antitrypsin is controlled at a single autosomal gene locus. Pi (protease inhibitor), genotypes and phenotypes can be identified by electrophoresis, the severe deficiency states associated with a Pi ZZ genotype and normal levels with the common Pi MM genotype. Heterozygotes for Z or M including several other genotypes are associated with intermediate levels of circulating antitrypsin blood levels. Early studies showed that the rare Pi ZZ genotype had a very high association with development of basal emphysema at an early age in smokers. A series of reports followed suggesting that the intermediate levels for α_1-antitrypsin found in mixed phenotypes was associated with an increase in the risk of developing emphysema but recently such a clear relationship has not been confirmed. Heterozygotes probably have normal airway function but minor loss of elastic recoil suggesting some loss of alveolar elasticity. The high incidence of heterozygotes, and the comparatively low incidence of patients with chronic obstructive bronchitis within this group, suggest that α_1-antitrypsin deficiency is not the only genetic marker for predisposition to lung disease. The rarity of Pi ZZ genotype and the conflicting evidence for heterozygote susceptibility, even in individuals smoking cigarettes, exclude this investigation as suitable for screening populations for emphysema. However, screening families of a

Table 5.3   Available tests for screening for small airways obstruction

Test	Comment
Frequency dependence of compliance	Reference test, difficult to perform in field
Residual volume	Not repeatable
Oxygen desaturation on exercise	Time consuming in field
Single breath test phase 4/$VC\%$ closing capacity	Can be difficult to interpret
$\triangle N_2/l$ alveolar plateau	Requires further investigation but promising
Forced expiratory manoeuvre forced expiratory volume in one second (FEV_1) forced vital capacity	Argument exists as to whether these detect early changes in small airway function
mean flow rates 25%–75% vital capacity	Simple but high coefficient of variation
instantaneous flow rates at 50% and 75% of expired vital capacity	High coefficient of variation and small number of reference values
flow rates with and without helium breathing	High coefficient of variation
volume of isoflow	Requires further investigation
mean transit time	Requires further investigation

patient with a homozygous deficiency and emphysema is mandatory to identify susceptible individuals and stop them from smoking.

5.9.1 Case finding for abnormal lung function

Although screening populations for early chronic obstructive bronchitis may not be profitable at the moment, the physician should always consider spirometry for individual patients with mild respiratory symptoms, or young male asymptomatic smokers. Premature abnormality of either FEV_1 or vital capacity probably has prognostic significance not only with respect to respiratory insufficiency but also early death from heart disease.

5.10 Screening for lung disease in industry

The association between certain industrial processes and lung disease is well known (see Chapter 17). The control of dusts is a problem for engineers and dust physicists and their efforts have been remarkably successful. The incidence of coal workers pneumoconiosis and asbestosis has been reduced by lowering airborne concentrations of coal dust and asbestos fibres in working areas. New industrial processes are now recognized as leading to various forms of lung disease. Allergic reactions leading to asthma have been reported with such varied processes as beer production and electronic flux soldering. The detection of an increased incidence of lung disease in new processes can be determined by questionnaires and simple respiratory function tests. The detection of airflow obstruction at an earlier stage in individuals may also be helped by using tests of small airway function as individuals can be then used as their own control in longitudinal studies. Many factories are now setting up screening programmes but there are few published longitudinal studies illustrating and measuring their value.

5.11 Screening asymptomatic subjects for lung cancer

Symptoms from lung cancer usually occur late in its natural history. The five-year survival is less than 10% and except for oat cell carcinoma, curative treatment is surgical and the prognosis is related to the stage of the disease at the time of detection. However, reports vary considerably as the total improvement in percentage survival with early detection, and little consideration has been given to morbidity. Lung cancer would still appear to be a disease suitable for screening at an asymptomatic stage especially in relation to its high prevalence and the existence of a 'high risk' subgroup can be easily defined in terms of age (over 45), cigarette consumption (more than 10 cigarettes/day) and to a lesser extent sex (males). At present three possible approaches are being evaluated; chest radiograph, sputum cytology and more recently the possibility of blood biochemical markers.

5.11.1 Chest radiograph

Most studies have shown only a small yield of patients with lung cancer compared with the number of normal radiographs taken. The detection of lung cancer in asymptomatic subjects with serial chest radiograph has so far had little effect on prognosis. Only recently has notice been given to the evidence showing that the genetic load from diagnostic irradiation will double the incidence of congenital abnormalities by 1990. A number of lung cancer screening trials have been set up mainly in the USA and early reports are now becoming available. These trials are using combinations of serial chest radiographs and sputum cytology in the high risk group. It is clear that serial chest radiographs in asymptomatic subjects tend to detect peripheral lung lesions which are usually adenocarcinoma which is not associated with cigarette smoking. Central lung lesions seen radiologically tended to be either unresectable or were identifiable earlier by sputum cytology.

5.11.2 Sputum cytology

The diagnosis of lung cancer is confirmed by sputum cytology of histology obtained either at bronchoscopy or thoracotomy. Sputum cytology in specialist laboratories will give a positive cell type in approximately 80% of cases when a central lesion is seen on chest radiograph and the sputum collections are supervised (see Chapter 13). Such high yields are frequently not attained in routine cytology in district hospitals. The yield is lower for peripheral lesions. The positive yield even with central lesions is poor on single sputum specimens and is only marginally increased with three sputum specimens on a single day, and therefore population screening requires sputum obtained on three separate days. Frequently, unsupervised sputum collections are of a poor quality and separate visits to the screening centre are required to obtain adequate material. A further problem which has arisen is the identification of abnormal sputum cytology in the presence of a normal chest radiograph. The logical next step is fibreoptic bronchoscopy but often this reveals no obvious carcinoma. Blind biopsies have occasionally revealed the site or worse, multiple sites. Segmental bronchial lavage and cytology has been reported as identifying the site of the carcinoma on some occasions. Such a train of events is frequently a disaster for the patient as rather than awaiting the symptomatic stage of his disease in blissful ignorance, he is awaiting his death for an increased length of time.

The supporters of screening for early lung cancer suggest four-monthly sputum cytology with chest radiographs every four or six months as effective in detecting early lung cancer in the high risk middle aged, male, heavy smoker. The combination of both radiograph and cytology is considerably more effective than either alone. The Mayo Clinic data suggests that high risk groups 'may' benefit from such screening. The author's view is that until clear benefit to the individual patient is shown from such surveys they should be limited to specialist centres, where the high costs and possible dangers can be both determined and observed. The possibility of screening for occupational lung cancer has been suggested but should be deferred until the Mayo Clinic and John Hopkins surveys have answered some of the questions posed earlier.

5.11.3 Blood biochemical markers

Biochemical markers associated with neoplasms have been reported with increasing frequency over the last few years (see Chapter 8). The value of biochemical markers in both diagnosis and management in some cancers such as chorioncarcinoma and gonadal tumours is well accepted. Bronchogenic carcinoma is associated with non-metastatic syndromes such as Cushings' syndrome and inappropriate antidiuresis and tumour-produced hormone has been detected. These hormones, however, are most commonly associated with oat cell carcinoma and are probably related to tumour bulk. Hypercalcaemia is more commonly associated with squamous cell carcinoma but usually with extensive unresectable disease. The other biochemical markers, the oncofoetal antigens (carcinoembryonic antigen or α-foetoprotein), the enzymes (placental alkaline phosphates), and the cell turnover products (polyamines) have not been tested in terms of their efficacy for screening for asymptomatic lung cancer but their lack of specifity, sensitivity and validity suggest they are unlikely to be sufficiently sensitive to detect early carcinoma.

5.12 Summary

The mass screening of large populations to detect individuals with early lung disease is still more of a dream than a cost effective or valid exercise. Although the procedures described in this chapter are often useful or essential in the management and diagnosis of an individual patient seeking help from a medical practitioner, they have yet to be fully evaluated in screening populations. The natural history of the diseases themselves and the effects of therapeutic intervention at an earlier stage in their natural history must also be estimated but not in terms of a few days longer of misery, but rather in useful, active happy life. Clearly cigarette smoking is a major aetiological factor in such diseases and changes in cigarette habit may well yield considerably greater therapeutic effects, but even here, the morbidity of such change should be accurately assessed.

The cottage industry of screening of early lung disease developed in the 1970s is now assessing its present position. Further expansion of screening programmes should not take place for diseases which are poorly amenable to therapy, such as lung cancer until considerable improvements in therapy are established. Long-term controlled studies are required to support the thesis of Fletcher and his co-workers that only FEV_1 is required to determine individuals at risk of developing severe airways obstruction, and such prospective studies should include the more hopeful tests of small airway function. Such studies should be collaborative so that the advances in thoracic medicine are linked with the greater understanding of epidemiological and statistical techniques. Data collection and calculation should be supervised by suitably trained scientists, so that a number of errors which have occurred over the last ten years may be avoided.

Further reading

Benatar, S. R., Clark, T. J. H. and Cochrane, G. M. (1975), Clinical relevance of the flow rate response to low density gas breathing in asthmatics, *Am. Rev. resp. Dis.*, **111**, 126–34.

Cochrane, G. M., Prieto, F. and Clark, T. J. H. (1977), Intra-subject variability of maximal expiratory flow volume curve. *Thorax,* **32**, 171–6.

Coombes, R. C., Ellison, M. L. and Neville, A. M. (1978), Biochemical markers in bronchogenic carcinoma, *Br. J. Dis. Chest*, **72**, 263–300.

Despas, P. J., Le Roux, M. and Macklem, P. T. (1972), Site of airway obstruction in asthma determined by measuring maximal expiratory flow breathing air and a helium-oxygen mixture. *J. clin. Invest.*, **51**, 3235–43.

Fontana, R. S. (1977), Early diagnosis of lung cancer, *Am. Rev. resp. Dis.*, **116**, 399–402.

Hutcheon, M., Griffin, P., Levison, H. and Zamel, N. (1974), Volume of isoflow. A new test in detection of mild abnormalities of lung mechanics. *Am. Rev. resp. Dis.* **110**, 458–65.

Melamed, M. *et al.* (1977), Preliminary report of the lung cancer detection program in New York. *Cancer*, **39**, 369–82.

Permutt, S. and Menkes, H. A. (1979), Spirometry analysis of forced expiration within the time domain. In: *The Lung in Transition between Health and Disease*, Vol. 12, Lung Biology in Health and Disease (eds. P. T. Macklem and S. Permutt), Marcel Dekker, New York and Basel, Ch. 6, pp. 113–51.

Pride, N. B. (1979), Analysis of forced expiration. A return to the recording spirometer. *Thorax*, **34**, 144–7.

Rose, G. and Barker, D. J. P. (1978), Repeatability and validity, *Br. med. J.*, **2**, 1070–1.

References

1. Illich, I., (1975), In: *Medical Nemesis*, Calder and Boyer.
2. Cochrane, A. L. (1972), The history of the measurement of ill health. *Int. J. Epidemiol.* **1**, 89–92.
3. Macklem, P. T. and Mead, J. (1967), Resistance of central and peripheral airways measured by a retrograde catheter, *J. appl. Physiol.*, **22**, 395–401.
4. McLean, K. H. (1958), The pathogenesis of pulmonary emphysema. *Am. J. Med.*, **25**, 62–74.
5. Hogg, J. C., Macklem, P. T. and Thurlbeck, W. M. (1968), Site and nature of airway obstruction in chronic obstructive lung disease. *New Engl. J. Med.* **278**, 1355–60.
6. Prieto, F. *et al.* (1978), Spirometry in healthy men: A correlation with smoking and with mild symptoms. *Thorax*, **33**, 322–7.
7. Woolcock, A. J., Vincent, N. J. and Macklem, P. T. (1969), Frequency dependence of compliance as a test of obstruction in the small airways. *J. clin. Invest.*, **48**, 1097–107.
8. Levine, G., Housley, E., MacLeod, P. and Macklem, P. T. (1970), Gas exchange abnormalities in mild bronchitis and asymptomatic asthma, *New Engl. J. Med.* **282**, 1277–82.
9. Fry, D. L. and Hyatt, R. E. (1960), Pulmonary mechanics. A unified analysis of the relationship between pressure, volume and gas flow in the lungs of normal and diseased human subjects. *Am. J. Med.* **22**, 672–89.
10. Fletcher, C. and Peto, R. (1977), The natural history of chronic airflow obstruction. *Br. med. J.*, **1**, 1645–8.
11. Becklake, M. R. and Permutt, S. (1979), Evaluation of tests of lung function for 'screening' In: *The Lung in the transition Between Health and Disease*, Vol. 12, Lung Biology in Health and Disease. (Eds. P. T. Macklem and S. Permutt), Marcel Dekker, New York and Basel, Ch. 16, pp. 345–81.

CHAPTER SIX

Radiology

I. H. Kerr

The purpose of this chapter is to discuss the various techniques available in diagnostic chest radiology, giving some guide to the best use of X-rays in chest disease. It is not a comprehensive survey, but includes the methods in general use in a chest hospital. No attempt has been made to discuss the interpretation of the examinations except in general terms, and reference to more detailed works on chest radiology should be made for description of the radiological appearances in various diseases.

The chest radiograph should be regarded as part of the clinical examination of a patient with chest disease. As such it behoves the clinician to be familiar with the interpretation of the radiograph and also to know the potential and limitation of the technique. The radiograph is such an integral part of the examination of the patient that many chest physicians look at the radiograph before examining the patient, and then study it again afterwards. The place for the chest radiograph is at the bedside or in the outpatient clinic and not filed away in an X-ray department with only a radiologist's report to hand when the patient is being examined. Similarly the report should not be made by the radiologist without full knowledge of all the clinical data either by consultation or by having the case notes available. This means that the clinician must have some knowledge of the basic principles of chest radiology.

6.1 The plain chest radiograph

The image on the film is produced by differential absorption of the X-ray beam by the structures in the body through which it passes. In broad terms in the human body there are four different naturally occurring absorption bands.

1. The most dense is calcium, including bone.
2. Fluids and soft tissues including muscle, blood vessels, cartilage and connective tissue.

3. Fat including adipose connective tissue, fat pads, lipomata and cholesterol.
4. Gases such as air, alveolar gases, etcetera.

Where there is an interface between these absorption bands an edge is
visible on the radiograph and structures become identifiable. Where there is
no interface between bands, i.e. where two structures of the same density lie
next to each other, no edge will be visible and the two structures will appear
as one (Fig. 6.1). The radiograph is a two-dimensional representation of a
three-dimensional structure and of course all parts from the back to the front
will be superimposed. Application of anatomical knowledge and use of
additional projections allows the trained observer to reconstruct a three-
dimensional picture in his mind. Stereoscopic radiographs are for most
radiologists unnecessary though in spite of the additional radiation and cost
this is a technique used by some. The overlying bony structures, the ribs and
spine, frequently obscure the portion of the thorax of most interest to the
physician, the lung. Newer techniques employed in radiography have done
much to reduce this difficulty. For many years the kilovoltage employed for
the standard radiograph has been between 60 and 80 kV. With the development of X-ray apparatus kilovoltages of a medium range 80 to 120 kV
or high kilovoltages from 120 kV upwards, are now employed. The higher
the kilovoltage the more energy there is in the X-ray beam and the less
effect there is in differential absorption. In simple terms the X-rays are
less affected by the structures through which they pass. The contrast produced on the film between air in the lungs, and soft tissues, and the bony
thorax is greatly reduced (Fig. 6.2).

In order to reduce scatter from secondary radiation with high kilovoltages
either a grid is used, or an air gap in which a space of 6 to 10 in is interposed
between the patient and film. If an air gap is used, the focus to film distance is
usually increased from the standard 6 ft (1.84 m) to 10 ft (3 m). This increases
magnification of the image. The person interpreting the radiograph should
know what technique has been employed. Radiographs taken at high kilovoltage show the pulmonary vessels and abnormalities in the lungs very well
yet at the same time there is good visualization of the mediastinum. Because
of the reduction in contrast the ribs interfere less with detail in the lungs.
This effect has some disadvantage in that lesions in the ribs such as fractures
or metastases may be difficult to identify; similarly calcification in tuberculous or other intrapulmonary lesions, in the pleura or in the heart may be
overlooked. With experience of this technique, however, one comes to
recognize the small increase in density which represents calcification.
Another advantage of the high kilovoltage technique is that there is greater
latitude in the exposure and therefore serial radiographs taken on different
days are much more similar in exposure and hence more comparable. In the

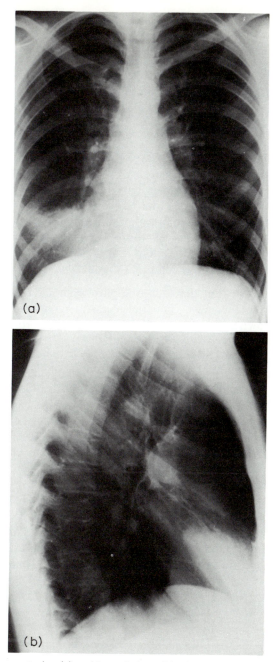

Fig. 6.1 Postero-anterior (a) and lateral views (b) of the chest showing consolidation in the middle lobe. The right heart border is lost in the PA projection due to air in the middle lobe being replaced by inflammatory cells and fluid of the same density as the adjacent heart – the silhouette sign.

X-ray department repeat examinations because of radiographic error are fewer.

The ideal chest radiograph should satisfy the following criteria.

1. The patient should be straight. The inner ends of the clavicles should be an equal distance from the upper dorsal vertebrae. These can be recognized by the rings of the pedicles on either side or by the spinous processes.
2. The film should include the lower cervical spine, the rib cage on both sides and the costophrenic angles.
3. The scapulae should not be projected over the lung fields. The patient's arms are pushed forward in order to achieve this.
4. The exposure should be short so that there is no movement.
5. The exposure should be such that the vessels in the lung fields are clearly visible and yet of sufficient penetration that the dorsal spine is faintly seen through the central mediastinal shadow.

The medial end of the left dome of the diaphragm should be visible through the heart shadow (Fig. 6.2). The translucency of the trachea should be visible at least down as far as the level of the arch of the aorta. These criteria will be affected to some extent by the build of the patient and of course, by disease in the chest.

The standard radiograph is obtained by the patient standing, the cassette containing the film close to the front of the chest and the X-ray beam passing from posterior to anterior (PA). Because this cannot always be achieved, mainly when the patient is in bed, the film may be taken with the beam passing anterior to posterior (AP) and the cassette behind the patient's back. Also, with the use of a mobile X-ray machine a distance of less than 6 ft may be necessary to give as short an exposure as possible. These two factors produce differences in the image so that structures in front of the chest, notably the heart, become more magnified than in the standard posterior–anterior (PA) projection. In a very ill patient the radiograph may be taken with the patient supine. This alters the position of fluid which may be present and air-fluid levels are now no longer visible as the beam is at right angles to the fluid surfaces. Hydropneumothorax may then not be appreciated.

6.1.1 The laterial chest radiograph

The lateral view of the chest is obtained by placing the patient with the saggital plane parallel to the film and at right angles to the X-ray beam. The side of the patient in which the main lesion is to be examined is placed closest to the film. This is because detail of structures closest to the film is slightly less affected by geometrical blurring than those further away. With

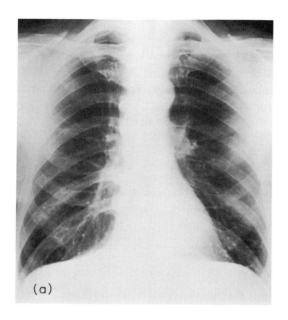

(a)

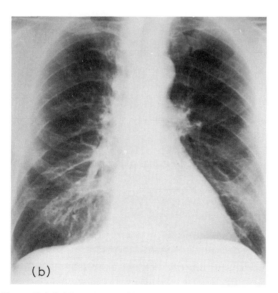

(b)

Fig. 6.2 The effect of high kilovoltage. (a) Postero-anterior projection of the chest at 65 kV; (b) the same patient at 150 kV. Note at the higher kilovoltage the loss of contrast of the ribs, yet the vessel pattern in the lungs is clearer.

fine focal spot X-ray tubes this is more theoretical than is found in practice and lesions on both sides of the chest are usually equally well seen. A stationary or moving grid is used to absorb scattered radiation. In the ideal lateral radiograph, exposure is such that the blood vessels in the lungs are visible at the lung bases and yet penetration is such that the dorsal spine and sternum are clearly demonstrated. The posterior ends of the ribs on the two sides should be almost superimposed (Fig. 6.3). When a lesion is seen in the PA view, a lateral view should be obtained to provide additional information regarding its shape, size and anatomical position. It is an essential preliminary to tomography or needle biopsy.

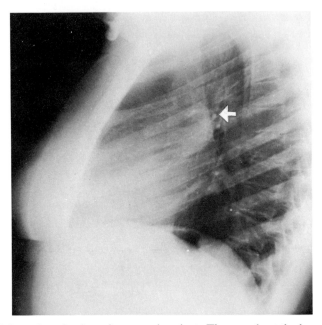

Fig. 6.3 A lateral projection of a normal patient. The vessels at the lung bases are visible, and yet the sternum and dorsal spine can be clearly seen. The posterior ends of the ribs are superimposed. The trachea (arrowed) and main bronchi can be identified.

Though some radiologists would regard the lateral projection as having little value claiming that all the diagnostic information is given by the PA view, especially using high kilovoltage technique, most advocate its use when there is an abnormality seen on the frontal view. In recent years, however, its routine use in screening patients has been mostly abandoned, because of the additional radiation hazard and cost.

6.1.2 Additional views

Oblique views of the chest have limited value in investigation of lung disease. A shallow 15° oblique view may be used to provide an additional view of the lung fields but does not often give much useful information. A 40 to 50° oblique projection is often of value in showing lesions in the mediastinum and has recently become popular in demonstrating lesions of the hila and the major bronchi. Traditionally this view was used for showing the outline of the heart but very few cardiac centres now use it as a routine. Oblique views are essential in investigation of diseases of the ribs and are to be preferred to linear tomography for this and for lesions in the lung or pleura close to the chest wall. In such lesions it is often of great help to obtain views in differing degrees of obliquity by using a fluoroscopic machine and taking spot films while observing the lesion on the television monitor.

6.1.3 Apical views

The apices of the lungs are often obscured on the frontal radiograph by the upper ribs and clavicle. Views obtained by angling the tube downwards by 30° in the PA projection or upwards by 30° in the AP projection, or by placing the patient in a lordotic position with the nape of the neck resting on the upper border of the cassette in the AP projection, allow the shadow of the clavicle to be projected outside the lung field. This may be of great assistance in deciding if an opacity lies within the lung apex or is due to soft tissues outside.

6.1.4 Lateral decubitus radiographs

Fluid free in the pleural space or in cavities shifts with change of position and can be demonstrated by radiographs taken by a horizontal X-ray beam with the patient lying down. The projection is not lateral and is usually AP or PA. Its greatest use is in delineating cavities in which there is an air fluid level and in pleural effusions particularly when subpulmonary (Fig. 6.4).

6.1.5 Expiration films

A posterior anterior radiograph on full expiration when compared with one taken at full inspiration will demonstrate diaphragm movement, demonstrate localized air trapping and help in showing a shallow pneumothorax. An extension of the technique involves a series of films taken on a film changer whilst the patient breathes into a spirometer. The first radiograph is taken on full inspiration and then the patient is requested to breathe out as rapidly as possible. The second radiograph is taken after one second, that is after a

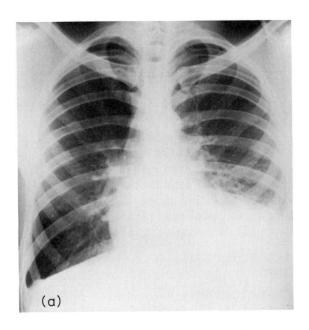

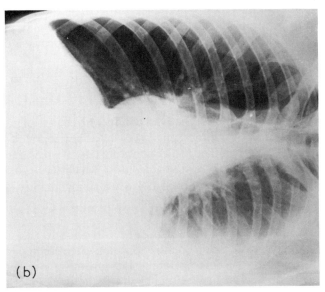

Fig. 6.4 (a) Pleural effusion which has collected between the lung and the diaphragm, i.e. subpulmonary, in the erect position. (b) The lateral decubitus projection shows that the effusion is free in the pleural space and is now lying along the lateral chest wall, which is the most dependent part of the pleura.

forced expiratory volume in one second (FEV_1) has been achieved. The third radiograph is exposed on full expiration, that is when the vital capacity has been reached. The three radiographs will then demonstrate regional differences in ventilation and the areas in which air is trapped.

6.1.6 Magnification radiography

Fine focal spot X-ray tubes which are now available allow the production of magnified images with as little geometrical blurring as possible and clear, well defined margins of structures. The patient–film distance is increased up to 50% of tube to film distance so that magnification is increased. In adults only a small part of the lung can be examined at any one time and the tube rating may be such that a long exposure may have to be given. Movement blur may then detract from the advantage produced by magnification. The technique, however, is of considerable value in infants and in young children and in some centres it is used routinely in neonates despite the higher radiation dose to the skin.

6.2 Special radiological procedures

6.2.1 Fluoroscopy

There was a time when every patient admitted to a chest hospital was routinely 'screened'. Fluoroscopic apparatus was relatively cheap but with the use of image intensification availability has become restricted. The diagnostic importance of fluoroscopy has been realized to be much less than was previously thought, and the higher radiation dose of fluoroscopy compared with radiography has been appreciated. Fluoroscopy is now used mainly in conjunction with other procedures such as barium swallow, aspiration needle biopsy, fibreoptic bronchoscopy and bronchography. It is indicated however for:

1. *Diaphragm movement.* The diaphragm moves normally at least 3 cm between inspiration and expiration. The left dome moves slightly more than the right under normal circumstances. Measurement of the movement may be made from radiographs taken on inspiration and expiration but movement itself is best observed on fluoroscopy. When one dome of the diaphragm is paralysed there is paradoxical movement. This may be enhanced by requesting the patient to sniff. Minor degrees of paralysis of the diaphragm may be difficult to see particularly when the outer rim of the diaphragm is supplied by intercostal nerves. In elderly patients the diaphragm, which is more lax than in younger patients, should be examined in both the erect and horizontal positions. Paradoxical move-

ment may be easier to see when the patient is horizontal particularly on the right side as the weight of the liver and abdominal organs will influence movement of the diaphragm more when the patient is erect. Restriction of diaphragm movement is seen when an inflammatory disease or its aftermath is present either immediately above or below the diaphragm.

2. *Positioning of patient for oblique radiograph.* Tangential views of lesions or oblique views of the chest wall may be obtained using fluoroscopy for positioning the patient (see above).

3. *To elicit pulsation.* It is extremely difficult, if not impossible, to decide during fluoroscopy whether pulsation of a lesion in the mediastinum is transmitted or expansile. Fluoroscopy is therefore a poor method of deciding if a lesion is an aneurysm or not. Some arteriovenous fistulae in the lung pulsate excessively and may be observed to get smaller with forced expiration against the closed glottis (Valsalva procedure).

4. *Observing localized obstruction of ventilation.* Obstructive emphysema of the lung or part of a lung may be diagnosed by fluoroscopy when the mediastinum will be seen to shift to the opposite side and the diaphragm on the same side will show restricted movement. This may be of particular value in infants when a pair of radiographs on inspiration and expiration is difficult to obtain.

6.2.2 Barium swallow

Many lesions in the mediastinum displace the oesophagus and their extent and position can be assessed by barium swallow with radiographs taken in the AP, lateral and both oblique projections. Displacement and indentation of the barium column may show the extent of spread of a tumour (Fig. 6.5). Fixation of the oesophageal wall and destruction of the mucosa of the oesophagus would indicate invasion by tumour. Hiatus hernia, achalasia, varices and tumours of the oesophagus would be revealed by barium swallow. Apart from the mediastinal shadows these lesions produce, obstruction of the oesophagus may cause chronic pneumonic consolidation in the lungs. Systemic sclerosis is also associated with changes in the oesophagus, and inflammatory lesions in the lungs.

6.2.3 Tomography (conventional)

The principle of tomography is co-ordinated movement of the X-ray source (the tube) together with movement of the film in an appropriate direction and distance so that the plane in the object being examined is stationary relative to the tube and film. The same effect can be obtained by movement of the object and film or the tube and object provided the ratio of the tube-to-film distance and the tube-to-object distance remains constant. The motion is about a pivot point and results in blurring the structures above and below. The position of the pivot determines the level of the layer to be examined. The angle through which it occurs determines the thickness of the layer examined. The larger the angle the thinner the layer of clarity. In computed tomography (CT) the procedure is more complex. The radiation detector is not a photographic film but a scintillation crystal. The information it obtains is fed into a computer which constructs the image, usually a transverse section of the body.

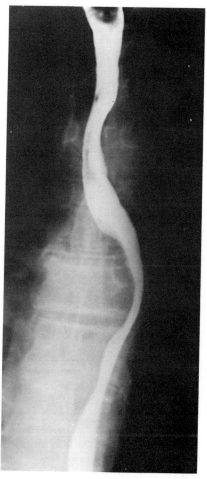

Fig. 6.5 Barium swallow. The oesophagus outlined by barium is deviated to the left by a mass of subcarinal lymph nodes in a patient with carcinoma of the bronchus.

The image produced in tomography is affected by the type of movement. The simplest and most commonly used is linear tomography when the tube and film move in a straight line usually in the long axis of the object – the patient. The exposure is usually about one second. Lesions in the lung are generally well shown by this method but linear shadows lying in the plane of movement will not be blurred and will be reproduced on many levels. The shadow cast by the dorsal spine causes a density overlying the mediastinum, as the dorsal spine, though blurred, always remains in the line of movement. The effect of this is a dense white shadow in the middle of the chest with darker lung areas on either side. It is not possible then to see detail in both mediastinum and lung at the same time unless an aluminium trough filter is used to even up the density in the lungs with that of the spine. Calcification in costal cartilages and the anterior ends of the clavicles may produce dense streaks on the tomograph and may be mistaken for pulmonary lesions (Fig. 6.6).

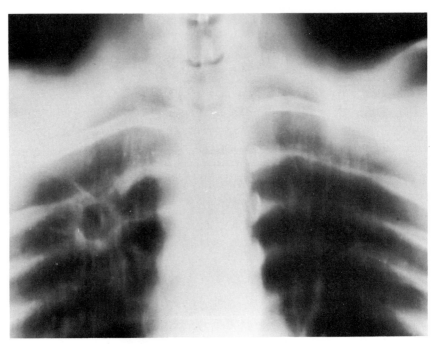

Fig. 6.6 Linear tomogram showing a cavitating tuberculous lesion on the right. The opacity at the left apex is due to blurring of the dense medial end of the left clavicle. As the patient is slightly rotated, the right clavicle is not projected over the lung to the same degree. Note there is no blurring of the medial aspect of the left apical shadow. The tube movement is in the saggital plane, which is the same plane as the surface of this medial end of the clavicle.

Rotational tube movement, which may be hypocycloidal, circular, or eliptical, blurs superimposed shadows in all directions. Suitable apparatus for this is expensive and not available universally. Well constructed apparatus is essential for the tube movement may rock the X-ray table and blurring of the selected plane may occur due to patient movement. Exposures are often long, 2–6 s, to allow for the movement of the tube, though in general they are much shorter than in CT. Patients with respiratory diseases may find difficulty in breath-holding for these longer exposures.

Inclined plane tomography is used for showing the trachea, main bronchi, and both hila on a single radiograph. This is achieved by tilting the film, usually 15°, so as to lie parallel to the plane of the trachea. This may be done using a standard linear tomography unit with the patient horizontal and the film inclined beneath the couch, or with a fixed tube, the patient erect and rotating in a cradle seat which is linked to an inclined film which also rotates. Blurring with the latter is in a horizontal direction reducing the effect of the density due to the spine. Because of its limited application the apparatus to achieve this is only available in a few centres.

The indications for conventional tomography are:

1. To define, more clearly than the plain radiograph, opacities in the lungs or to show minimal lesions either not visible on the plain radiograph, or suspected because of minimal shadowing.
2. To define anatomical localization.
3. To show lesions in the hila and mediastinum and to define the major airways.

In general, there has been a decline in the use of conventional tomography in recent years. The need for clarification is less because the quality of the plain film has altered, especially with the use of high kilovoltage. But the main reason for the decline is a change in emphasis in diagnosis. The prime indication for tomography in the past was the demonstration of cavitation in tuberculosis because of the importance of its presence in management. Tuberculosis is much less common and the presence of cavitation of less importance. The main indication for tomography now is in the diagnosis of pulmonary masses and the differentiation of carcinoma from other diseases.

After an opacity in the lungs is discovered on the plain radiograph, the next step in diagnosis is to obtain cytological, histological or bacteriological evidence of its nature. Many radiological signs have been described to distinguish carcinoma from other lesions in the lungs including such characteristics as umbilication, satellite shadows, spiculation, irregular edges, peribronchial linear shadows, etc. These may be best seen by tomography but none is reliable and there is little to be gained in most cases from tomography before cytological and bacteriological testing of the sputum, bronchoscopy or other biopsy examination. Even the presence of calcification in a lesion does not exclude, though it greatly reduces the chances of, carcinoma which may have occurred in a tuberculous scar. One exception is when arteriovenous fistula (Fig. 6.7) is suspected when tomography may be needed to show the feeding artery and draining veins. Once the diagnosis of carcinoma is made then tomography of the hilum and mediastinum to assess spread may be valuable.

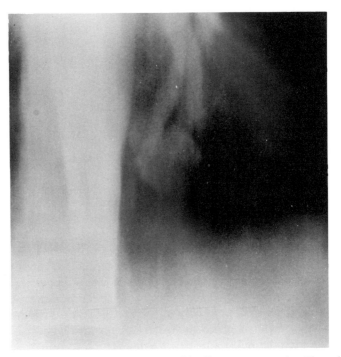

Fig. 6.7 Arteriovenous fistula demonstrated by linear tomography. Note the large feeding and draining vessels.

This is not to say that there are no indications for tomography before bronchoscopy or other more invasive examinations. It may be of great value in deciding if a prominent hilar shadow is due to normal vessels or due to a possible sinister lesion; in deciding whether there is a lesion in the lung at all, when the plain radiograph is ambiguous; or in the search for metastases when whole lung tomography may be undertaken. Before embarking on tomography a recent plain radiograph should be available together with a lateral view. The lateral view helps to decide what tomographic cuts should be taken. It is all too easy to take innumerable tomographic cuts in the search for an opacity which has cleared in the interval between the initial radiograph and the examination. The other catch is the lesion seen only in one projection not due to an intrapulmonary lesion at all but due to the shadow cast by a polypoidal tumour or wart on the skin. Satisfactory tomography may not be easy to achieve in lesions near to the heart due to transmitted pulsation, or near the diaphragm and chest wall due to the difficulty in blurring dense structures in close proximity to opacities of lower density. Tomograms may be obtained in more than one projection. AP and lateral projections are those most frequently used though oblique tomography of the hilum is of great help. Reference to the anatomy of the lungs is important in deciding which projections are likely to be most useful. The trachea, the main bronchi, upper lobe bronchi and intermediate bronchi are best shown in AP and oblique projections. The middle lobe and lower lobe bronchi are best seen in the lateral projection and the lingula and middle lobe bronchi in the oblique projections. The hila are often best examined in at least two projections, PA and lateral or oblique.

6.2.4 Computed tomography (CT)

The invention of the whole body computerized scanner has provided a new dimension in the radiological investigation of diseases of the thorax. The principle involved in this technique is similar to conventional tomography in that an X-ray source and a radiation detector make a co-ordinated movement around the patient. In this case the detector is not a photographic film but a scintillation crystal (sodium iodide, bismuth germinate or calcium fluoride). The signals received by this detector are processed by a computer and depend on the variations in the amount of absorption of the X-ray beam as it passes through the subject. By a mathematical process of image reconstruction the computer forms a picture representing a cross-sectional slice of the body 3 to 13 mm thick. The resolution of the system is extremely good and lesions as small as 3 mm can be identified in the lungs. The exposure time varies with different machines from 2–20 s. The patient is usually examined with breath holding at maximal inspiration, though if it is unlikely that this position can be maintained during the exposure, and cannot be achieved with consistency when further exposures are made at different levels in the chest, the exposures can be made at resting end volume. The patients must be able to breath-hold for up to 20 s depending on the CT machine used, for movement blurring will occur if this is not achieved. Lesions near the heart and great vessels may be blurred by transmitted pulsation and line artefacts may be produced which, though annoying, do not seriously interfere with interpretation. The development of apparatus with exposure times of fractions of seconds or 'gated' programmes timed by the cardiac cycle, is required to provide pictures of the heart.

A useful part of CT is the ability to provide a measurement of the attenuation coefficient of an area of interest on the scan. This gives an estimate of the density of the lesion or area of the body. This is known as the CT number and water has been arbitarily assigned a CT number of zero. For other tissue its CT number is determined by the computer and using EMI units air has a CT number of −500, bone +500, fat −40 to −50 and other soft tissues +5 to +40. If a contrast medium is injected intravenously the CT number will increase in vascular lesions such as aneurysms and in very vascular tumours but will remain constant in avascular lesions such as fluid-containing cysts.

After the introduction of CT apparatus for whole body sections initial reports were promising for scanning of the abdomen but were pessimistic about its value in the thorax. However, though still not fully evaluated, definite indications for the use of this technique in diseases of the chest have emerged. There is little doubt that it is of help in the diagnosis of lesions in the chest particularly using the CT number and contrast enhancement.

The indications for CT are:

(a) Mediastinum

1. To elucidate doubtful opacities in the mediastinum seen on a plain radiograph.
2. To determine the nature of a lesion in the mediastinum by rough determination of its tissue density (CT number). Lipomas, dermoid cysts, fat pads, have a negative CT number (Fig. 6.8). Soft tissue lesions, tumours, fluid containing cysts have a positive CT number. Contrast enhancement will increase this number if the lesion is vascular and the great vessels can be identified with confidence.
3. To evaluate spread of malignant disease by showing mediastinal lymph nodes (Figs 6.9 and 6.11). It seems unlikely that CT will be found to be superior to good conventional mediastinal tomography in the demonstration of mediastinal lymph nodes in most cases, but one group of nodes around the pleura of the diaphragm have been found to be shown by CT far better than by conventional tomography.
4. To evaluate the abnormal hilum. This has been advocated by some to be an indication for CT but it is doubtful again if the method is superior to good conventional tomograms in the AP, lateral and oblique projections.

(b) The lungs

1. The primary indication for CT of the lung fields is to demonstrate nodules not apparent on the plain radiograph or on whole lung tomograms. It has

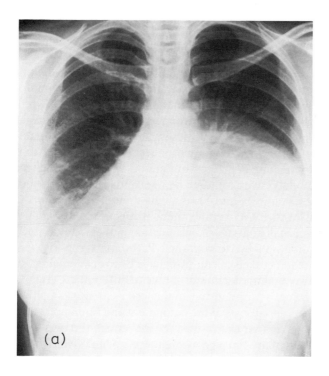

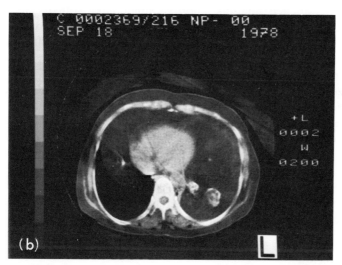

Fig. 6.8 (a) Plain chest radiograph. (b) Computed tomogram (CT) of a large fat containing tumour with some calcification, previously diagnosed as tuberculous pericarditis. Note the lower density of the tumour compared with the heart which it surrounds. (By permission of Professor I. Isherwood.)

been shown that about 20 to 25% of patients with nodules seen on plain radiography will have further lesions shown by whole lung tomography. CT will detect smaller lesions and more sub-pleural lesions than conventional tomography so that in about 30 to 50% of patients additional nodules, mostly 3 to 10 mm in size are found. The detection of multiple nodules is of greatest value in metastatic lung disease (Fig. 6.10). The chances that further nodules are metastases are high though it must be realized that not all such opacities will be due to malignant disease. In an NIH study in the USA thoracotomies were performed to excise such nodules in the lung in a group of patients with known malignant disease [1]. The nodules were found to be a second primary carcinoma in 9.3%, metastases in 74.3%, and benign inflammatory lesions in 16.4%. Techniques using the CT number may distinguish the benign lesions by identifying small amounts of calcification in them, not visible on conventional radiographs or tomograms. Preliminary reports, using the CT number to detect such calcification have been encouraging, though other reports deny that this technique is able to differentiate granulomata from small metastases especially when the lesions are very small. CT is expensive both in capital costs of the equipment and running costs. Its use must therefore be limited to those patients in which the result will affect the management of the case and where there is a high chance of success in the demonstration of an abnormality. It is therefore indicated in patients who have primary tumours which commonly metastasize to the lungs such as testicular tumours, chorionepitheliomas, soft tissue sarcomas, primary bone tumours and melanomas in the search for possible metastases, and in any tumour in which a metastasis is found in the lung in looking for further lesions particularly if surgery is being considered for the treatment of the metastasis.

2. Interstitial fibrosis is shown by CT at an earlier stage than by conventional radiography [2]. An early sign of this is loss of the normal gravity-dependent perfusion seen on CT scans. The gravity-dependent parts of the lungs are normally denser so that in the supine position the posterior parts appear whiter than the anterior. The density difference is seen to alter with position, so that when the patient is lying on the side, or prone, the whiter area moves to the lower side, or anteriorly respectively. These gravity dependent changes are less marked if the CT scans are performed on deep inspiration than at resting volume.

(c) The pleura

The cross-sectional view of the chest provided by the CT scan is an excellent method of detecting and assessing pleural disease (Fig. 6.11). Plaques of thickened pleura or diffuse pleural thickening can be seen with ease. The

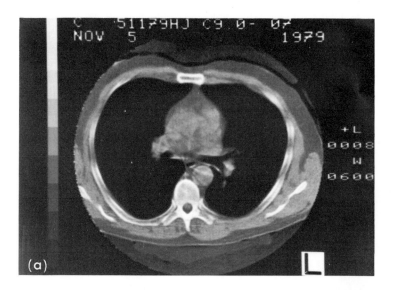

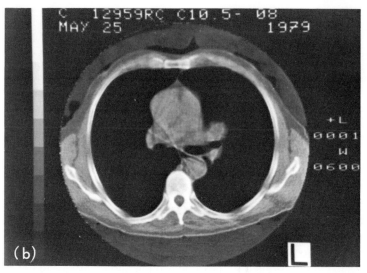

Fig. 6.9 Computed tomogram. (a) Normal patient at the level of the left main bronchus. The image is conventionally projected as if one is viewing the chest from below. The descending aorta is seen just to the left and in front of the vertebral body, and the left main bronchus with its upper lobe branch in front of the aorta. (b) A tomographic 'cut' at the same level as (a). Enlarged lymph nodes are present at the left hilum just in front of the left upper lobe bronchus in a patient with malignant disease.

extent and size of pleural tumours, malignant deposits or mesothelioma can be seen well, much better than with conventional tomography. Loculated pleural effusions can be distinguished from tumours.

(d) Radiotherapy

CT is valuable in planning radiotherapy of the lung and mediastinum.

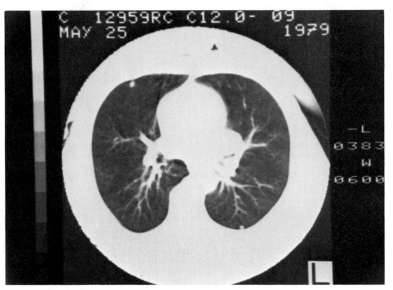

Fig. 6.10 CT of the same patient as Fig. 6.9 (b), showing two small metastases at the periphery of the lungs, one anteriorly on the right and the other, posteriorly on the left. The image on this scan is produced by a wider window setting than that of Fig. 6.9 reducing the contrast.

6.2.5 Bronchography

The prime indication for bronchography has always been bronchiectasis and this is still the main indication for this investigation. The reduction in incidence of bronchiectasis has followed the decline in severe respiratory diseases in childhood such as whooping cough and measles and the prompt treatment by antibiotics of complicating bronchopneumonia. Together with the doubt of the efficacy of surgery in many cases of bronchiectasis, this has greatly diminished the importance of anatomical localization of the disease. However, it is still the definitive method of diagnosing bronchiectasis. (Fig. 6.12). It must be remembered particularly if surgery is contemplated for localized bronchiectasis that the exclusion of the disease may also be an

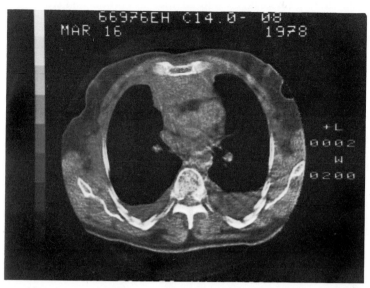

Fig. 6.11 CT of a patient with a malignant mass in the anterior mediastinum. Compare the appearances behind the sternum with Fig. 6.9. Bilateral plural effusions are seen. As the examination has been performed with the patient supine these are in the most dependent part of the chest, in the paravertebral gutters posteriorly.

important aspect of bronchography. Thus, if localized bronchiectasis is displayed by a bronchogram of one lung it is of great importance to exclude the disease in the contralateral lung.

The second most important indication for bronchography is recurrent haemoptysis where the cause has not been discovered by bronchoscopy. With the advent of fibreoptic bronchoscopy this indication is becoming less frequent. Unsuspected 'dry' bronchiectasis, endobronchial tumours and healed granulomata are found in about 5% of such cases, but about 50% show bronchographic evidence of chronic bronchitis, presumably the cause of the haemoptysis. Carcinoma and solitary nodules in the lung have been suggested as indications for bronchography but the yield is poor and a histological diagnosis obtained by transbronchial biopsy or percutaneous aspiration is more rewarding. Selective bronchography through a fibreoptic bronchoscope may be of some help in showing patent bronchi, in a distal inflammatory lesion as opposed to the blocked bronchus due to a neoplasm which may be beyond the range of the scope. Occasionally, unsuspected localized bronchiectasis may be shown this way.

Other diseases in which it may occasionally be of value to perform bronchography are chronic bronchitis, bronchopulmonary aspergillosis to show the characteristic type of proximal bronchiectasis, bronchitis obliterans, foreign bodies, chronic cavities and bronchial fistulae. Anomalies and congenital lesions of the bronchial tree may be diagnosed by bronchography.

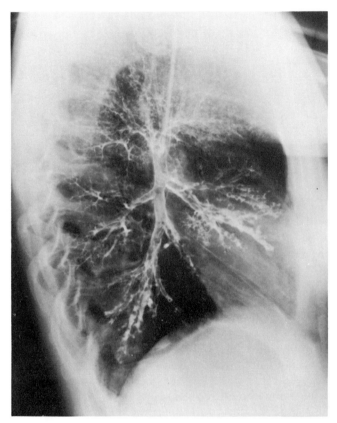

Fig. 6.12 Bronchogram, right lateral projection, showing bronchiectasis in the middle lobe, and to a lesser degree in the basal segments of the right lower lobe. The remainder of the bronchial tree, is normal. The left side examined subsequently was also normal.

There are three main ways of performing bronchography:

1. Injection into the mouth or nasopharynx.
2. Per oral or per nasal intubation into the trachea or major bronchi.
3. Cricothyroid injection.

The cricothyroid method is now performed by introducing a catheter over a guide wire inserted through the cricothyroid membrane under a local anaesthetic, down the trachea into the main bronchi. The advantage of this method is that it is more certain of success than the other methods but has the complications of possible damage to the larynx, surgical emphysema of the head and neck and possible infection in the soft tissues. It is therefore a method for the experienced bronchographer and should be resorted to only when one of the other methods has failed.

Success of bronchography depends on patient co-operation, mainly in restraining cough, and on good anaesthesia. The pharynx and larynx should be sprayed with local anaesthetic using a fine atomizer. An atomizer which produces large drops will only successfully anaesthetize the back of the tongue. Injection of local on to the larynx either through a tube in the nasopharynx or directly through the mouth is also advisable. An authoritative confident manner on the part of the operator together with alacrity will do much to allay the fears of the patient. In patients with restricted respiratory reserve it is advisable to examine one side only at a time, and examine the contralateral side on another day. The right side is best examined first when a bilateral study is being performed so that a lateral view of the right bronchial tree may be obtained without superimposed contrast in the left bronchial tree. A left posterior oblique view will adequately display the left bronchial tree. The contrast medium now used universally is propylio-done (Dionosil; Glaxo), usually suspended in an oily solution. The aqueous suspension of Dionosil is more irritant and more viscous. Barium carboxy-methyl-cellulose mixture may be used in patients known to be iodine-sensitive but can produce other undesirable side-effects, and coating is not as good as with Dionosil. Reactions to Dionosil, usually mild, are however not infrequent. The mucosa of the airways may show mild inflammatory change and there may be a fever. Wheezing with breathlessness and a chemical bronchopneumonia are fortunately rare. Even when there is no obvious reaction the airways are obstructed by the contrast medium and after a bilateral bronchogram the vital capacity is reduced by 30 to 40% and the FEV_1 by 25%. The diffusing capacity may be reduced by 50%. These respiratory function tests may take up to 72 hours to return to normal. Thus bronchography should not be undertaken immediately prior to surgery and similarly, because of irritation to the larynx by instrumentation, broncho-graphy should not be undertaken for several days after bronchoscopy.

As a result of these disadvantages of Dionosil a search has been made for other contrast media. The only substance which has great promise is tanta-lum powder. This is an inert, dense metal which gives excellent coating in the bronchi and is non-toxic. Coughing does not dislodge tantalum from the mucosal surface unlike Dionosil. The tantalum is cleared by the mucociliary blanket within two to four days. Like all finely powdered metals there is a danger of combustion and explosion especially in pure oxygen. Tantalum oxide may be used as a safe substitute. The difficulty with tantalum, and the reason it has not received universal acceptance, is its injection into the bronchial tree as it has to be blown into each part of the lung to be examined making the procedure long and tedious. It is excellent for laryngography but injection into the smaller airways has to be done by selective catheterization. It is therefore an excellent tool for research purposes to outline bronchi under study but has limited value in the clinical field.

Bronchography under general anaesthetic should be undertaken with care. The restriction of pulmonary function by the contrast medium should be remembered by the anaesthetist and a careful watch made on the amount of contrast injected. It is in children that general anaesthetics are most frequently used for bronchography and because of the small size of the lungs the dose of contrast becomes more critical. An adult requires about 30 to 36 ml of Dionosil for a bilateral bronchogram, 20 ml for the right side and 16 ml for the left. The dose for children is 0.75 to 1 ml/lung/year of age. Under the age of one bronchography should be performed with extreme caution because of the danger of anoxia.

6.2.6 Arteriography

(a) Aortography

Because of the difficulty of separating opacities in the mediastinum different methods to define the structures, normal or abnormal, may have to be employed. One of the common problems is that of deciding if a mass arises in the mediastinum or in the lung, and opacification of vessels, arterial or venous, or of the oesophagus may help in anatomical localization. Another problem is in deciding if a mass is arising from the aorta, i.e. an aneurysm, or is due to some other pathology before undertaking a biopsy procedure, such as needling, bronchoscopy or mediastinoscopy. Because of the obvious hazard of haemorrhage it is prudent to perform aortography to confirm or exclude the diagnosis of arterial aneurysm, though it has been claimed by some that needle aspiration biopsy with a fine 21 or 23 gauge spinal needle can be performed in these circumstances without danger if the aorta is punctured. Other indications for aortography include congenital anomalies, such as vascular rings, pseudocoarctation or true coarction and pulmonary sequestration, and acquired diseases such as aortic dissection, trauma and giant cell arteritis (Takayasu's disease). The diagnosis of aortic aneurysm can be made by contrast enhancement using the CT-scanner, though as yet it does not replace aortography in showing the extent of the lesion.

(b) Pulmonary arteriography

The prime indication for pulmonary arteriography is pulmonary embolism. If there is doubt in minor cases of pulmonary embolism after radio-isotope studies have been performed, pulmonary arteriography may need to be undertaken as it is the definitive method of diagnosis. In acute massive pulmonary embolism there may not be time to perform radio-isotope scanning or it may not be available, and pulmonary arteriography again is a quick and reliable method of diagnosis.

Pulmonary arteriovenous fistula is best diagnosed by pulmonary arteriography and the importance of this examination is not only in showing the suspected lesion but also in showing other similar lesions in the lung, as multiple fistulae are present in 30 to 50% of patients. Other vascular abnormalities demonstrated by arteriography include anomalous left pulmonary artery where the left branch passes around the right main bronchus which it compresses before reaching the left lung, abnormalities of the venous drainage such as the 'scimitar' syndrome, and pulmonary varices.

Though there is some increase in hazard of pulmonary arteriography in patients with pulmonary hypertension it may be of great value for diagnosis and management to show the cause of the disease. Pulmonary arteriography has a very limited place nowadays in the preoperative assessment of carcinoma of the bronchus though it may be of value in deciding if the left pulmonary artery or main pulmonary trunk is invaded by a carcinoma in the left hilum.

(c) Bronchial arteriography

Selective injection of the bronchial arteries for diagnostic purposes has proved to be disappointing. There is little difference in appearance between benign and malignant lesions and even between tumours and inflammatory conditions. Recently, however, catheterization and embolization of the bronchial arteries has been employed with encouraging results in patients with repeated haemoptysis in such conditions as bronchiectasis, and cystic fibrosis, in which the bronchial arteries enlarge.

6.2.7 Venography

Though obstruction of the superior vena cava may be well shown by venography, propagation of thrombus proximal to the obstruction may give rise to difficulty in interpretation. However, it may be of great help in showing the site of the lesion particularly if the lumen of the superior vena cava is narrowed and not obliterated. It is a simple procedure performed by injection of contrast medium into the antecubital veins in each arm simultaneously and obtaining serial radiographs of the upper part of the chest.

Opacification of the azygos vein and its tributaries is more difficult and involves either intraosseous injection of contrast medium into the lower ribs of the posterolateral wall of the chest under general anaesthesia or the introduction of a catheter through the femoral vein, to the right atrium and superior vena cava, into the azygos vein retrogradely. This investigation is indicated in the rare abnormalities of varicosities of the azygos system which cause posterior mediastinal opacities. It has been used in the preoperative assessment of spread of lung carcinoma but it is of doubtful value as the information can be obtained by simpler means.

Selective retrograde injection of the thymic vein outlines the thymus and the presence of a tumour in the thymus is demonstrated by a displacement of these veins. This is of particular value in patients with myasthenia gravis and has the advantage over mediastinal pneumography of not restricting ventilation in these patients whose respiratory reserve may already be reduced by a muscular weakness. The thymic veins drain into the innominate vein and can be selectively injected by a catheter inserted through a left arm vein.

6.2.8 Mediastinal pneumography

This investigation is mainly employed for demonstration of tumours of the thymus. It may also be used for showing lymph nodes in the mediastinum in the staging of carcinoma and other neoplasms. Various routes have been used for the introduction of the gas. The most favoured are the retrosternal route in which the needle and catheter are introduced alongside the trachea, the trans-sternal where the needle is inserted through the manubriosternal joint, and the substernal where the needle is inserted into the mediastinum from below. The catheter may be inserted during mediastinoscopy or scalene node biopsy and the insufflation performed later in the day. In view of the danger of air embolism an initial injection of carbon dioxide is usually made followed by a larger injection of oxygen to delineate the mediastinal structures. The method will almost certainly be superceded by CT scanning in the future.

6.2.9 Sinograms and pleurograms

The extent of an empyema may be demonstrated by the percutaneous injection of contrast medium into the infected cavity after aspiration. Lipiodol, an oily contrast medium which is heavier than pus, is used and films taken in the erect position. The lowermost point of the cavity is then demonstrated, this being the most suitable place for insertion of a surgical drain.

A sinus may occur spontaneously or following surgical drainage of an empyema. The extent of the sinus and whether it communicates with the bronchial tree through a fistula may be outlined by the injection of contrast medium, Lipiodol or Dionosil, into the sinus. This should be achieved by the introduction of a catheter along the sinus track. Injection under pressure into a closed system should be avoided as it is possible to force air or pus into a vein with resultant embolization. The examination is best performed under fluoroscopic control so that a bronchopleural fistula can be identified early and suitable radiographs can be taken to show the limit of the sinus cavity.

6.3 Mass miniature radiography (MMR)

Miniature radiographs can be obtained on film 35 mm to 100 mm in size by photographing a fluorescent screen through a lens system. This method was introduced for mass survey work as film handling is reduced to a minimum and thus many more patients can be examined in a given time. The clarity of the films is excellent for this type of work but if there is any doubt about an abnormality a standard radiograph is taken. Because of the small size of the film and the need to magnify the image minor degrees of nodular shadowing in the lungs cannot be accurately assessed. Miniature radiography is therefore not suitable for most industrial survey work. It was best used for the detection of pulmonary tuberculosis in the 1940s and 1950s when the incidence of new cases in the general population in Great Britain was approximately 7 per 1000. By the 1970s, although figures of 4 to 40 per 1000 radiographs could be found in developing countries, in industrial countries such as Great Britain the incidence of pulmonary tuberculosis was about 0.6 per 1000 in the general public attending mass survey units. Though the incidence in patients referred by general practitioners in urban areas has been reported as high as 5.8 per 1000, the incidence of pulmonary tuberculosis in rural areas is about half that in urban areas. Other diseases of importance are rare and even lung cancer without symptoms is detected in only 0.2 to 0.3 per 1000 routine chest radiographs.

The cost of detecting tuberculosis or cancer in patients without symptoms by mass surveys using mass miniature radiographs, together with the disadvantage that this type of apparatus in general requires a higher radiation dose to the patient than standard technique, has led to mass miniature surveys being abandoned in this country and very few units are now in use.

6.4 Viewing and interpreting

Good radiographs should be viewed under good conditions. Time, effort and expense put into the production of a good quality radiograph is often wasted by the clinician or radiologist looking at it under poor conditions. Holding a radiograph up to the light at a window is to be abhorred. Viewing boxes should be used and these should be well illuminated by modern fluorescent tube lights. Side and background lighting should be reduced to a minimum. All too frequently in outpatient clinics and wards sunlight pours in on the viewing boxes making it extremely difficult to study the radiograph and it is not surprising that abnormalities are missed. Even under ideal conditions there is an astonishingly high incidence of error in both the identification and interpretation of the abnormalities amongst experienced observers shown by many studies into the accuracy of diagnostic procedures. Interobserver error in the identification of an abnormality has been reported from 10 to 25% and intraobserver error from 3 to 30%.

In the examination of a radiograph it has been shown that there are two methods of inspection, directed search and free search. In directed search the observer follows a pattern of inspection. The chest wall, and soft tissues, diaphragm, heart and mediastinum and finally the lungs are inspected in order. This is the method which the inexperienced and trainee should adopt until the pattern of the normal is imprinted on the mind. In free search, the radiograph is examined in a random manner and without a preconceived plan. It has been shown that this is the method used by most experienced radiologists though a combination of both methods is probably the ideal.

Interestingly, studies have shown that viewing the chest radiographs at a distance of 6 to 8 ft or using diminishing lenses improves the perception of lesions with indistinct margins. The perception of an image depends upon the rate of change in illumination across the retina. Thus a lesion with a sharp edge will be well seen at the standard viewing distance. Increasing the distance and hence decreasing the angle projected on the retina will increase the rate of change in illumination across the retina of a less well-defined lesion. Magnification on the other hand will have the opposite effect and it is therefore only of use in shadows of relatively high contrast. Films therefore should be observed at standard distance and at 6 to 8 ft. If a disease with diffuse shadowing of relatively high density is present magnification may be of assistance.

Perception of lesions in certain parts of the lung is not as good as elsewhere. The periphery of the lung is overshadowed by the ribs and chest wall and pathological studies and CT scanning have shown lesions up to 1 cm in diameter can be missed in these areas. Also close to the heart, aorta, mediastinum and spine and diaphragm, the adjacent dense shadows make small lesions difficult to identify. With a well-defined margin non-calcified lesions as small as 3 mm can be seen in the central parts of the lung fields, but with poorly defined margins they may be much larger before they can be perceived. A carcinoma less than 1 cm in diameter is seldom identified. With calcification, however, lesions smaller than 3 mm can be seen.

6.5 Summary

An essential element in the diagnosis of chest diseases lies in the plain chest radiograph which should be viewed under good conditions. The image obtained when an X-ray beam passes through the body depends on the differential absorption of the different structures bone, soft tissues, fat and air. Improved visualization of the lungs can be obtained by using high kilovoltages which reduce the density of the overlying ribs and spine. Additional projections, and fluoroscopy may provide useful diagnostic information. Tomography, by blurring structures superimposed on the area of interest and computed tomography which provides an image of a cross sectional slice of the body are more sophisticated methods of investigation enhancing the information provided by plain radiography. Materials containing substances of higher atomic number, i.e. denser, than the tissues of the body, may be used to show various structures in the thorax. These contrast media are used to show the oesophagus, bronchi, pulmonary arteries and pulmonary veins, bronchial arteries, systemic veins and pathological spaces.

Miniature radiography is a useful method for surveying large numbers of the population, but its use in developed countries no longer seems justified and it is unfortunately of little value in surveys of workers in industry exposed to dusts.

Further reading

Fraser, R. G. and Paré, J. A. P. (1979), *Diagnosis of Diseases of the Chest*, 2nd edn, Vols I–IV, W. B. Saunders Co., Philadelphia.
Kreel, L. (1978), Computed tomography of the thorax. *Radiol. Clinics N. Am.*, **16**, 575–84.
Sagel, S. S. (1976), *Special Procedures in Chest Radiology*, W. B. Saunders Co., Philadelphia.
Siegelman, S. S., Stitik, F. P. and Summer, W. R. (eds.) (1979), *Multiple Imaging Procedures* Volume I, *Pulmonary System*, Grune and Stratton, New York.

References

1. Neifeld, J. P., Michaelis, L. L. and Doppman, J. L. (1979), Suspected pulmonary metastases – correlation of chest x-ray whole lung tomograms and operative findings. *Cancer*, **39**, 383–7.
2. Katz, D. and Kreel, L. (1979), Tomography in pulmonary asbestosis. *Clin. Radiol.*, **30**, 207–13.

CHAPTER SEVEN

Radioisotope Imaging

F. Fazio

7.1 General principle of radioactive measurements of regional perfusion and ventilation

The standard chest radiograph is probably the most useful – and used – instrumental technique for the clinical investigation of pulmonary disorders. It shows a detailed map of the regional distribution of lung densities, which therefore provides information on lung anatomy *in vivo*. Similar information is provided by CAT scanning, which is a tridimensional, quantitative measurement, of organ density (see Chapter 6).

It is evident that, in addition to the information on lung anatomy, an assessment of regional lung function would be valuable for the diagnosis and the staging of patients with chest disease.

The most important function of the lung (aside from its role in metabolism and in providing a biologic barrier between man and environment) is gas exchange. This depends to a great extent on the distribution of perfusion and ventilation. Attempts to detect macroscopic changes in regional perfusion and ventilation from the chest radiograph can be made, mainly from consideration of the size and distribution of pulmonary vessels and changes in lung parenchyma [1]. These indirect measurements rely on the fact that variations of blood flow and ventilation are sometimes associated with variations of blood and air volumes, respectively. However, this is not always the case [2] and specific techniques are now available for obtaining a functional map (or image) of the distribution of both perfusion and ventilation. These techniques are based on the use of radioactive isotopes.

The general principle of *in vivo* radioactive measurements is to introduce into the body a radioactive tracer and to follow its distribution externally with radiation detectors. In the case of perfusion and ventilation, the functional parameter measured is flow, which can be defined as the amount of air or blood passing through a given lung cross-sectional area in a given time. An ideal assessment of regional ventilation (or perfusion) would be a functional, quantitative image representing the turnover of radioactive air (or blood) within the lungs.

The first measurements of regional lung function were obtained in 1955 [3] following with single counters the arrival (for perfusion) or the washout (for ventilation) of respectively injected or inhaled radioactive gases. These measurements have the advantage of being quantitative, that is, yielding values for regional perfusion (or ventilation) per alveolus or per gram of tissue [4]. On the other hand, they offer a rather poor spatial resolution, yielding information on a limited number (usually four or six) of lung regions. With this technique, functional images of ventilation and perfusion can be obtained by following with a gamma camera and a digital computer the washout of inhaled 133 Xe (for ventilation) or the arrival of injected 133 Xe (for perfusion) and by displaying the spatial distribution of transit times from multiple small regions of the lung [5]. These measurements are quantitative but require a relatively long time, are obtained only in one view and demand considerable expertise and technical resources.

A technique to be used in a clinical context should be simple, quick and yield good spatial information; ideally a functional image which could directly be compared with the corresponding anatomical image, the chest radiograph.

This chapter will deal only with methods which could be applied in a routine clinical context for obtaining functional images of regional ventilation and perfusion. These will be referred to as ventilation and perfusion scans. It will not consider other techniques useful for quantitative physiological studies but not having the requirements of being simple and of high spatial accuracy.

7.2 Instrumentation

Two devices are now currently being used for obtaining images of the *in vivo* distribution of radioactive isotopes: the rectilinear scanner and the γ-camera. The rectilinear scanner, invented in 1951, consists of a metal gantry which carries a detector made of a sodium iodide crystal and a focusing collimator. The detector head moves at a constant speed across the object, then stops and moves forward (or backwards) a small distance; it then starts another transverse motion in the opposite direction. Thus, the detector explores point by point and a dot is printed on paper every time a pulse is received; the number of pulses are proportional to the number of γ-rays hitting the crystal at each point and, therefore, to the radioactivity of that point of the object. The rectilinear scanner has been widely used for nuclear medicine imaging in the sixties and is still in use in several nuclear medicine departments. However, it has now been largely replaced by a stationary device, the γ-camera, developed in 1965.

Modern cameras have a diameter of 10–16 inches, and contain collimated crystals with an electronic circuitry capable of locating the point where a γ-ray has impinged on the crystal. By accumulating enough counts it is therefore possible to obtain an image of the distribution of radioactivity in an object. As for rectilinear scanners, the accuracy of the image and thus of the information obtained mainly depends on the statistical accuracy of the radioactive counting procedure, that is, on the number of events collected. At least 300 000 counts should be, in general, collected for a good γ-camera image of the lungs. The major advantage of this latter device over the rectilinear scanner is the much shorter time (about a fifth) required for obtaining an image of comparable statistical accuracy. This is due to the larger amount of crystal available for recording radioactive events.

Both γ-cameras and rectilinear scanners are equipped with movable 'windows' which can detect and record, under optimal conditions, isotopes emitting γ-rays of different energy and can also detect individual isotopes one at a time when more than one isotope is present in the body.

7.3 Lung perfusion scanning

Lung scanning following the intravenous injection of labelled particles is the procedure for obtaining functional images of regional pulmonary perfusion. This technique, developed in 1964, is now routinely used in virtually every department of nuclear medicine [6–8].

Human serum albumin particles of 10 to 30 μm in the polydispersed (macroaggregates) or the monodispersed (microspheres) form, are now commercially available from a number of manufacturers and can be labelled with a variety of isotopes [technetium-99m (^{99m}Tc) is commonly used]. These particles are injected in a peripheral vein and mix uniformly with blood during their passage through the right heart and then reach the pulmonary capillary bed where they are trapped in a way proportional to the regional blood flow through the capillary network. External recording of their distribution with a rectilinear scanner or a γ-camera will, therefore, yield a functional image of pulmonary perfusion. The proportion of capillaries which are blocked by the particles is small and the procedure has been shown to be safe: for the perfusion scan, less than half a million particles are injected, while it has been estimated that there are about 280 billion pulmonary capillaries. Their safety has been confirmed by experiments in animals. Within a few hours from the injection the particles are broken down, freed into the circulation and metabolized as albumin. The only, remote, potential danger of these particles is that they have, on occasion, caused reflex pulmonary vasoconstriction and one should be careful in administering the injection to patients with severe pulmonary hypertension (particularly if primary pulmonary hypertension is suspected). In these patients and in patients with right-to-left shunt (in whom some of the microspheres will reach the systemic arterial circulation) care must be taken not to inject more than 50 000 – 100 000 microspheres. An injection of about 2 mCi per test is given when modern γ-cameras are used. This results in a dose of 500 mrad to the lungs (target organ), 20 mrad to the whole body and 40 mrad to the bone marrow (the marrow dose from a standard two-view chest radiograph is 25 mrad). The particles can be injected with the patient either erect or in the supine posture. The choice of posture is important because blood flow is not uniformly distributed throughout the lungs, being gravity dependent. Injection with the patient erect is useful in order to detect a shift of perfusion toward the apices (inversion of the normal base to apex perfusion gradient) which can occur in patients with disease of the left heart. The advantage of injecting in the supine posture is a better view of the apices. Both methods are acceptable but it is convenient that once the choice is made, the same procedure is then always used.

Following the injection, the patient is asked to sit in front of the γ-camera (in unconscious or unco-operative patients, as in babies, supine scans can be obtained), the window is set for the energy of ^{99m}Tc (140 keV) and 300 000 or more counts are collected. The patient is then repositioned and the procedure is repeated in order to obtain another view. Six views (anterior, posterior, right and left laterals, right and left posterior obliques) are recommended. Right and left anterior obliques can also be performed in the suspicion of lesions to the middle lobe and the lingula respectively. Lateral and oblique views are important because of the front-to-back stratification of segments within the lung, segmental differences being more obvious from the lateral than from the anterior or posterior views (Fig. 7.1). Lateral views should be interpreted carefully because of the spillover or shine-through effect: in a subject of normal size approximately 20–30% of the counts recorded in a straight lateral position following intravenous injection of ^{99m}Tc-labelled particles are due to radioactive events originating in the contralateral lung. This percentage can be even greater when using isotopes emitting more energetic γ-rays, such as ^{113m}In. Oblique views allow one to inspect part of the external surface of the homolateral lung and part of the internal surface of the contralateral lung without artefacts due to spillover.

7.4 Lung ventilation scanning

Perfusion scanning using the technique described above is now an established diagnostic procedure routinely used in the clinical context, as it is simple, safe, does not require co-operation of the patient and it provides functional images in multiple views of the pulmonary perfusion of high statistical accuracy.

In order to produce comparable images for ventilation, different techniques are now being used in different centres. Indeed, none of these techniques can yet be regarded as satisfactory as the lung perfusion scan, which therefore in many centres is still used alone, not supplemented by ventilation measurements.

Techniques for ventilation scanning involve the use of either radioactive gases or aerosols.

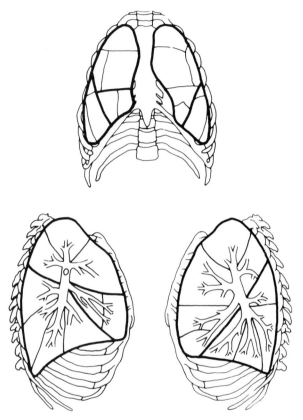

Fig. 7.1 Drawing of lung segment.

7.4.1 Radioactive gas methods

(a) *Single breath/washout of radioactive xenon* [9, 10]

Xenon-133 (^{133}Xe) is a chemically inert gas with a half life of 5.3 days. The patient is asked to take a deep breath of ^{133}Xe (10–15 mCi) and then to breath-hold for 30 s. During this time up to 100 000 counts can be collected on a γ-camera (this method cannot be used with a rectilinear scanner). The image recorded on the γ-camera will be proportional to the regional *arrival* of the radioactive gas, which in turn is proportional to regional ventilation (Fig. 7.2a, bottom). Rebreathing of ^{133}Xe can then be carried out in a closed circuit for 3–5 min until equilibrium is reached and another image can be obtained, which is representative of lung volume rather than ventilation (Fig. 7.2b, top). The patient is then switched to room air and serial pictures (every 60s) are taken while ^{133}Xe is washed out. In a normal subject, the lung empties in a uniform manner and all the activity should have washed out within one minute. Areas of reduced ventilation will be seen during the wash-out phase as areas of abnormal ^{133}Xe retention (Fig. 7.2b, bottom). Washout images are useful in detecting localized areas of reduced or absent ventilation but are not directly comparable to the perfusion images obtained with ^{99m}Tc-HAMM. On the other hand, the images obtained in the first part of the procedure (single breath–breath-holding) require manoeuvres which are not physiological and are impracticable in dyspnoeic patients. These images are usually obtained in only one projection (due to dosimetric problems and to the build-up of ^{133}Xe background in the chest wall). They are generally of poor quality, owing to the low counting statistics achievable during the breath-holding.

Another problem is the unfavourable physical characteristics of [133]Xe. Its significant solubility ($\sim15\%$) may introduce errors in the washout phase due to uptake of tracer in the blood and in the chest wall. Its low γ-ray energy (80 keV) is not optimal for imaging and cannot be compared directly with lung perfusion images obtained with ^{99m}Tc-HAMM (140 keV). The low energy of ^{133}Xe also prevents inhalation scans from being done after the perfusion study, which is regarded as a limitation in the diagnostic strategy of pulmonary embolism, one of the most important clinical applications of lung scanning.

For these reasons, ^{133}Xe has been recently replaced, in some centres, by xenon-127 (half-life 36.4 days) [11]. This isotope has more favourable physical characteristics, having an emission energy of 200 keV, which is good for imaging with the γ-camera and can easily be separated from the 140 keV of ^{99m}Tc, thus making it possible for the ventilation study to be performed *after* the perfusion study. The procedure recommended when using [127]Xe is as follows: the perfusion study is first performed in multiple views; then a ventilation study (single breath–breath-holding–washout) is obtained in the view in which a perfusion defect was best seen in order to increase the chances of differentiating between pulmonary embolism (impaired perfusion, normal ventilation) from chronic obstructive lung disease (defects of both perfusion and ventilation). Disadvantages of the [127]Xe technique are those already mentioned for [133]Xe (apart from the γ-emission): need of co-operation (breath-holding) from the patient, ventilation study limited to one view only, relatively poor counting statistics.

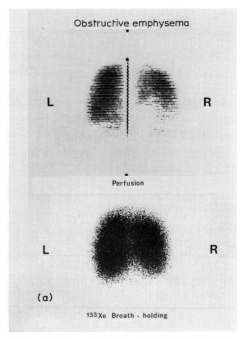

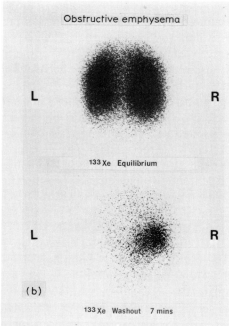

Fig. 7.2 ^{99m}Tc perfusion/^{133}Xe ventilation studied in a patient with obstructive emphysema.
(a) ^{99m}Tc perfusion (top); ^{133}Xe single breath (bottom).
(b) ^{133}Xe equilibrium (top); ^{133}Xe washout (bottom). (Courtesy of Dr D. Ackery.)

Another disadvantage of [127]Xe is that it is expensive and difficult to obtain, since for its production a very high proton energy (over 100 MeV) is needed, which is not available in medical cyclotrons (including machines for commercial production) but requires higher energy physics research facilities such as a linear accelerator. However, [127]Xe can, in part, be recovered and reused with specially devised systems. A system for recovery and waste disposal is, in any case, required for using long-lived radioactive gases such as ^{133}Xe or [127]Xe.

(b) *Continuous inhalation of [81m]Kr* [2, 12, 13]

Krypton-81m is a 190 keV γ-emitting radioactive gas with a very short half-life (13 s). This gas can be continuously produced by passing air through a generator made of its parent [81]Rb [14]. [81]Rb has a half-life of 4.6 h and can be efficiently produced on a medium-energy medical cyclotron. The half-life of the parent enables [81m]Kr to be continuously available all day after a morning (or late evening) production of [81]Rb. When [81m]Kr is continuously added to the inspired air during normal breathing, equilibrium of the isotope with alveolar gas is never reached because of the short half-life; thus the distribution becomes representative of ventilation rather than volume, unlike longer-lived radioactive gases such as ^{133}Xe or [127]Xe. Thus, continuous recording with a γ-camera of the activity over the chest when [81m]Kr is simply added to the inspired air yields a functional image of ventilation. The technique can be combined with an injection of ^{99m}Tc-labelled macroaggregates in order to perform ventilation/perfusion studies in multiple views; ventilation and perfusion can be sequentially obtained for each view by adding [81m]Kr to the inspired air for recording of ventilation only. Thus, [81m]Kr will no longer be present while recording ^{99m}Tc; when recording ventilation, the 190 keV of [81m]Kr can easily be discriminated from the 140 keV of [99m]Tc. Both perfusion and ventilation images can be obtained in 2–4 min for each view, the patient being unaware of the switching from perfusion to ventilation. No waste disposal is required for [81m]Kr, due to the short half-life of the isotope and its low concentration in the expired air.

[81m]Kr yields functional images of pulmonary ventilation under physiological conditions, i.e. during quiet tidal breathing. These images can be directly compared to the standard lung perfusion scan with ^{99m}Tc-HAMM: perfusion and ventilation scans can be recorded in rapid succession without moving the patient, contain the same number of counts and have almost identical resolution. [81m]Kr scans can also be used for recording a rapid sequence of physiologic events, such as the response of regional ventilation distribution to bronchodilator treatment. The major practical disadvantage of the method is the relatively short half-life of the parent, [81]Rb (4.6 h), which requires considerable planning and interest on the part of the user. As

^{81m}Kr can only be used within 16–18 h from the shipment of the ^{81m}Kr generator, the location and availability of cyclotrons will determine the use of this valuable technique.

7.4.2 Aerosol methods [6, 15]

Following the inhalation, during normal tidal breathing, of aerosolized radioactive solutions, deposition of the aerosol within the lungs will take place by (a) sedimentation to the lower respiratory tract according to regional ventilation and (b) impaction in the large airways. If all particles would sediment to the lung periphery, the images obtained following their nebulization would be representative of regional ventilation. Therefore the potential advantage of this method is to obtain images of regional ventilation of good statistical quality in multiple views and without requiring a great deal of co-operation from the patient. In fact, if the particles are sufficiently small (mass median diameter less than 2–3 μm), deposition occurs mainly by sedimentation in small airways and, at least in subjects free from airways disease, little is retained in the throat, trachea or large bronchi. However, bronchial stenosis due to excessive mucus or bronchial inflammation can induce local turbulence of airflow which in turn increases deposition of particles for impaction and leads therefore to a preferential distribution of the inhaled aerosol in the large airways. Indeed, in patients with chronic airflow obstruction the distribution of inhaled particles is more central than that of inhaled gases, although by and large areas of lack of peripheral penetration of aerosol particles correspond to areas of decreased ventilation assessed by radioactive gas methods (Fig. 7.3) [16]. Thus, aerosol techniques may not be adequate for assessing regional ventilation in patients with severe chronic airflow obstruction. On the other hand, deposition of particles by impaction in the large airways can be minimized by reducing the mass median diameter of the inhaled particles [17].

An ideal aerosol method for the clinical assessment of regional ventilation should have the following requirements: (a) be simple and quick to prepare and to administer; (b) be labelled with a short-lived isotope with energy over 180 keV; this would allow a perfusion scan with ^{99m}Tc to be obtained first, the 140 keV of ^{99m}Tc not interfering in higher windows; ideally, the energy should be not more than 250 keV, because energies above this threshold are suboptimal for the γ-camera; (c) the mass median diameter of the particles inhaled should be between 0.5 and 1.0 μm. Larger particles tend to deposit in central airways of patients with airflow obstruction. Smaller particles tend to be re-exhaled, therefore minimizing the fraction of particle deposited. For an aerosol with a mass median diameter of 1.0 μm less than 10% of the particles inhaled are retained in the lungs, more than 90% being recovered in the expired air. This results in a considerable waste of radioactivity and in increased radioactive risk to the operator; with the breathing circuitry commonly used (nebulizer connected to the inspiratory line and a filtre for trapping the particles to the expiratory line), in order to get 1–2 mCi of a tracer into the lungs of a patient, the operator has to start off with 20–30 mCi.

In order to optimize the particle size, different aerosols have been proposed by different laboratories. Simple nebulization of a radioactive solution (even with ultrasonic nebulizers) yields particles of relatively large size (3–5 μm) and therefore suboptimal for ventilation scanning. Better results are achieved by nebulizing presized radioactive particles (human albumin micospheres). These can be labelled with ^{99m}Tc and nebulized with a Venturi nebulizer, yielding, at the outflow of the nebulizer, particles with a mass median diameter of 1.0–1.5 μm. By comparing the images obtained with those particles with ^{81m}Kr ventilation scans, it has been found that this aerosol provides satisfactory ventilation images in patients with chronic airflow obstruction provided their FEV_1 is not less than 50% of the predicted value.

Excellent results are also obtained using a simple and ingenious approach proposed by George Taplin [15]. A solution of ^{99m}Tc-labelled DTPA is nebulized via a disposable low volume nebulizer (operated by compressed air at a flow rate of 8–10 l/min) in a reservoir settling bag placed in the delivery line between the nebulizer and the patient's mouthpiece. This bag removes most particles and/or droplets larger than 2 μm in size by sedimentation or impaction. By using, instead of ^{99m}Tc-DTPA, ^{113m}In-labelled human serum albumin, the aerosol ventilation scan can be performed following the ^{99m}Tc-perfusion scan. This is preferable for the diagnostic strategy of pulmonary embolism (the perfusion scan should be obtained first as a normal perfusion would rule out the presence of thromboembolic disease). Although systematic comparisons with other aerosols or with ^{81m}Kr are, as yet, not available, this method seems to provide, in patients with chronic airflow obstruction, less central deposition than other particle methods, including presized aerosols. The technique which is currently being evaluated in our laboratory is to perform first the perfusion scan with ^{99m}Tc (140 keV) and to subsequently obtain a ventilation scan with ^{113m}In (390 keV), using a high-energy collimator. It should be kept in mind that the two images (perfusion and ventilation) are not strictly comparable, as the coefficient of attenuation within the body for the two isotopes is different. There are also differences in resolution (even using a high-energy collimator), the energy of ^{113m}In being not optimal for the γ-camera. When using ^{113m}In, only the anterior, posterior and oblique views should be obtained, lateral views being meaningless due to the high penetration coefficient (and therefore the significant shine-through) of the highly energetic γ-rays of ^{113m}In.

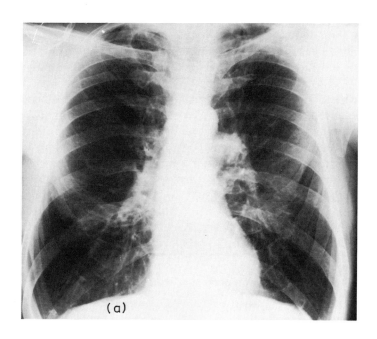

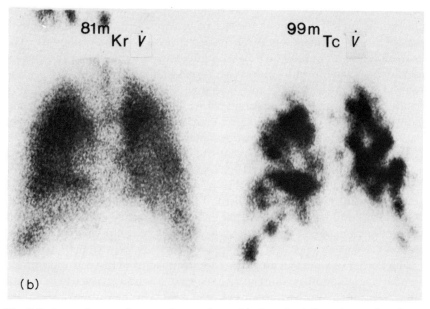

Fig. 7.3 Aerosol versus krypton in a patient with chronic airflow obstruction showing central spots in the aerosol.

7.5 Clinical applications of lung scanning

In this section patterns of ventilation/perfusion scanning in various disease states will be described, as obtained on a large field γ-camera using the ^{99m}Tc-labelled microspheres technique for perfusion and continuous inhalation of [81m]Kr for ventilation. While the former technique is now routinely used in virtually every nuclear medicine department, [81m]Kr is, as yet, only available in relatively few centres. As continuous inhalation of [81m]Kr provides images of pulmonary ventilation in multiple views and directly comparable to the ^{99m}Tc-HAMM lung perfusion scan, this technique is used in this chapter for describing the patterns of regional ventilation in disease as compared to ^{99m}Tc-HAMM lung perfusion scans. Knowledge of ventilation/perfusion relationships in disease states will serve as a guideline to interpret ventilation/perfusion scans also when ventilation scanning is performed with more available but less accurate or specific techniques (such as single breath-washout of ^{133}Xe or inhalation of radioactivity aerosols).

7.5.1 The normal ventilation/perfusion scan (Fig. 7.4)

It has now been shown, using the washout of radioactive gases, that in normal individuals in the upright posture (sitting or standing), there is a gradient of both blood flow and ventilation down the lung, with greater perfusion and ventilation per unit volume in the lower zones [18]. This gradient is mainly due to the effect of gravity on the hydrostatic blood pressure (for perfusion) and the pleural pressure (for ventilation). The distribution of air and blood flow from the bottom to the top of the lungs is more even when the patient is supine. A quantitative evaluation (in terms of ventilation or perfusion per unit of volume) of these gradients is difficult to obtain from routine lung scanning; a lung scan is not an absolute measurement of perfusion or ventilation per unit lung volume, but rather a map of the regional distribution of these parameters within the lungs.

Thus, a normal lung perfusion scan obtained in the upright position shows a gradient of perfusion towards the bases which might be exaggerated by geometry because the base of the lung is thicker than the apices; more activity would be recorded from the bases even if perfusion per unit of volume was uniform. A similar (but less obvious) gradient is present in the ventilation scan. These gradients should always be found on a normal lung scan.

The border of a normal lung scan should appear well defined and convex. The cardiac silhouette should only be seen in the anterior view where the left lung base appears to be thinner than the right. On the posterior view, the lungs appear symmetrical, with straight and parallel medial borders. Lack of symmetry or convex medial borders in the posterior view are usually indica-

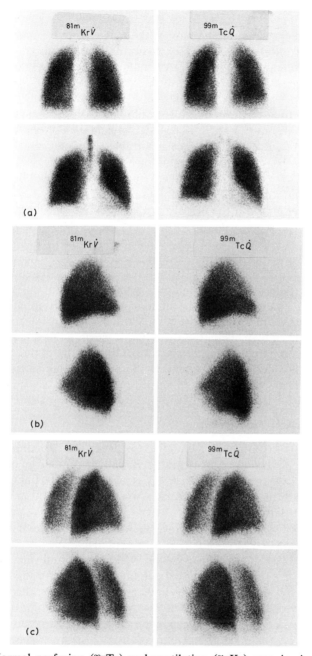

Fig. 7.4 Normal perfusion (^{99m}Tc) and ventilation (^{81m}Kr) scan in six views. (a) Posterior (top); anterior (bottom); (b) right lateral (top); left lateral (bottom); (c) right posterior oblique (top); left posterior oblique (bottom).

tive of pathology of the lower lobes. Lateral and oblique views are essential in showing the segmental anatomy of the lung, as lung segments are stratified in the frontal plane (Fig. 7.1). In normal erect subjects, lateral views show that ventilation and perfusion are not only following a gravity gradient but are preferentially distributed to the lower lobes (Fig. 7.4).

Both lateral and oblique views normally show convex and smooth borders with the exception of the costophrenic angles which should have a sharp, triangular appearance. A rounded appearance of one costophrenic angle in an oblique or a lateral view and in absence of pleural effusion on the chest radiograph may indicate pathology of the posterior segment of the lower lobe. However, a rather convex, round, appearance of the costophrenic angles (on both sides) can be found in obese patients due to increased attenuation of γ-rays at the bases. For the same reasons obese patients, or females with large breasts, can show less evidently the normal preferential distribution of perfusion and ventilation to the lower lobe.

Oblique views are now increasingly used, as, unlike laterals, they are virtually free from contribution from the contralateral lung. This is important in thin patients and in children, where lateral views have, for this reason, very limited value. The oblique views allow one to inspect the external surface of the lung closer to the γ-camera and the internal surface of the contralateral lung. The posterior oblique views, however, provide little information on pathological changes of the lingula and of the middle lobe, which are best detected on lateral or anterior oblique views (the latter should be always preferred in children).

7.5.2 Pulmonary embolism

The diagnosis of pulmonary embolism is generally considered the most important application of lung scanning. Pulmonary embolism is a relatively common condition, estimated to affect as many as 500 000 patients per year in the United States, where it causes some 50 000 deaths per year [19]. Prognosis of pulmonary embolic disease is good following diagnosis and early and appropriate therapy. Nevertheless, pulmonary embolism can be very difficult to diagnose clinically. Common diagnostic procedures (chest radiograph, blood tests, electrocardiography) are often unhelpful in the diagnosis of this disease. The most definite procedure for the diagnosis of pulmonary embolism is pulmonary angiography. However, this is a complex and expensive procedure, which is associated with some morbidity and is difficult to carry out in emergencies, even in specialized centres. In addition, it is also subject to interpretative limitations such as the inability to demonstrate obstruction in small pulmonary arterial branches [20]. The perfusion lung scan is an ideal technique for this purpose, as it provides a map of pulmonary blood flow. A negative lung perfusion scan (if properly performed in multiple views) excludes the presence of a significant embolus [21]. However, its specificity is rather low, perfusion defects being also present in other pathological conditions such as airways disease. The typical lung scan of a patient with pulmonary embolism shows multiple, segmental or subsegmental defects of perfusion throughout both lungs, in presence of a normal chest radiograph and normal ventilation (Fig. 7.5). Unfortunately, the lesions are not always segmental, particularly if the scan is not performed immediately after the embolization and the embolus has partially resolved. The specificity of the perfusion scan is improved by combining it with a ventilation scan. This will show a normal ventilation with impaired perfusion in pulmonary embolism but a combined perfusion/ventilation defect in parenchymal lung disease. Ventilation scanning with ^{133}Xe is now extensively being used for that purpose. The specificity of this combined technique is nearly 100% for patients with multiple large defects and normal ventilation, but less than 50% for patients with smaller defects and with defects corresponding to known radiographic abnormalities [22].

The reason for this is probably that ^{133}Xe ventilation scanning, as discussed previously, requires co-operation from the patient, cannot be performed in multiple views and does not yield images of good statistical quality which would be required for detecting small ventilation defects. These problems are overcome by the use of [81m]Kr; although a systematical comparison with angiography has yet to be made, it is possible that using the combined [81m]Kr/^{99m}Tc technique the specificity of lung scanning for the diagnosis of pulmonary embolism would approach 100%, even in patients with small defects and abnormal chest radiograph.

The importance of obtaining a complete ventilation/perfusion study in multiple views is shown in Fig. 7.6, where the diagnosis of pulmonary embolism is made from the lateral view. This patient with embolism without infarction shows defects in lung perfusion with normal ventilation and clear lung fields on the chest radiograph. In patients with radiological evidence of infarction, perfusion is always absent or reduced in correspondence to the infarcted area seen on the chest film, whereas the [81m]Kr ventilation scan is variably impaired, ventilation being in any case less impaired than perfusion. Fig. 7.7 shows the correlation between the scintigraphic and the radiological estimate of regional lung perfusion and ventilation in patients with pulmonary embolic disease; standard chest radiographs are usually unable to detect defects of perfusion due to embolic disease [2]. In half of the patients shown in Fig. 7.7, perfusion was judged to be normal (100%) and in one-third only minimally altered (>93%) at the radiographic assessment, whereas perfusion defects were always present on lung scans.

Once the diagnosis of pulmonary embolism is made, the patient should be followed up with ventilation/perfusion scans in order to monitor the effect of treatment. Blood flow is (at least in part) restored to the affected region in about one-third of the patients, particularly if young [23]. However, follow-up perfusion scans often show a marked redistribution of blood flow within the lungs, with restoration of perfusion to previously non-perfused or badly perfused areas and new perfusion defects in areas previously well perfused. This can be due to (a) the breaking up of large emboli into smaller fragments, or (b) to new emboli; sometimes it can be difficult to distinguish between these two possible causes of redistribution, as the lung perfusion scan is no more than a qualitative map of pulmonary blood flow. Follow-up studies are essential in that pulmonary thromboembolism only rarely presents as an isolated episode; rather, it should be regarded as a recurrent disease, usually associated with the presence of deep vein thrombosis. Thus, it is also important to identify the site of origin of thrombi; 95% of pulmonary emboli originate from deep vein thrombosis of the legs. This can be diagnosed, apart from the clinical signs, in many ways (contrast venography, positive thrombi imaging with radiolabelled fibrinogen, radionuclide venography).

Radionuclide venography can be performed at the time of the perfusion scan without additional injections or administration of radioactivity or contrast medium to the patient; the labelled macroaggregates are injected in a calf vein and their arrival is recorded by collimating the γ-camera over the pelvis. When deep thrombosis of the leg or of the pelvic veins is present, the arrival of the radioactive tracer is delayed; sometimes the patterns of collateral venous flow are shown. On occasions, 'hot' spots can be seen, resulting from labelled particles stuck to thrombotic areas. When ventilation scanning is not available, routine radionuclide venography is recommended, as it has been shown to add specificity to the lung perfusion scan [24].

7.5.3 Airways disease

Regional ventilation and perfusion can be severely impaired in both acute and chronic airways disease, even in the presence of clear lung fields on the chest radiograph.

(a) Asthma

Lung scans can be grossly abnormal in asthma. During acute exacerbations, while the chest radiograph is normal or only shows large volume lungs, ^{81m}Kr ventilation scans reveal large, segmental or even lobar areas of reduced ventilation, with a distribution similar to that observed for perfusion in pulmonary embolism [25]. Bronchodilators induce immediate improvement of ventilation defects and reduction of lung size but full restoration of normal ventilation can usually be achieved only following prolonged treatment.

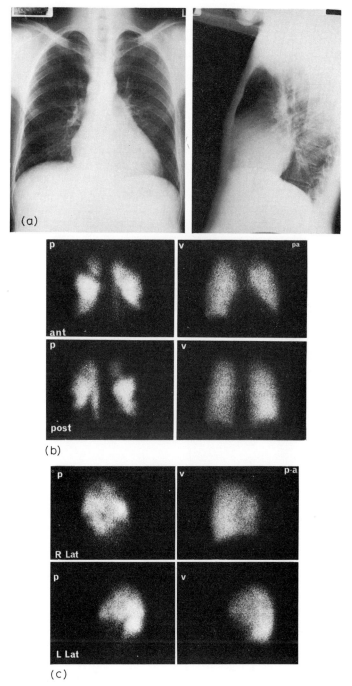

(a)

(b)

(c)

Fig. 7.5 Perfusion/ventilation study in a patient with pulmonary embolism showing impaired perfusion and normal ventilation.

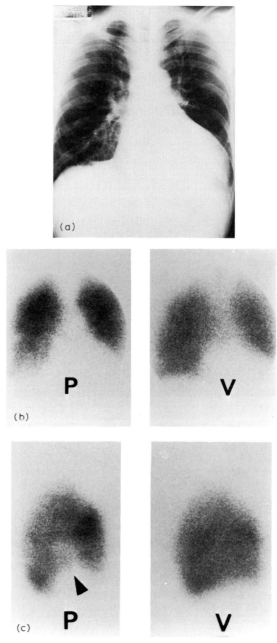

Fig. 7.6 Perfusion/ventilation study in a patient with pulmonary embolism. Segmental perfusion defects are seen only in the lateral view.

The relationships between regional ventilation and perfusion (on a macroscopic basis) in asthma have, as yet, been poorly studied. The ventilation abnormalities can be accompanied by parallel changes of perfusion to the same areas. This perfusion impairment to poorly ventilated areas could be explained either by hypoxic vasoconstriction [26] or by mechanical factors (blood being squeezed out of the hyperinflated areas). On other occasions, however, ventilation and perfusion can be mismatched, showing preferential perfusion distribution to badly ventilated areas and vice versa. The mechanisms responsible for these changes are, as yet, unclear.

(b) Acute bronchitis

Patients with acute bronchitis, either isolated or superimposed to chronic bronchitis, often show large, sometimes segmental, defects of both ventilation and perfusion with clear lung fields at the chest radiograph. In these patients, ventilation is usually more impaired than perfusion. Normal patterns can be restored following treatment with antibiotics and physiotherapy (Fig. 7.8). The alteration of ventilation seen in asthmatics and bronchitics can be explained on the basis of functional and morphological alteration of the bronchial wall (bronchospasm, bronchial oedema, inflammation) or of the bronchial lumen (mucus plugging), resulting in a reduced air flow to part of the bronchial tree. This is confirmed by the fact that these alterations can

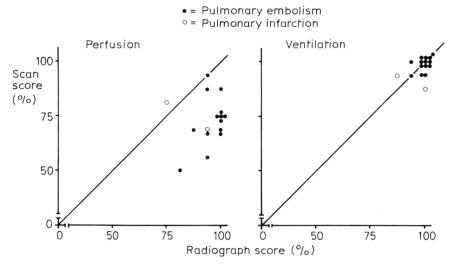

Fig. 7.7 Assessment of perfusion and ventilation from scans and radiographs in pulmonary embolism. Assessment of perfusion from radiographs underestimates perfusion defects. (Reproduced from the *Am. J. Roentg.*)

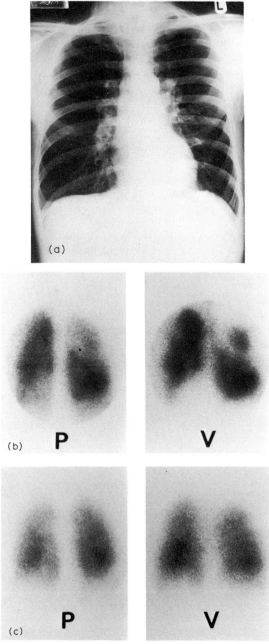

Fig. 7.8 (a) Acute bronchitis showing segmental defects of both perfusion and ventilation. The perfusion scan alone would have been compatible with pulmonary embolus (b). (c) Same patient following treatment with antibiotics and physiotherapy. (Reproduced from *Am. J. Roentg.*)

sometimes be partially reversed by coughs (Fig. 7.9). The alteration of perfusion can be attributed to functional mechanisms induced by the ventilation impairment (hypoxic vasoconstriction, lobar shrinkage, etc.), or to direct involvement of blood vessels by inflammatory processes.

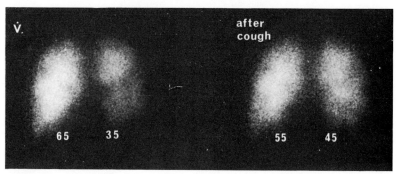

Fig. 7.9 Segmental defect of ventilation (left) which subsides following a cough manoeuvre. (It was probably due to a mucus plug). (Reproduced from *Br. J. Radiol.*)

(c) Consolidation, atelectasis

Patients with an acute respiratory illness and consolidation seen on the chest radiograph, usually show an impairment of perfusion and ventilation corresponding to the radiological opacity. These alterations can follow different patterns according to the pathology underlying the consolidation. In the case of pulmonary infarct, perfusion appears to be *more* impaired than ventilation. On the other hand, in the presence of consolidation due to pneumonia or bronchopulmonary infection, ventilation appears to be more impaired than perfusion (Fig. 7.10). Knowledge of these typical appearances can be useful for the differential diagnosis of acute chest disease with and without the presence of consolidation of the chest radiograph. Lung ventilation/perfusion scanning can also be of value in assessing combined pathologies, such as the association, in the same patient, of thromboembolic and infective processes (Fig. 7.11).

In the presence of the radiological appearance of collapse or atelectasis of a lobe or a portion of lung, the characteristic appearances on the lung scan are those of an absent or reduced ventilation to the collapsed area with normal or only slightly reduced perfusion (Fig. 7.12).

Why, in cases of pneumonia and collapse/atelectasis, ventilation can be almost absent whilst perfusion is only slightly reduced, is not clear. Atelectasis may occur as a result of bronchial plugging and subsequent disappearance of air from the distal portions of the lung. Apparently, in these cases, hypoxic vasoconstriction is not highly effective.

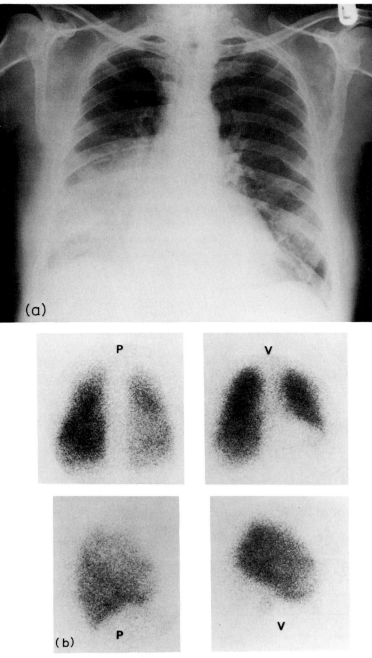

Fig. 7.10 Patient with pneumonia showing perfusion less impaired than ventilation.

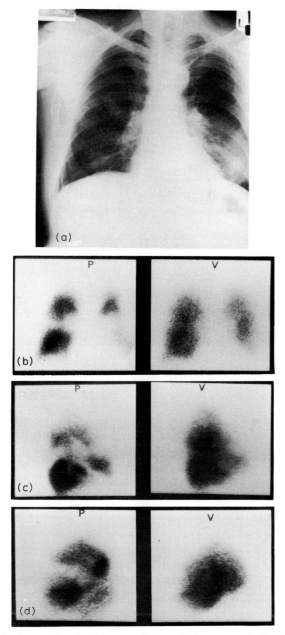

Fig. 7.11 (a) Patient with mixed lung pathology (infarct + embolus in right middle zone; pneumonia left lower zone). Scans show impaired perfusion with slightly abnormal ventilation in the right lung (infarct + embolus). However, ventilation is absent in the left lower lobe (b) where some perfusion is still present (pneumonia).

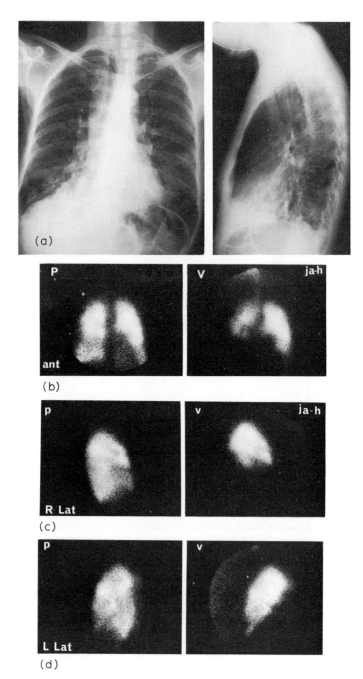

Fig. 7.12 Partial collapse of right and left lower lobes. Perfusion is still preserved while ventilation is absent. (Reproduced from *Recent Advances in Radiology* T. Lodge and R. E. Steiner.)

(d) Chronic airways disease

In patients with chronic airways disease, predominantly of the emphysematous type (diffuse emphysema), both perfusion and ventilation show multiple, patchy areas of reduced or absent activity, the ventilation scans showing a pattern similar to that of perfusion down to the finest structural level resolved by the γ-camera. In contrast to the lung scan, only diffuse abnormalities rather than regional alterations are usually seen in these patients on the chest radiograph, the typical picture being that of large volume lungs with low diaphragms and overall reduction of the vascular markings. In bullous emphysema, the areas of reduced activity on the scans usually correspond to the bullae seen on the chest radiograph, but additional defects, presumably due to focal emphysema, can be present.

Ventilation/perfusion scans can be particularly useful when pulmonary embolism is suspected in patients with chronic airways disease; it is often difficult from the perfusion scan alone to separate areas of reduced or absent perfusion due to parenchymal lung disease from perfusion defects due to pulmonary emboli (Fig. 7.13). A correct diagnosis can usually be obtained with an ^{81m}Kr/^{99m}Tc ventilation /perfusion scan while alternative methods for ventilation scanning can be inadequate. These patients can be ill and cannot hold their breath long enough to perform the ^{133}Xe-single breath inhalation procedure. Only one view can routinely be obtained with this method, which reduces the chances of detecting ventilation/perfusion mismatching.

Aerosol techniques can provide a satisfactory measurement of regional ventilation in patients free from airways disease, as previously mentioned (p. 178). In the presence of airways obstruction, however, there is a significant deposition of the inhaled particles in central airways, probably due to impaction of particles in stenotic airways with turbulent airflow regimen (Fig. 7.3). When particles with a mass median diameter between 1.0 and 1.5 μm are used, a reasonably good peripheral distribution of the tracer can be obtained in patients with FEV_1 more than 50% of the predicted value.

Using smaller particles a better peripheral penetration of the aerosol might be achieved even in patients with severe airways obstruction. This might be the alternative solution for ventilation scanning when ^{81m}Kr is not available.

7.5.4 Bronchogenic carcinoma

In peripheral tumours, ventilation and perfusion are usually absent in correspondence with the mass seen on the chest film. Similar findings are observed in the case of pulmonary metastases.

In central tumours, however, both perfusion and ventilation are often grossly reduced to the side affected by the tumour, to an extent unpredictable from the chest radiograph. The finding of absent ventilation and perfusion to the affected side is not uncommon (Fig. 7.14). Ventilation is often less impaired than perfusion, probably because the impairment of perfusion is at least in part due to involvement of pulmonary vessels, particularly low pressure pulmonary veins. These alterations of regional ventilation and perfusion can, in part, be relieved by radiotherapy, unlike tests of overall lung function like FEV_1 and FVC [27]

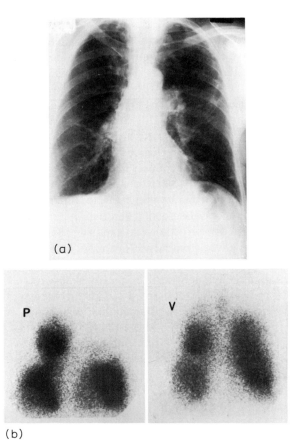

(a)

P   V

(b)

Fig. 7.13 Mixed pathology patient with scar and parenchymal disease in the middle and right lung (both ventilation and perfusion impaired) and pulmonary embolus at the left apex (perfusion absent, ventilation normal). (Reproduced from *Recent Advances in Radiology*, eds T. Lodge and R. E. Steiner.)

7.5.5 Heart disease

Patients with long-standing left heart disease show a variable degree of redistribution of regional pulmonary blood flow toward the apices [18]. The lateral views of the lung scan show that blood flow appears in these patients to be shifted not only toward the apices, but also toward the anterior regions of the lung. In particular, whereas in normal sitting subjects the main bulk of perfusion is in the lower lobes, in patients with heart disease it can be predominant in the anterior segments of the upper lobes. These changes of the regional distribution of pulmonary perfusion are due to several mechanisms. Blood flow redistribution can be induced by mechanical compression from an enlarged heart. Patients with cardiomegaly show markedly reduced perfusion to the lung bases on the anterior (and sometimes on the posterior) view, although, in the lateral views, perfusion to the costophrenic angles is usually preserved. In fact, redistribution of blood flow *per unit of lung volume*, is largely due to factors other than heart compression, such as the increase in left atrial pressure and the increase in pulmonary vascular resistances. Together with a redistribution of perfusion, some redistribution toward the apices of regional ventilation has also been observed in patients with left heart valvular disease [28].

A practical application of lung scanning in patients with heart disease is the qualitative detection of right-to-left shunts in congenital heart disease. Care should be taken, in this case, to administer not more than 50 000–100 000 particles. Presence of activity over the kidneys is indicative of right-to-left shunt whilst activity over liver and spleen usually indicates presence of free pertechnetate ($^{99m}Tc–O_4^-$) due to a suboptimal labelling of the albumin particles. Quantitative techniques have also been proposed to evaluate the fraction of blood shunted from the right to the left heart, but these are, as yet, still rather cumbersome and inaccurate.

Apart from shunt detection, ventilation perfusion scanning can be valuable in patients with congenital heart disease, for the non-invasive assessment of the congenital abnormality; for instance, children with congenital absence of a pulmonary artery show lack of perfusion and normal ventilation on the affected side.

7.6 The value of lung ventilation/perfusion scanning

In a radiology department, the chest radiograph constitutes about one-third of the work load. This is, in part, due to prevalence of pulmonary and cardiac disease and also to the large amount of information present in the standard chest film. However, this information is primarily anatomic rather than functional, as the chest radiograph essentially detects increased or reduced density of lung structures. Lung scanning provides now an accurate

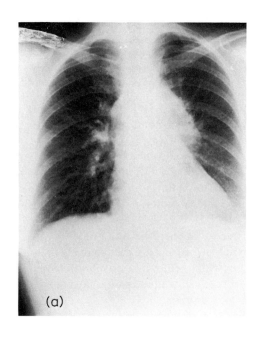

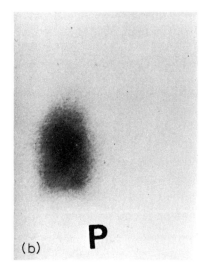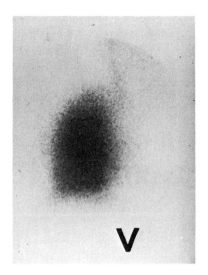

(b)   P   V

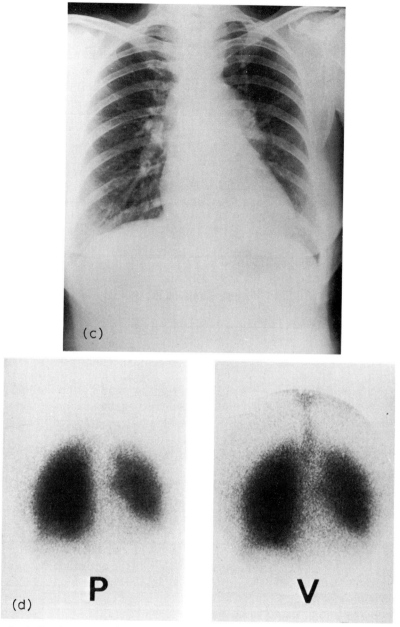

Fig. 7.14 Carcinoma of the main left bronchus (a, b). Perfusion and ventilation are absent in the right lung despite the persistence of vascular markings on the radiograph. Following radiotherapy, the radiograph is virtually unchanged (c) but perfusion-ventilation scans show clear improvement to the left-lung (d).

means to assess regional lung function, in particular regional perfusion and ventilation; despite the claim that inferences concerning regional lung perfusion and ventilation can be derived from consideration of the size and distribution of pulmonary vessels and changes in lung parenchyma, there is now experimental evidence that the degree to which regional perfusion and ventilation are impaired is difficult to predict from the chest radiograph [2].

Regional function can be impaired with and without the presence of structural abnormalities seen on the chest radiograph. Therefore, a lung scan should never be interpreted without the corresponding chest radiograph, which should be taken *on the same day as the scan*. The combination of these two techniques provides a powerful diagnostic tool for differential diagnosis. By adding a lung ventilation/perfusion scan to the routine chest radiograph, it is possible to separate acute vascular (pulmonary embolism) from bronchial (acute bronchitis, asthma) disease, to assess whether the radiological finding of a consolidated lung is due to pneumonia or to infarction, and accurately to describe the pathological processes at work in patients with mixed pathologies.

However, diagnosing disease is not the only aim of lung ventilation/perfusion scanning. On occasions, lung scans can be useful to attract attention to a particular lesion on the chest radiograph or to localize a lesion exactly; it should be remembered that lung scanning allows one separately to study both right and left lung in multiple views, which cannot be obtained with standard radiology. Another important application of lung scanning is the staging and follow-up of lung disease. A functional evaluation of the patient's condition is nowadays as important as knowing the pathological and anatomical nature of the disease. The functional evaluation of patients with chest diseases rests on tests of overall and regional lung function.

Spirometric measurements (for the assessment of overall function) and lung scanning techniques (for assessing regional function) are not in competition but complementary. Spirometry can be impaired in the presence of normal perfusion/ventilation scans, as these provide a qualitative assessment of relative differences of ventilation and perfusion between lung regions, rather than absolute quantitative measurements of ventilation and perfusion. On the other hand, tests of overall lung function may be relatively insensitive to detect small changes in function and are by definition incapable of detecting regional differences. With lung perfusion and ventilation scanning one can have a visual insight into the lungs, which can uncover alterations not predictable from radiological or spirometric measurements.

Follow-up lung scan can be very useful in lung disease, to assess if a treatment is effective or whether a patient is steady, improving or deteriorating.

To this aim, it is important to obtain both perfusion and ventilation scans, although a great deal of information can also be provided by the perfusion scan alone. Perfusion scanning with ^{99m}Tc-macroaggregates or microspheres is now routinely available in any hospital with nuclear medicine facilities. As far as ventilation scanning is concerned, ^{133}Xe is still widely used in the United States, although this tracer is admittedly inadequate. ^{81m}Kr would probably be the agent of choice but its availability is, as yet, limited. Aerosol ventilation scanning with ^{113m}In is very promising and warrants further consideration.

7.7 Future developments

Future developments of lung scanning rest on the development of new recording devices for improving spatial resolution and of new radiopharmaceuticals for functional studies.

Although in the last ten years rectilinear scanners have been virtually replaced by γ-cameras, conventional γ-cameras are not likely to be the ultimate instrument for radionuclide imaging. This is because both scanners and gamma cameras provide an image in two dimensions of a tridimensional distribution of a radionuclide (as a standard chest radiograph provides a bidimensional image of a tridimensional distribution of densities). Thus, however good the resolution* in the frontal plane, the resolution in the plane perpendicular to the detector will be very poor, being of the order of magnitude of the object thickness.

This concept can be explained with an example. Consider external recording of lung activity following inhalation of a radioactive gas using a γ-camera with a spatial resolution (in the frontal plane) of 0.5 cm. Suppose the recording is obtained in the anterior view (e.g. with the γ-camera positioned in front of the patient's chest). The image obtained (provided the statistics of radioactive counting are good) will have a spatial resolution in the frontal plane of 0.5 cm. This means that two small areas of different radioactivity 0.5 cm apart or more *in the frontal plane* will be seen as different. However, *each of the two areas could be anywhere in the anteroposterior plane*, where the resolution of our measurement will be more than 15 cm, for a chest thickness of 20 cm.

In order to overcome this problem, images are, in nuclear medicine procedures, currently taken in multiple views and it is then left to the reporting physician's brain mentally to reconstruct a tridimensional distribution of activity from a series of images in two dimensions taken from different angles.

A more direct approach is that of building a device for obtaining images in three dimensions of the distribution of radioactivity within the body. This can now be achieved by a new technical development called emission

---

* Resolution: the smallest distance apart at which two radioactive point sources can be separated by an imaging device.

computerized tomography, which differs from transmission computerized tomography (known as CAT-scanning) in that the radiation source is internal (rather than external) to the body.

Different instruments have been devised for obtaining tomographic images of the *in vivo* distribution of radioactive isotopes. These can generally be divided into two categories: tomographs for counting isotopes emitting positrons and tomographs for counting isotopes emitting single γ-photons. Both approaches have advantages and disadvantages [29]. From a technical standpoint, systems for counting positrons are more accurate. A positron is a positively charged β-particle which annihilates on interacting with an electron, emitting two 511 keV photons in opposite directions. These can be detected by coincidence circuits which, relative to conventional circuits for counting single γ-rays, are more accurate for localizing where a radioactive event has originated. The major advantage of counting positrons is that the most suitable biological tracers are positron emitters (^{15}O, ^{11}C, ^{13}N, ^{18}F, etc.). Recent advances in radiopharmaceutical science have made it possible to label, with these isotopes, a number of biological compounds (Table 7.1) (aminoacids, hormones, polysaccharides, mediators and drugs). The major disadvantage of positron-emitting isotopes is that, due to their very short half-life (minutes), they require the presence of a cyclotron on site plus a purpose-built tomograph which would make positron emission tomography only available in a few highly specialized research centres.

Single photon emission tomography can be obtained with a γ-camera mounted on a gantry which allows a 360° rotation around the patient (180° if a two-headed system is used). During the rotation, data are recorded on a digital computer and then reconstructed in both transaxial and longitudinal

Table 7.1 Positron emitting radiopharmaceuticals available from a medical cyclotron

---

$^{15}O_2$, $C^{15}O_2$, $H_2^{15}O$, $C^{15}O$

$^{13}N_2$, $^{13}NH_3$, ^{13}N-alanine, ^{13}N-glutamine, ^{13}N-asparagine, ^{13}N-valine, ^{13}N-leucine, ^{13}N-glutamate

^{18}F-phenylalanine, ^{18}F-tryptophan, ^{18}F-tyrosine, ^{18}F-oestradiol, ^{18}F-haloperidol, ^{18}F-DL DOPA, ^{18}F-deoxyglucose

^{11}CO, ^{11}C-RBC, ^{11}C-glucose, ^{11}C-fructose, ^{11}C-galactose, ^{11}C-glycerol, ^{11}C-mannitol, ^{11}C-palmitate, ^{11}C-Acetate, ^{11}C-Oxaloacetate, ^{11}C-Citric Acid, ^{11}C-Tryptophan, ^{11}C-Valine, ^{11}C-Phenylalanine, ^{11}C-thymidine, ^{11}C-acetyl phosphate, ^{11}C-acetyl CoA, ^{11}C-DL DOPA ^{11}C-chlorpromazine, ^{11}C-thioproperazine, ^{11}C-imipramine, ^{11}C-diazepam, ^{11}C-caffeine

---

sections. The cost of a rotating γ-camera is only slightly higher than the cost of an ordinary γ-camera with dedicated computer. This could also be used in the bidimensional mode. It is therefore possible that these instruments will have a wide use in the future. Single photon emission tomography has the advantage that readily available isotopes (such as ^{99m}Tc, ^{81m}Kr, ^{113m}In, ^{123}I, etc.) can be used, thus avoiding the need for a cyclotron on site. With these isotopes it is only possible, at present, to obtain tomographic reconstructions of the distribution of regional ventilation and perfusion. However, it is conceivable that further developments in radiochemistry will provide means of using these more available isotopes for labelling drugs and biological markers of organ function and metabolism. The association of new tracers with computerized emission tomography could provide, in the not too distant future, a non-invasive, quantitative, tridimensional assessment of a number of functions and metabolic processes of the lungs and other organs.

Further Reading

Fazio, F., Lavender, J. P. and Steiner, R. E. (1978), Radioisotopes, chest radiology and lung physiology. *J. belge Radiol.* **61**, 219–28.

Giuntini, C. *et al.* (1974). Factors affecting regional pulmonary blood flow in left heart valvular disease. *Am. J. Med.* **57**, 421–36.

Lavender, J. P., Irving, H., Fazio, F. and Jones T. Radioisotope lung scanning using Krypton-81m in acute respiratory disease. *Am. J. Roentg.* (submitted for publication).

Taplin, G. V., Johnson, D. E., Dore, E. K. and Kaplan, H. S. (1964), Lung photoscans with macroaggregates of human serum radioalbumin. *Hlth. Phys.*, **10**, 1219–27.

References

1. Simon, G. (1973), The plain radiograph in relation to lung physiology. *Radiol. Clinics N. Am.*, **11**, 3–16.
2. Fazio, F., Lavender, J. P. and Steiner, R. E. (1978), ^{81m}Kr ventilation and ^{99m}Tc perfusion scans in chest disease: comparison with standard radiographs. *Am. J. Roentg.*, **130**, 421–8.
3. Knipping, H. W. *et al.* (1955), Eine neue Methode zur Prüfung der Herz-und Lungen-funktion: die regionale Funktionsanalyse in der Lunger- und Herzklinik mit Hilfe des radioaktiven Edelgases xenon-133 (Isotopen-Thorakographie). *Dt. med. Wschr.*, **80**, 1146–7.
4. Ball, W. C. Jr., Stewart, P. B., Newsham, L. G. S. and Bates, D. V. (1962), Regional pulmonary function studied with Xenon^{133}. *J. clin. Invest.* **41**, 519–31.
5. Secker-Walker, R. H. *et al.* (1975), The measurement of regional ventilation during tidal breathing: a comparison of two methods in healthy subjects, and patients with chronic obstructive lung disease. *Br. J. Radiol.* **48**, 181–9.

6. Taplin, G. V., Poe, N. D. and Greenberg, A. (1966), Lung scanning following radioaerosol inhalation. *J. nucl. Med.* **7**, 77–87.
7. Wagner, H. N. Jr. *et al.* (1964), Regional pulmonary blood flow in man by radioisotope scanning. *J. Am. med. Ass.*, **187**, 601–3.
8. Quinn, J. L. III, Whitley, J. E., Hudspeth, A. S. and Prichard, R. W. (1964), Early clinical applications of lung scintiscanning. *Radiology*, **82**, 315–17.
9. Loken, M. K., Westgate, H. D. (1968), Using Xenon-133 and a scintillation camera to evaluate pulmonary function. *J. nucl. Med.*, **9**, 45–50.
10. Newhouse, M. T., Wright, F. J. and Ingham, G. K. (1968), Use of scintillation camera and [135]Xenon for study of topographic pulmonary function. *Resp. Physiol.* **4**, 141–53.
11. Goddard, B. A. and Ackery, D. M. (1975), Xenon-133, [127]Xe and [125]Xe for lung function investigations: a dosimetric comparison. *J. nucl. Med.*, **16**, 780–6.
12. Fazio, F. and Jones, T. (1975), Assessment of regional ventilation by continuous inhalation of radioactive Krypton-81m. *Br. med. J.*, **3**, 673–6.
13. Goris, M. L. *et al.* (1977), Applications of ventilation lung imaging with [81m]Krypton. *Radiology*, **122**, 399–403.
14. Clark, J. C., Horlock, P. L. and Watson, I. A. (1976), Krypton-81m generators. *Radiochem. radioanalyt. Letters*, **25**, 245–54.
15. Taplin, G. V. and Chopra, S. K. (1978), Lung perfusion-inhalation scintigraphy in obstructive airway disease and pulmonary embolism. *Radiol. Clinics N. Am.*, **16**, 491–513.
16. Fazio, F. *et al.* (1978), Lung imaging following inhalation of ^{99m}Tc-labelled microspheres: a comparison with the [81m]Kr ventilation technique. In: *Clinical and Experimental Applications of Krypton-81m* (ed. J. P. Lavender) British Journal of Radiology, Special Report No. 15, Ch. 17, pp. 130–140.
17. Muir, D. C. F. (1972), Deposition and clearance of inhaled particles. In: *Clinical Aspects of Inhaled Particles*, William Heinemann Medical Books Limited, London, Ch. 1, pp. 1–20.
18. West, J. B. (1977), *Regional Differences in the Lung* (ed. J. B. West), Academic Press, New York, San Francisco, London.
19. Moser, K. M. (1977), Pulmonary embolism. *Am. Rev. resp. Dis.*, **115**, 829–52.
20. Dalen, J. E. *et al.* (1966), Pulmonary angiography in experimental pulmonary embolism. *Am. Heart J.*, **72**, 509–20.
21. Greenspan, R. H. (1974), Does a normal isotope perfusion scan exclude pulmonary embolism? *Invest. Radiol.*, **9**, 44–6.
22. McNeil, B. J. (1976), A diagnostic strategy using ventilation-perfusion studies in patients suspect for pulmonary embolism. *J. nucl. Med.* **17**, 613–6.
23. Secker-Walker, R. H., Jackson, J. A. and Goodwin, J. (1970), Resolution of pulmonary embolism. *Br. med. J.*, **4**, 135–9.
24. Ahmad, M. *et al.* (1979), Radionuclide venography and lung scanning: concise communication. *J. nucl. Med.*, **20**, 291–3.
25. Fazio, F. *et al.* (1979) Studies of regional ventilation in asthma using [81m]Kr. *Lung*, **156**, 185–94.
26. Von Euler, U. S. and Liljestrand, G. (1946), Observations on the pulmonary arterial blood pressure in the cat. *Acta physiol. Scand.*, **12**, 301–20.

27. Fazio, F., Pratt, T. A., McKenzie, C. G. and Steiner, R. E. (1979), Improvement in regional ventilation and perfusion after radiotherapy for unresectable carcinoma of the bronchus. *Am. J. Roentg.*, **133**, 191–200.
28. Fazio, F. *et al.* (1979), Regional lung ventilation and perfusion in patients with left heart valvular disease. In: *Cardiac Lung*, (eds. C. Giuntini and P. Panuccio) Piccin, Padova, pp. 85–96.
29. Phelps, M. E. (1977), Emission computed tomography. *Sem. nucl. Med.* **7**, 337–65.

Acknowledgements

I wish to thank the whole staff of the MRC Cyclotron Unit for constant co-operation through the years and particularly for the development and supply of ^{81m}Kr generators. Amongst my colleagues, I acknowledge especially the active, positive support and co-operation of Dr J. P. Lavender in the Department of Radiology, where most of the scans shown in this review were obtained. I would also like to express here my strong feelings of gratitude to Mr T. Jones of the MRC Cyclotron Unit for his stimulating friendship. In addition, I thank Dr J. M. B. Hughes of the Department of Medicine for his support throughout the years and Mr Tim Pratt and Mrs M. M. Barr for their dedicated skill. Mrs H. Creed typed the manuscript.

CHAPTER EIGHT

Biochemistry

D. M. Geddes

Until recently non-respiratory functions of the lung have attracted little attention. This has been partly because of the overwhelming importance of gas exchange but also because the metabolic and biochemical properties of the lung are particularly difficult to study.

There are two fundamental problems: firstly, the lung is made up of over forty different cell types and so studies on lung slices or homgenates are difficult to interpret; secondly, the lung receives the whole cardiac output and so only gross metabolic changes can be detected by measuring arterio-venous differences. This approach is further complicated by the separate bronchial circulation.

Over the past ten years these problems have been largely overcome by the development of techniques for isolating single cell types and the use of isolated lung preparations. As a result, a mass of information on the biochemical and metabolic functions of the normal lung has accumulated.

This knowledge has led to a better understanding of the pathogenesis of many lung diseases but has not yet found much application in routine clinical practice. It is, however, inevitable that further work on lung metabolism in disease will lead to advances in diagnosis, treatment, prognosis and screening. This chapter is therefore intended to draw attention to a fast developing field of research in pulmonary medicine which will undoubtedly play a useful role in investigation in the future. A number of comprehensive reviews [1–4] of lung metabolism and biochemistry have recently appeared; only those aspects which are obviously relevant to human disease are discussed here.

8.1 Surfactant [5, 6]

The alveoli and terminal bronchioles are coated by an alveolar lining layer. This surfactant layer prevents alveolar collapse by keeping the surface tension very low. The surfactant film is composed of lipids with a small quantity of protein and carbohydrate and is separated from alveolar cells by the hypophase, a thin aqueous layer containing mucopolysaccharides. Within the surfactant layer there are lamellar structures called 'tubular myelin'.

These probably represent material recently ejected from the lamellar bodies of the type II alveolar cells. Surfactant can be obtained by lavage or isolated from type II cells. Its constituents are listed in Table 8.1.

Table 8.1   Surfactant constituents

Dipalmitoyl phosphatidyl choline (DPPC)	50%
Monoenoic phosphatidyl cholines	20%
Phosphatidyl ethanolamine	10%
Phosphatidyl glycerol	<10%
Cholesterol	<10%
Sphingomyelin	<10%
Non-serum protein	<10%

The most important constituent both in quantity and in surface activity is DPPC which can lower alveolar interfacial surface tension to < 10 dynes/cm. The other lipids may influence the rate of absorption of the film to the interface and may increase molecular mobility within the film. The proteins appear to be specific for surfactant and may have a structural role.

As alveoli enlarge during inspiration the surface film becomes spread more thinly and surface tension increases. During expiration surfactant coalesces and this reduces surface tension and prevents alveolar collapse. A part of alveolar enlargement is by uncrumpling and surfactant may also act as an antiglue allowing two opposed surfaces to separate easily [7].

8.1.1 Synthesis

The formation of surfactant has been studied by supplying labelled precursors to the lung and following their progress radiographically. The radioactivity appears first in the rough endoplasmic reticulium of the type II alveolar cells and then moves via the Golgi apparatus to the lamellar bodies. These bodies store the surfactant before it is released onto the alveolar surface. Some synthesis may also take place in the Clara cells of the bronchioles. DPPC is synthesized from fatty acid, triose phosphate and choline. The fatty acids come from three sources: plasma, intracellular synthesis and intracellular triglyceride breakdown. The triose phosphate is derived from glucose. Choline is preformed and then incorporated by the CDP-choline pathway; a little DPPC may be synthesized by serial methylation of phosphatidyl ethanolamine. A number of synthetic pathways exist but the relative importance of each is uncertain; for detailed review see Mason [8]. Factors controlling surfactant synthesis are not known although secretion of surfactant into the alveoli is increased by pilocarpine (blocked by atropine) and isoprenaline (blocked by propanolol). Neurohumoral control of secretion is further suggested by the presence of nerve endings close to the type II cells which resemble those found in some endocrine organs.

8.1.2 Clearance

The site of breakdown of surfactant is unknown. The best hypothesis is that alveolar macrophages engulf old surfactant which is then broken down by phospholipase A. Other possibilities are *in situ* degradation, transepithelial absorption, and loss by mucociliary clearance. The half-life of DPPC in the lung is about fourteen hours.

8.1.3 Maturation

Shortly before term a number of enzymes involved in DPPC synthesis increases in the lung. At the same time the production of DPPC increases rapidly. This process can be accelerated by corticosteroids and the fetal lung is singularly rich in cortoid receptors which suggests that steroids have an important physiological role. Surfactant from premature infants is low in DPPC and has relatively more C_{18} (oleic) and C_{20} (arachidonic) phosphatidyl cholines than mature surfactant [9].

8.1.4 Surfactant and lung disease

(*a*) *Neonatal respiratory distress syndrome*

This syndrome affects dysmature neonates and is probably due to a deficiency of surfactant. Surface tension is therefore high in a number of alveoli and many of these collapse. The result is patchy atelectasis visible on chest radiograph with increased shunting of mixed venous blood. Not only is the surfactant deficient in quantity but it also contains relatively less DPPC than mature surfactant and so its surface activity is less. Within the collapsed alveoli a hyaline membrane with a high muco-polysaccharide content is formed.

Treatment is by artificial ventilation using positive and expiratory pressure to prevent alveolar collapse. Attempts at surfactant replacement using aerosols of DPPC have been unsuccessful to date. However, lung washes from adults can successfully treat the respiratory distress syndrome in rabbits and this is a promising line of future research. Neonatal lung immaturity can be detected and predicted by analysis of fluids for surface activity. Before term, amniotic fluid is used while after delivery gastrin aspirates can be analysed. Two tests have been developed: the lecithin: sphingomyelin

ratio [10] and the shake test [11]. In the former, sphingomyelin and saturated phospholipid are extracted and assayed by chromatography. When
the fetus is mature and lecithin production adequate the ratio varies from 2
to 10. When the ratio is below 2 there is relative lack of lecithin and this
implies immaturity and a risk of development of fetal distress. The shake
test is simpler but less precise. The amniotic or gastric fluid is diluted with
ethanol and shaken, a stable foam implies the presence of surface active
lipids and correlates well with fetal maturity and the lecithin:sphingomyelin
ratio.

(b) Adult respiratory distress syndrome

A wide variety of pulmonary insults can result in non-cardiogenic pulmonary oedema and surfactant deficiency may often be a contributory factor.
Hyperoxia, volatile anaesthetics, cigarette smoking and hypercarbia may all
alter surfactant production. Pulmonary artery occlusion elevates the surface
tension of the lung and so pulmonary embolism is likely to lead to local
abnormalities of surfactant. Atelectasis itself may interfere with surfactant
production and this may be prevented by mechanical inflation. Finally,
pulmonary oedema fluid may lead to a loss of surfactant from the alveoli as
well as contamination of the surface active layer by plasma lipids. All these
events will tend to increase the surface tension of the alveolar air interfaces
so favouring the development of pulmonary oedema and alveolar collapse.
The pulmonary oedema which occasionally develops with rapid reinflation
of a collapsed lung following drainage of a pleural effusion or chronic
pneumothorax may be due to surfactant deficiency.

(c) Alveolar proteinosis

Lavage fluid from patients with this disease contains large amounts of lipids,
chiefly lecithins. Interestingly, although the DPCC content is high, the
surface activity is less than in normal surfactant. The pathogenesis of alveolar proteinosis is unknown but the hypothesis of an abnormality of surfactant production either in quantity or quality is attractive.

8.2 The pulmonary circulation

The whole cardiac output passes through the lungs and is in contact with
70 m^2 of capillary endothelium. The endothelial cells are metabolically
active and so a number of circulating substances are altered during passage
through the pulmonary circulation. There are basically three mechanisms:

1. Intraluminal metabolism by endothelial cell surface enzymes.

2. Uptake with subsequent intracellular metabolism.
3. Uptake by endothelial cells without metabolism.

These properties and the substances affected are summarized in Table 8.2.

Table 8.2 The effect of the lungs on circulating substances

1. *Intraluminal metabolism*
   Bradykinin $\longrightarrow$ Inactive fragments
   Angiotensin I $\longrightarrow$ Angiotensin II + fragments
   ? Insulin
   ? Gastrin $\longrightarrow$ Reduction in immunoreactive levels
   ? Glucagon

2. *Endothelial cell uptake and metabolism*
   5-Hydroxytryptamine
   Noradrenaline
   Prostaglandins E, F
   ? Dopamine

3. *Endothelial cell uptake without metabolism*
   Basic lipophilic amines (see Table 8.3)

8.2.1 Possible clinical implications

Clinical relevance has been established for only a few of these properties of the pulmonary circulation. The following summary includes current areas of active research, the importance of which has yet to be established.

(a) Blood pressure control

Angiotensin II, a potent vasoconstrictor is formed in the lung while bradykinin, a potent vasodilator, is inactivated. Other vasodilators, e.g. 5-hydroxytryptamine (5-HT) and prostaglandin E (PGE) are also inactivated. Although these changes also occur in other capillary beds, the lung is unique in three respects. Firstly, it is situated immediately upstream of the high pressure systemic circulation in an ideal site to modify levels of vasoactive substances; secondly, the lung receives the whole cardiac output and finally in contrast to other capillary beds the pulmonary circulation does not inactivate angiotensin II. While these factors suggest a real role for the lung in blood pressure control the fact that blood pressure is maintained during cardiopulmonary bypass indicates that the lung is not essential.

Recent evidence suggests that the renin-angiotensin system modifies blood flow to different organs and to different parts of the same organ. This raises interesting possibilities about the role of the system in hypoxic pulmonary vasoconstriction.

(b) Tests of pulmonary capillary damage

A predictor for the development of shock lung or pulmonary oxygen toxicity would be valuable in clinical practice. 5-HT uptake by the lung diminishes as a result of hyperoxia in the rat [12] and this may form the basis of a clinical test of endothelial cell function in the future.

(c) Pulmonary hypertension

Little is known about the pathogenesis of primary pulmonary hypertension in man although there are some suggestions that pulmonary concentration of a circulating substance may be important. There is an association between pulmonary hypertension in young women and the ingestion of appetite suppressants and so the pulmonary concentration of dextroamphetamine and chlorphentermine in rats may therefore indicate an important pathogenic mechanism. Similarly, the association of severe liver damage with pulmonary hypertension led to the idea that some substance which is normally inactivated by the liver is able to reach the lungs in liver disease, lodging there and causing hypertension.

8.3 Drug disposition and metabolism

Many drugs accumulate in the lungs following oral or intravenous administration (see Table 8.3) [13]. Some compounds are taken up into endothelial cells by active transport mechanisms (e.g. imipramine) while others appear to bind non-specifically to endothelial cell membranes as a result of their physicochemical properties. The majority of the latter are basic lipophilic

Table 8.3 Drug accumulation in the lungs (for full list see [13])

Chlorpromazine
Dextroamphetamine
Imipramine
Lignocaine
Mepacrine
Methadone
Morphine
Propranolol

amines (e.g. propranolol, chlorpromazine). Lung uptake occurs rapidly and is probably complete within a few circulations after intravenous drug administration. Following uptake some compounds are metabolized (5-HT, impramine) while others return to the circulation unchanged to be metabolized and excreted by the liver or kidney (e.g. propranolol).

The lung also contains many drug metabolizing enzymes. Most of these are present in much larger quantities in the liver, but some enzymes are present in the lung and liver in comparable quantities and others are present in the lung in a slightly different form from that found in the liver. The overall contribution of the lung to drug metabolism is therefore small but may be significant in certain specific instances. Inhaled drugs encounter the lungs before the gut or liver and so initial metabolism depends on pulmonary enzymes, e.g. the circulating metabolites of salbutamol are different when the drug is inhaled as compared with oral ingestion.

8.3.1 Clinical implications

The accumulation of drugs in the lung is probably an important factor in causing local drug toxicity (see Chapter 16). Many compounds can produce pulmonary fibrosis following chronic administration (e.g. busulphan, bleomycin). Paraquat accumulates in the lung and causes tissue damage by local production of superoxide radicles. Bleomycin toxicity is unusual as it is due to unusually slow clearance of drug from the lung as compared with other tissues which therefore causes tissue damage because of persistence rather than concentration. Since lung uptake is relatively non-specific it may be possible to limit the toxicity of one drug by prior administration of another which shares the same mechanism of lung uptake. This approach has been used in paraquat poisoning when *d*-propranolol has been given in an attempt to reduce lung levels of paraquat.

8.4 Carcinogen metabolism [14]

Many of the chemicals in tobacco smoke need to be metabolized by host tissues before they are able to cause cancer.

Benzo-(*a*)-pyrene (B(*a*)P) is a potent carcinogen of this sort present in cigarette smoke and is also produced by burning of fossil fuels; its metabolism by human lung has been well studied and is summarized in Fig. 8.1. This metabolism is important in its own right but has attracted special interest since differences between individuals in their capacity to metabolize the carcinogen might result in marked differences in their susceptibility to smoking-induced lung cancer. A smoker who is able to metabolize B(*a*)P only slowly or who preferentially produces non-carcinogenic metabolites might be expected to be at low risk of the disease. Another individual with the ability to metabolize B(*a*)P actively and especially to the 7–8 diol metabolite might be particularly susceptible. This theory is attractive since it might help to explain why nine out of ten heavy smokers do not get lung cancer and why the disease tends to run in families independently of smoking habits.

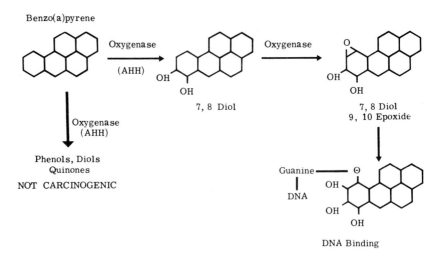

Fig. 8.1

Attempts at identifying metabolic differences between individuals for carcinogen metabolism have used two approaches: measurements of levels of enzymes involved in the metabolic pathway, and measurements of binding of carcinogen to DNA.

8.4.1 Enzymes

Aryl hydrocarbon hydroxylase (AHH) is the enzyme system responsible for much of the metabolism of B(*a*)P and forms part of the microsomal mixed function oxygenases which use cytochrome P450 for electron transport. Some early studies showed a high inducibility of AHH in the lymphocytes of patients with lung cancer as compared with controls and suggested a simple genetic basis of increased susceptibility to lung cancer. Unfortunately, these promising results have been discounted [15]. The techniques used in these studies are difficult and tend to give unreproducible results especially when measurements are made in lymphocytes. More promising work is proceeding using circulating monocytes or alveolar macrophages obtained by lavage.

8.4.2 DNA binding

The binding of a carcinogen to DNA correlates well with its carcinogenicity in many animal systems. It is likely that the resulting damage to DNA or to some related macromolecule is an important event in producing malignant change. DNA binding of B(a)P to human bronchial epithelial cells has therefore been studied in tissue culture systems. Preliminary results from a large series of patients with and without lung cancer have shown a tendency for higher levels of binding to occur in patients with the disease [14]. This is consistent with an increase in susceptibility to lung cancer related to increased metabolism of B(a)P to the ultimate carcinogenic metabolite.

These results are encouraging and further large scale studies in patients are being undertaken. The goal of this work is to develop a test simple enough to be used for screening large populations of smokers in order to identify those most likely to develop cancer. These people could then be subjected to intensive antismoking propaganda and also be examined regularly to detect early disease.

8.5 Tumour markers and ectopic hormones

Small cell carcinoma of the lung originates from the neuroectodermal cells in the basal layers of the bronchial epithelium. These are a part of the APUD (Amine Precursor Uptake and Decarboxylation) cell system which is often associated with peptide synthesis and release. Oat cell cancers have been shown to release a wide range of compounds (Table 8.4) and this has led to a search for a circulating tumour marker substance. The subject has been comprehensively reviewed [16, 17].

No single tumour marker has emerged but the following are encouraging:

8.5.1 ACTH

Raised serum ACTH levels have been reported in as many as 67% of patients with lung cancer, but in many of these the hormone was probably being secreted from the pituitary in response to stress. More promising is the finding of elevated levels in 70% of patients with oat cell-cancers [16] since in many cases the ACTH molecule was larger than normal. This big ACTH is probably a precursor of the normal circulating hormone and with the development of more specific and sensitive assays it may prove a valuable marker of oat cell cancer. It is particularly interesting that smoking causes a rise in the ACTH concentrations of the lungs in dogs.

Table 8.4   Biochemical markers in lung cancer (Modified from [17])

Tumour Derived Products

Hormones:	Adrenocorticotrophin, growth hormone antidiuretic hormone, parathyroid hormone calcitonin, placental hormones and many others
Oncofetal antigens:	Carcinoembryonic antigen, α-fetoprotein, ferritin and others
Enzymes:	Sialyl transferase, galactosyl transferase, placental alkaline phosphatase
Cell turnover products:	Polyamines, nucleosides

Tumour Associated Changes

Glycoproteins, globulins, acute phase proteins
Hydroxyproline
Liver enzymes

Tumour Associated Antigens

8.5.2 Calcitonin

A large form of calcitonin has been detected in the serum of 62% of 26 men with lung cancer. This hormone is immunologically distinct from the normal monomeric circulating form. Secretion of calcitonin by oat cell tumours *in vitro* correlates with the secretion of ACTH.

8.5.3 ADH

In one report 35% of 49 patients with oat cell cancer had raised ADH levels in association with the syndrome of inappropriate ADH secretion. One limitation of this hormone is that it is secreted in response to stress and in non-malignant lung disease (see below). By itself ADH is likely to be too non-specific to be a valuable tumour marker.

8.5.4 Carcinoembryonic antigen (CEA)

Early reports of high levels in as many as 70% of patients with lung cancer have been discounted since the normal range has turned out to be wider than first thought. Many patients with non-malignant lung disease have slight elevation of serum CEA levels. If levels > 50 µg/l are considered abnormal then only 6% of lung cancer patients have raised CEA. Nevertheless there is some correlation between CEA level and tumour burden and the measurement has been used to assess operability with some success.

8.5.5 Other substances (see Table 8.5.3)

Many other circulating substances are elevated in lung cancer and there is often correlation between tumour bulk and measured level. However, none appear to be specific for lung cancer and they are not as yet sensitive enough to detect preclinical disease.

8.5.6 Conclusions

Unlike chorioncarcinomas where raised chorionic gonadotrophin levels can detect a tumour bulk as little as 10^4 cells, no marker in lung cancer approaches this sensitivity. Nevertheless, specific and sensitive assays for big hormone variants are promising. There are, however, two major limitations: first, all the progress is in oat cell cancers which make up only about a fifth of total lung cancers and second there is good evidence that metastases may not all have the same metabolic properties as the primary [18]. Thus, a marker may give information about the primary tumour but ignore a large mass of secondaries.

8.6 Emphysema [19, 20]

Excessive breakdown of lung structural protein appears to be important in the pathogenesis of emphysema. Abnormalities of proteases, antiproteases and lung protein itself have all been implicated.

8.6.1 Proteases

Proteolytic enzymes capable of degrading lung collagen and elastin are present in neutrophils, alveolar macrophages and some bacteria. The relative importance of the various enzymes is uncertain but at present neutrophil elastase holds the centre of the stage. Tobacco smoke and other irritants favour the accumulation of neutrophils in the lung as well as inducing enzyme activity and promoting enzyme release.

Studies which have attempted to associate differences in leucocyte proteases with disease have produced conflicting results. Some workers have found that low levels of enzyme appear to protect against emphysema while others have found no correlation. A qualitative difference has also been suggested since leucocyte elastase of slow electrophoretic mobility has been found in patients with chronic airflow obstruction. At present, tests of protease activity are difficult and have no place in the routine investigation of patients with emphysema.

8.6.2 Antiproteases

There are at least six serum proteins (e.g. α_1-antitrypsin, α_2-macroglobulin) which are capable of inhibiting a wide range of proteolytic enzymes. The importance of α_1-antitrypsin in emphysema is shown by the association between α_1-antitrypsin deficiency and young onset panacinar emphysema as well as by the fact that α_1-antitrypsin can prevent the development of emphysema in animals following intratracheal instillation of proteolytic enzymes. At present there is little evidence to incriminate the other antiproteases. α_1-Antitrypsin may also be important in inactivating neutrophil chemotactic factors and so limiting the accumulation of protease carrying cells. Furthermore cigarette smoke condensate suppresses its antiproteolytic activity. The α_1-antitrypsin level and activity are inherited. The phenotype of the protein is controlled by over 26 codominant alleles of which one is inherited from each parent. Each allele has been given a letter describing its electrophoretic mobility (F = fast, M = medium, S = slow, Z = immobile). An individual's phenotype is therefore designated Pi (protease inhibitor) MM, Pi MZ, Pi ZZ etc. The commonest phenotype is Pi MM which is found in 85–90% of a caucasian population. Only Pi ZZ and Pi SZ are definitely associated with disease. These phenotypes occur in less than 0.3% of the normal population. Population screening for abnormal phenotypes in order to detect pre-symptomatic emphysema does not appear to be worthwhile.

8.6.3 Structural protein

Emphysema is associated with some generalized disorders of connective tissue such as cutis laxa. Lysyl oxidase, an enzyme which forms crosslinkages between tropoelastin chains during the synthesis of elastin is deficient in some patients with primary emphysema. Study of the protease antiprotease system has shed much light on the pathogenesis of emphysema. At present this knowledge has not led to effective treatment.

8.7 Sarcoidosis

Some serum enzymes are often raised in sarcoidosis. These may be helpful in diagnosis and management.

8.7.1 Serum angiotensin converting enzyme (SACE) [21, 22]

Angiotensin converting enzyme is a carbopeptidase which splits the terminal two amino acids from angiotensin I to convert it to angiotensin II. The enzyme is situated on cell surfaces and especially on capillary endothelial cells both in the lung and elsewhere. The enzyme is also found in association with macrophages and a little exists in a free state in the serum. Because the enzyme was originally thought to come from the lungs, an investigation of SACE levels and blood pressure was carried out in patients with lung disease by Lieberman. He found an increased level of SACE in patients with sarcoidosis as compared with normal controls and patients with other lung diseases. This has since been confirmed by two large studies and these are summarized in Table 8.5. SACE levels are often raised in sarcoidosis both in acute and chronic progressive disease. The high levels are reduced by steroid therapy. The SACE is increased in sarcoid granulation and the epithelioid cell seems to be producing the enzyme which then leaks into the blood.

The clinical value of SACE in sarcoidosis is uncertain. For diagnosis a high level appears to be relatively specific for sarcoidosis and is unusual in tuberculosis. However, the differential diagnosis of sarcoidosis includes extrinsic allergic alveolitis and silicosis and no large series of SACE levels in these conditions has been reported. Since 60% of patients with sarcoidosis have normal levels, SACE is at best a very insensitive diagnostic test. A second possible use is in assessing the activity of the disease and in monitoring steroid therapy. Steroids certainly reduce SACE levels but this could be due to a direct effect on the enzyme rather than to control of the sarcoidosis.

Table 8.5 Serum angiotensin converting enzyme (SACE) in sarcoidosis [21, 22]

	n	Mean SACE	Normal range	Raised values (%)
Normal	138	33	14–52	5
Sarcoidosis	206	55		40
Active tuberculosis	62	37		8
Other chest diseases*	353	33		7
Other granulomatous diseases†	85	37		7

* Inactive tuberculosis, asthma, bronchitis, lung cancer, chronic airflow obstruction.
† Primary biliary cirrhosis, inflammatory bowel disease, leprosy, liver granuloma.

It would seem reasonable, however, to increase the steroid dose in a patient whose SACE level remains high on treatment.

8.7.2 Serum lysozyme

This is an enzyme found in monocytes and polymorphs. Serum and urinary levels are raised in a wide range of disorders which involve these cells, notably monocytic leukaemias and bacterial infections as well as in a renal failure. Serum lysozyme is also raised in sarcoidosis presumably due to an increase in the number and activity of tissue macrophages.

The diagnostic value of high lysozyme level in sarcoidosis is small. Although the test is more sensitive than SACE with as many as 70% of patients having raised levels it is much less specific, with 20% false positives which include active tuberculosis. The enzyme may be a valuable measure of disease activity and since steroids reduce the lysozyme level it may be useful in monitoring therapy. Lysozyme and SACE levels measured at the same time are likely to be more valuable than either alone.

8.8 Miscellaneous

8.8.1 Syndrome of inappropriate antidiuretic hormone (SIADH)

This is a syndrome of low serum sodium and osmolality with inappropriately high urine osmolality in the presence of normal renal and adrenal function. The syndrome has many causes but the majority of cases have central nervous system or intrathoracic disease. The commonest chest disorders are oat cell carcinoma and pneumonia, but mesothelioma and pneumothorax may also give rise to SIADH. The mechanism is by secretion of ectopic ADH in oat cell cancers and may be due to stimulation of left atrial or pulmonary venous baroreceptors with reflex release of ADH in other conditions. SIADH may respond to treatment of the underlying disease but early recovery of mental state and serum electrolytes follows oral demeclocycline up to 1.2 g daily. This drug interferes with the action of ADH on the renal tubule.

8.8.2 Lavage fluid [24]

Bronchoalveolar lavage fluid contains protein, lipids, carbohydrates and electrolytes. These have been analysed in normals as a basis for studies in disease. This is still at an experimental stage but may yield useful information. The presence of IgM may support a diagnosis of extrinsic allergic alveolitis.

8.9 Summary

There are many other aspects of lung metabolism which have not been dealt with in this chapter. For example, the biochemistry of lung collagen, elastic fibres and other connective tissue components are being actively studied, and this is leading to a greater understanding of the processes involved in pulmonary fibrosis and emphysema. Individual lung cells are being isolated and cultured and much fundamental knowledge of their metabolic properties is accumulating. This may lead to a better understanding of the way the lung reacts to damaging stimuli. In particular, the alveolar macrophage, which is easily isolated by bronchoalveolar lavage, is being extensively investigated to elucidate its protective and tissue-damaging role in infection and lung fibrosis. Much research is also being done into the formation, release and inactivation of inflammatory and allergic mediators and the area of overlap between lung metabolism and immunology and this is dealt with in Chapter 10. These topics have been omitted since this brief review is intended to highlight those areas of lung metabolism which are likely to become important in the investigation and treatment of patients with lung disease. The possible applications of this knowledge are summarized in Table 8.6.

The more fundamental research work has not yet found great clinical application. However, the study of the biochemical properties of the lung is relatively new and normal processes need to be defined and understood before extending the work into pathological abnormalities. Inevitably, these studies will throw much light on normal lung function and then on the pathogenesis of many lung diseases. When this has been done, diagnostic and therapeutic applications of an understanding of lung metabolism will naturally follow. The most likely applications will be in the development of screening tests for susceptibility to disorders such as lung cancer, emphysema, fibrosis and bronchitis with a view to prevention or early diagnosis. However, the discipline is expanding so fast, that it is difficult to predict the likely advances and their applications. Undoubtedly, lung metabolism will be one of the most active and fruitful areas of research in pulmonary medicine for the next few decades.

Table 8.6 Summary of possible clinical applications referred to in each section of text

	Surfactant	Pulmonary circulation	Drug disposition and metabolism	Carcinogen metabolism	Tumour markers	Emphysema	Sarcoidosis	Inappropriate ADH secretion
Diagnosis	Gastric aspirate shake test	? Tests of altered 5-HT metabolsim in oxygen toxicity			Lung cancer	α_1-Antitrypsin deficiency	Serum ACE and lysozyme	
Treatment	? Surface active aerosols		d-Propranolol treatment in paraquat poisoning		? Lung cancer			Demeclocycline
Screening	Amniotic fluid lecithin: Sphingomylin ratio			? Screening tests for susceptibility to lung cancer		? Protease/ antiprotease profiling		

References

1. Crystal, R. G. (1976), *The Biochemical Basis of Pulmonary Function*. Marcel Dekker, New York.
2. Bakhle, Y. S. and Vane, J. R. (1978), *The Metabolic Functions of the Lung*. Marcel Dekker, New York.
3. Hyman, A. L., Spannhake, E. W. and Kadowitz, P. J. (1978), Prostaglandins and the lung. *Am. Rev. resp. Dis.*, **117**, 111.
4. Van Golde, L. M. G. (1976), Metabolism of phospholipids in the lung. *Am. Rev. resp. Dis.*, **114**, 977.
5. Goerke, J. (1974), Lung surfactant. *Biochim. Biophys. Acta*, **344**, 241.
6. Morgan, T. E. (1971), Pulmonary surfactant. *New Engl. J. Med.*, **284**, 1185.
7. Sanderson, R. J., Paul, G. W., Vatter, A. E. and Filley, G. F. (1976), Morphological and physical basis for lung surfactant action. *Resp. Physiol.*, **27**, 379.
8. Mason, R. J. (1976), Lipid metabolism. In: *The Biochemical Basis of Pulmonary Function*. Marcel Dekker, New York, Ch. 5.
9. Shelley, S. A., Kovacevi, M., Paciga, J. E. and Balis, J. U. (1979), Sequential changes in surfactant in hyaline membrane disease. *New Engl. J. Med.*, **300**, 112.
10. Borer, R. C., Gluck, L., Freeman, R. K. and Kubovich, M. V. (1971), Prenatal prediction of the respiratory distress syndrome, *Pediat Res.*, **5**, 655.
11. Tanswell, A. K., Sherwin, E. and Smith, B. T. (1977), Single step gastric aspirate shake test. *Archs Dis. Child.*, **52**, 541.
12. Block, E. R. and Fisher, A. B. (1977), Depression of serotonin clearance by rat lungs during oxygen exposure. *J. appl. Physiol.*, **42**, 33.
13. Brandenberger Brown, E. A. (1974), The localisation, metabolism and effects of drugs and toxicants in the lung. *Drug Metab. Rev.*, **3**, 33.
14. Harris, C. C. (1978), *The Pathogenesis and Therapy of Lung Cancer*. Marcel Dekker, New York.
15. Paigen, B., Gurtoo, H. L. and Minowada, J. (1977), Questionable relation of AHH to cancer risk. *New Engl. J. Med.*, **297**, 346.
16. Rees, L. H. (1975), The biosynthesis of hormones by non-endocrine tumours – a review. *J. Endocr.*, **67**, 143.
17. Coombes, R. C., Ellison, M. L. and Neville, A. M. (1978). Biochemical markers in bronchogenic carcinoma. *Br. J. Dis. Chest*, **72**, 263.
18. Baylin, S. B., *et al.* (1978), Variable content of Histaminase, L-Dopa, Decarboxylase and Calcitonin in small cell carcinoma of the lung, *New Engl. J. Med.*, **299**, 105.
19. Morse, J. O. (1978), Alpha l-antitrypsin deficiency. *New Engl. J. Med.*, **299**, 1045, 1099.
20. Karlinsky, J. B. and Snider, G. L. (1978), Animal models of emphysema. *Am. Rev. resp. Dis.*, **117**, 1109.
21. Silverstein, E., Friedland, J., Kitt, M. and Lyons, H. A. (1977), Increased serum angiotensin converting enzyme activity in sarcoidosis. *Israel. J. med. Sci.*, **13**, 995.
22. Studdy, P., Bird, R., James, D. G. and Sherlock, S. (1978), Serum angiotensin-converting enzyme in sarcoidosis and other granulomatous disorders. *Lancet*, **ii**, 1331.

23. Turton, C. W. G. *et al.* (1979), Value of measuring serum angiotensin I converting enzyme and serum lysozyme in the management of sarcoidosis, *Thorax*, **34**, 57.

24. Low, R. B., Davis, G. S. and Giancola, M. S. (1978), Biochemical analyses of bronchoalveolar lavage fluids of healthy human volunteer smokers and non-smokers. *Am. Rev. resp. Dis.*, **118**, 863.

CHAPTER NINE

Microbiology

J. M. Grange

9.1 The changing face of clinical microbiology

Man is not an island: throughout his life he is surrounded by, and interacts with, an environment containing large numbers of micro-organisms. Over the ages, non-specific and specific immune mechanisms have developed to ensure a happy balance between man and his microbiological environment. The discipline of medical microbiology is concerned principally with this balance and the various ways in which it may be upset. Consequently, the medical microbiologist's role is not just to isolate and identify pathogenic organisms but to investigate the patient's immune responses, or lack of such responses, to invading micro-organisms.

In the early days of bacteriology, a number of organisms were recognized as causing specific diseases, e.g. diphtheria, cholera, tuberculosis and plague. This led to the formulation of Koch's well-known postulates, namely that to qualify as the aetiological agent of a disease, an organism must be regularly isolated from cases of the disease and be obtainable in pure culture, and that this culture should produce the disease in experimental animals. Subsequently it was found that potentially pathogenic bacterial species were sometimes recovered from healthy people and, conversely, that some organisms which normally exist as saprophytes in the environment, or commensals within the human body, can cause disease when given the opportunity. Such 'opportunities' include the accidental or intentional exposure of closed systems of the body to the environment or the suppression of the normal specific and non-specific immune defence mechanisms either by disease or by its treatment. In recent years the range of surgical procedures and invasive diagnostic techniques, and the use of immunosuppressive therapeutic regimens, have greatly increased and so have, therefore, the 'opportunities'. Indeed, in the hospital environment, the classical distinctions between pathogens and saprophytes have become very blurred and almost any organism may, under suitable conditions, be the cause of disease. A fatal case of endocarditis, following heart surgery, due to *Coprinus cinereus* (a common toadstool) is a typical example [1]. As a consequence, the microbiologist of the future will need to be very clinically orientated and as well versed in immunology relating to host defence as in microbiology itself.

9.2 The clinical investigation of infection

The examination of a patient suspected of having an infective agent as a cause of, or a complicating factor in, a disease process may be considered under the following headings:

1. Clinical history and examination.
2. Obtaining suitable specimens.
3. 'Bedside' examination of specimens.
4. Transport of specimens to the laboratory.
5. Demonstration of micro-organisms in specimen.
   (a) direct microscopy.
   (b) culture.
   (c) chemical or immunological methods.
6. Determination of significance of isolated organisms.
7. Determination of susceptibility or resistance of significant organisms to antimicrobial agents (where relevant).
8. Other investigations, including
   (a) radiological examinations.
   (b) histological studies on biopsies.
   (c) haematological studies.
   (d) immunological studies, which include the detection of immune responses as an aid to diagnosis and a determination of the patient's ability to respond immunologically to an infection.

Microbiological investigations play an important role in the management of infectious diseases not only by determining suitable antimicrobial agents but also by monitoring the levels of such agents in the patient to ensure destruction of the organism without exposing the patient to unnecessarily high doses of potentially toxic agents.

9.2.1 The organization of clinical microbiological services

In view of the large number of different micro-organisms which infect man, it is clearly not practical for each hospital or clinic to have facilities for the complete range of investigations. The actual services offered by each laboratory depend on the local needs as well as on financial and manpower resources. Many countries have a number of reference laboratories to which cultures and sera may be sent for specialized studies. In Great Britain this facility is provided by the Public Health Laboratory Service, which consists of a number of reference and specialist units at the Central Public Health Laboratory at Colindale, London, as well as several regional and area laboratories. The regional laboratories perform routine investigations for the diagnosis of viral infections, including viral hepatitis B and perform phage typing of *Staphylococcus aureus* for epidemiological purposes. In addition there is an extensive facility for specialized tests in the reference laboratories as listed in the directory of the Service.

In the United States of America the equivalent service is provided by the Center for Disease Control, at Atlanta, in Georgia, and its dependent laboratories. In France the various branches of the Institut Pasteur provide reference services and similar institutes are located in most other developed countries.

Many hospitals issue handbooks listing the tests performed in their laboratories, the specimen required and the usual time required for completion of the test. In addition, the staff of the microbiology department will advise on the availability of specialized investigations.

9.2.2 Clinical history and examination

Laboratory investigations are no substitute for a careful history taking and clinical examination. Certain aspects of the clinical history are of importance not only in diagnosis but in the selection of, and interpretation of, laboratory investigations. In particular, details of recent travel abroad, antibiotic therapy, vaccinations and contact with cases of infectious diseases should be obtained. A history of recent antibiotic therapy is of particular importance if serum antibiotic levels are required as the presence of even small amounts of one antibiotic may interfere with the assay of others. Details of the patient's occupation may give clues as to the infectious agent or predisposing factors. Anthrax, as a rare occupation-associated pulmonary infection should not be overlooked.

The clinical examination should include a careful search for localized or generalized lymphadenopathy and rashes. Extrapulmonary manifestation of tuberculosis should be sought. In some cases miliary tuberculosis and retinitis associated with cytomegalovirus infection may be detected by ophthalmoscopy.

Factors in the history and examination likely to dispose to opportunistic infection should be noted. These include extremes of age, recent major surgery, severe injuries or burns, inhalation of foreign bodies or toxic vapours, cytotoxic or immunosuppressive therapy and autoimmune diseases.

9.3 Specimens

The collection of specimens is the most crucial step in the microbiological examination of a patient. It is the clinician's responsibility to see that suitable specimens are obtained and transported without delay to the laboratory.

9.3.1 Anterior nasal swabs

These are used principally to detect carriers of *Staphylococcus aureus*. The tip of the swab is inserted into the anterior nares and rotated firmly against the mucosa. It is advantageous to moisten the tip of swab in sterile nutrient broth before taking the specimen.

9.3.2 Posterior nasal swabs

The nasopharynx is swabbed either pernasally or by passing a curved swab behind the soft palate. The procedure is used to obtain specimens for the isolation of *Bordetella pertussis* (whooping cough) and for the detection of meningococcal carriers. The pernasal swab is made from thin copper or nichrome wire tipped with a small piece of cotton wool wrapped tightly on the wire. The swab is passed carefully along the floor of the nasal passage and rotated gently on the posterior wall of the nasopharynx. Alternatively a flexible wire swab may be placed inside a hockey-stick shaped glass or metal tube which is passed into the mouth and behind the soft palate. The tip of the swab is then extended out of the tube into the nasopharynx.

9.3.3 Throat swabs

These are used to diagnose upper respiratory tract infection which are usually due to β-haemolytic streptococci or viruses and occasionally to Vincent's angina, candidiasis or diphtheria. The pharynx should be visualized by the use of a tongue depressor and a good light. The swab should be rubbed fairly firmly on the tonsil or posterior pharyngeal wall, particularly against any membrane or exudate. This will cause the patient to gag. Indeed if the patient does not gag, the specimen has almost certainly not been taken properly.

9.3.4 Throat washings

This is a useful alternative to the throat swab for diagnosis of viral infection. The patient is given 10 ml of phosphate buffered saline and is asked to gargle and spit the fluid into a sterile container.

9.3.5 Laryngeal swabs

Principally used to diagnose tuberculosis in patients who do not expectorate sputum. This investigation requires a clear visualization of the vocal cords and should only be attempted by clinicians trained in this technique.

9.3.6 Gastric aspiration

This procedure is also used to obtain material for the diagnosis of tuberculosis. The stomach contents are aspirated through a Ryle tube after overnight fasting and after a period of coughing and swallowing. The mycobacteria survive the gastric acidity but not indefinitely. Thus the specimen should be taken to the laboratory immediately or neutralized with sodium hydroxide. Neither laryngeal swabs or gastric aspirates are as useful as sputum, even if scanty, for the diagnosis of tuberculosis.

9.3.7 Sputum

This material is the most inconsistent of all specimens and marked variation may be observed in specimens obtained from the same patient at close intervals of time. The specimen should always be collected directly into sterile containers and this applies also to sputum for the culture of *Mycobacterium tuberculosis*. On one occasion an apparent outbreak of *M. xenopi* infection was traced to the practice of collecting sputum in pots rinsed with contaminated tap water. In non-urgent cases, early morning sputum should be obtained. It is important to make sure that the specimen really consists of sputum as some patients, in order to please their medical attendants, produce specimens liberally diluted with saliva with its complement of oral commensal organisms. It is equally important to obtain the specimen *before* administering any antibacterial agent.

9.3.8 Blood cultures

Acute bacterial pulmonary infection, notably *Streptococcus pneumoniae* (pneumococcus) infection, may be accompanied by a bacteraemia or septicaemia. Blood cultures should be taken as soon as possible. 10 ml venous blood is distributed between two blood culture bottles which usually contain about 50 ml of nutrient broth containing an anticoagulant. If the patient has been receiving penicillin or a sulphonamide the culture medium must contain penicillinase or para-aminobenzoic acid respectively to neutralize the antibacterial agent. It is recommended that blood cultures should be taken in all cases of acute pneumonia.

9.3.9 Invasive procedures

In the vast majority of circumstances the above simple procedures are, if performed properly, adequate for a microbiological investigation. Occasionally it is necessary to resort to more invasive procedures, notably in cases of suspected anaerobe or opportunist infections.

Opportunist organisms may cause generalized or localized lung lesions. As a broad generalization, *Pneumocystis carinii* and viruses tend to cause bilateral homogeneous infiltrations (interstitial pneumonias) while fungi and bacteria are more likely to give rise to unilateral or bilateral localized lesions. In many cases of opportunist infections, a positive diagnosis is only obtainable by microscopic or cultural examination of lung tissue obtained by open lung biopsy, transcutaneously (needle or trephine biopsy) or through a fibreoptic bronchoscope. These procedures are not without risk to the patient and should not be undertaken lightly. On the other hand, such procedures may enable life-saving therapy to be commenced.

Open lung biopsies offer the best chance of reaching a definite diagnosis but require major surgical procedures. Needle and trephine biopsies are simpler and less traumatic but are much less likely to yield a positive diagnosis. Fibreoptic bronchoscopy enables secretions to be aspirated and small biopsies to be taken. In addition alveolar lavage may be performed by flushing in 50 ml of sterile normal saline, prewarmed to 37°C, during inspiration and aspirating it during expiration. Any type of lung biopsy may be complicated by haemorrhage or pneumothorax. A prothrombin time and platelet count should be routinely performed on all patients prior to any invasive procedure.

Anaerobic organisms may be the cause of localized abscesses in which case aspiration of the abscess cavity is required for their diagnosis. Alternatively, the infectious process may involve the pleural cavity causing an empyaema in which case drainage has a therapeutic as well as diagnostic purpose. In the event of the abscess draining into a bronchus, the organisms will appear in the sputum.

Unfortunately, the mouth contains many commensal anaerobes so that expectorated sputum is unsuitable for culture of anaerobes. In America specimens are often obtained by means of transcutaneous tracheal aspiration in which a catheter is passed into the trachea through a needle inserted directly through the skin into the trachea. This technique has not gained much popularity in Great Britain. Alternatively, secretions may be aspirated through a tube in a fibreoptic bronchoscope. It is, however, possible that upper respiratory tract commensals may be carried down into the lungs by such a procedure, thereby contaminating the specimen, but this appears to be a theoretical rather than practical objection.

9.3.10 Pleural fluid

Pleural effusions due to inflammation frequently coagulate on standing. Specimens should therefore be placed in bottles containing sterile sodium citrate as an anticoagulant.

9.4 Transport of specimens to the laboratory

This prosaic sounding topic is in fact of considerable importance. Many valuable specimens are ruined and much information is thereby lost by delays, which are mostly avoidable, in getting the material to the laboratory. In some cases organisms may perish either as a result of their inherent susceptibility to the changed environment or due to the presence of antibiotics present in the specimen. Other specimens are spoilt by an overgrowth of commensal organisms. Certain anaerobes, particularly those encountered in the respiratory tract, are extremely sensitive to oxygen so no time must be wasted between their collection and their delivery to the laboratory. When delays are unavoidable, swabs for culture of anaerobes should be placed in Stuart's transport medium and pus or sputum should be injected into a rubber-sealed bottle containing pure carbon dioxide.

When delays in transport are inevitable specimens for culture should be kept at a temperature between 2 and 4°C. Most viruses especially poxviruses and enteroviruses, are unstable above this temperature. On the other hand some, especially respiratory syncytial virus (RSV), are killed by freezing.

Certain transport media are available to protect pathogens. Pike's and Stuart's media [2, p. 781], are particularly useful for upper respiratory tract swabs as they maintain β-haemolytic streptococci. Transport media is usually dispensed as a soft agar in a tube. The swab is inserted into the tube so that the tip of the swab is stabbed into the medium.

Blood specimens for serology should never be frozen as this causes haemolysis. Separated serum may be frozen but repeated freezing and thawing should be avoided.

9.5 Examination of specimens in the laboratory

9.5.1 Microscopical examination

Direct microscopy has the advantage of speed but lacks the sensitivity and specificity of cultural procedures. Microscopy is used either to demonstrate the presence of micro-organisms in normally sterile specimens, e.g. cerebrospinal fluid and pleural fluid, or to indicate the possible nature of a pathogen in specimens which are not usually free of contamination, e.g. pneumococci or *Mycobacterium tuberculosis* in sputum. Opinions vary as to the usefulness of direct microscopy of sputum for the diagnosis of non-acute bacterial infections other than tuberculosis, but it is generally agreed that it is pointless to perform microscopy routinely on sputum from patients with chronic bronchitis or other chronic chest diseases. On the other hand, it frequently enables a rapid provisional diagnosis of acute pneumonia due to *Staph. aureus*, streptococci including *Strep. pneumoniae* or *Haemophilus influenzae*. Sputa will usually be prepared for microscopical examination in the laboratory although it is possible to prepare the slides in the clinic. Unless the sputum is first homogenized, a purulent portion of the specimen should be pipetted out and spread thinly on three slides which are clearly labelled by means of a diamond marker. After drying, the slides are fixed by passing them slowly, specimen upwards, three times through a Bunsen flame. Over-heating should be avoided and the specimen should not be fixed until it is dry. One of the slides is stained for non-acid fast bacilli by Gram's method of which there are several modifications. The other two slides are stained for mycobacteria and eosinophils respectively. The principle of the Gram staining technique is to determine whether the bacteria are resistant to decolourization by acetone after staining with a metachromatic stain such as crystal violet. The fixed slide is first treated with the crystal violet and then with Lugol's iodine which has a mordant action, thus fixing the dye to the bacteria. At this stage everything on the slide is stained blue. Acetone is then poured on the slide; this elutes the dye from some bacteria. To visualize the unstained bacteria, a counterstain, usually a red stain such as safranin, is then applied. On examination of the slide, Gram positive organisms will appear dark blue, while gram negative organisms and other materials, including cells, will appear red. Table 9.1 lists the common pathogenic bacterial genera according to their gram staining characteristics and their shape (elongated rods or circular cocci). Mycobacteria are gram positive although *M. tuberculosis* stains weakly and irregularly by this method.

Staphylococci and streptococci may usually be differentiated by the arrangement of the bacterial cells. Staphylococci are arranged in clumps like bunches of grapes, whereas the streptococci are arranged as chains. *Streptococcus* (Diplococcus) *pneumoniae* cells are often seen as pairs with the adjacent ends flattened and the distal ends somewhat pointed. This appearance led to the older term 'lanceolate diplococci'. The Gram negative bacilli are much less readily differentiated microscopically.

The *Brucellaceae*, including the genus *haemophilus*, are smaller than the *Enterobacteraceae* and are thus sometimes referred to as the Parvobacteria.

Direct microscopy is widely used to detect mycobacteria in clinical specimens, especially sputum. Microscopical detection of bacteria in this genus is particularly useful as cultures require several weeks incubation before

Table 9.1 Gram staining properties of the principal pathogenic bacteria

Gram positive	*Gram negative*
1. Cocci	1. Cocci
Staphylococcus	Neisseria
S. aureus	N. meningitidis
S. albus	N. gonorrhoeae
Streptococcus	
S. pyogenes	
S. viridans	
S. pneumoniae	
2. Rods	2. Rods
Corynebacterium	Enterobacteria
C. diphtheriae	Escherichia coli
Bacillus	Proteus spp.
B. anthracis	Salmonella spp.
Clostridia	Shigella spp.
C. perfringens	Klebsiella spp.
C. botunlinum	Serratia spp.
C. tetani	Pseudomonads
Actinomycetales	Pseudomanas aeruginosa
Actinomyces spp.	Vibrio cholerae
Mycobacteria spp.	Brucellaceae
Nocardia spp.	Brucella spp.
	Bordetella pertussis
	Pasteurella spp.
	Yersinia pestis
	Haemophilus influenzae
	Haemophilus parainfluenzae
	Other Haemophilus spp.
	Bacteroides
	B. fragilis
	B. melaninogenicus
	Legionella
	L. pneumophila

growth is discernable. Fortunately, mycobacteria resist decolourization by acid after staining by carbol fuchsin – a property known as 'acid fastness'. This staining technique, the Ziehl-Neelsen technique, is similar in principle to the Gram stain. The fixed slide is stained with hot carbol fuchsin (heating greatly accelerates the staining process) and is then treated with acid, e.g. 3% suphuric acid. The slide is then counterstained, usually with malachite green. The mycobacteria which resist decolourization by the acid are then seen as bright red organisms on a green background. Auramine O may be substituted for carbol fuchsin, enabling mycobacteria to be detected by means of fluorescence microscopy. Mycobacteria are much easier to detect by fluorescence microscopy than by the conventional Ziehl-Neelsen stain but the equipment is not so widely available. It must be emphasized that microscopy is a rather insensitive means of detecting mycobacteria in sputum. Even 5000 organisms per millilitre of sputum are easily missed. However, epidemiological studies have shown that infectious cases of tuberculosis are virtually limited to those patients who have microscopically detectable organisms in the sputum.

Viruses cannot be visualized directly by light microscopy but cells infected with viruses may be detected by means of fluorescence microscopy using specific antiviral antibodies conjugated with fluorescein isothiocyanate. This technique requires some technical expertise but often enables a specific virus diagnosis to be made very rapidly. Electron microscopy has at the present time little application in respiratory virology but, in conjugation with high speed centrifugation of specimens and ferritin-conjugated antisera, it may prove to be a useful diagnostic tool in the future.

9.5.2 Examination of specimens by culture

As summarized above, specimens received in the laboratory will fall into two main categories:

1. Specimens of normally sterile material e.g. tissue biopsies, blood, CSF.
2. Specimens very likely to be contaminated by commensal organisms, e.g. throat swabs and sputum; the majority of specimens for the investigation of respiratory infection will be in this group.

Any organism isolated from specimens in the first group need to be investigated fully. Ideally, all organisms from the second group of specimens should also be studied in detail, but this would greatly overburden the resources of the routine clinical laboratory. It is, therefore, unfortunately necessary in most cases to make a compromise and perform a limited number of investigations that will isolate or exclude known pathogens. Organisms which may be isolated by cultural techniques are:

Aerobic bacteria
Anaerobic bacteria
Mycobacteria
Mycoplasma
Fungi
Chlamydia (Psittacosis-LGV and TRIC agents), rickettsia and coxiella
Viruses

The techniques required for culturing these seven groups of organisms are quite different and indeed are often performed in different laboratories, thereby requiring separate specimens. Normally, the 'routine' examination of a specimen from the respiratory tract consists of a report on its macroscopic appearance (mucoid, purulent, blood-stained etc.), a culture for aerobic bacteria, antibiotic sensitivity testing of recognized pathogens, and usually a Ziehl-Neelsen stain or similar technique for mycobacteria. Cultures for the anaerobic bacteria and the other micro-organisms listed above are, in most centres, only undertaken when specifically requested.

(a) Aerobic bacteria

Various techniques have been introduced to attempt to distinguish organisms causing diseases in the lower respiratory tract from organisms, including potential pathogens, occurring as commensals in the upper respiratory tract. These techniques include elution of organisms adhering to the surface of lumps of sputum by washing with saline and aspiration of distinctly purulent parts of the specimen by means of a Pasteur pipette. Neither technique has met with much success or popularity. Likewise quantitation of pathogens is of limited value because of the marked variation in the composition of sputum. This variation within a specimen or between pooled specimens is overcome by homogenization, either by digestion with pancreatin or by the use of a mucolytic agent such as *N*-acetylcystein. A rather crude form of quantitation is attempted in some laboratories by making a 1:10 000 dilution of the homogenized sputum and inoculating this, as well as the undiluted homogenate, on to the media.

The aerobic pathogens of principle interest include:

Streptococcus pneumoniae (pneumococci)
β-haemolytic streptococci
Staphylococcus aureus
Haemophilus influenzae
Pseudomonas aeruginosa (particularly in cystic fibrosis)
Legionella pneumophila (causative agent of Legionnaire's disease)
Bordetella pertussis

Gram negative rods of the enteric group (*Escherichia, Klebsiella, Proteus, Serratia* etc.) are not infrequently isolated from sputum and pose a particular problem of interpretation. It is doubtful if any of this group of organisms is a primary pathogen in otherwise healthy people but they can colonize the respiratory tract following viral infections, when the lung is otherwise damaged as in chronic bronchitis or bronchiectasis or following inappropriate chemotherapy.

The extent to which bacteria are primary pathogens is not known, even so-called primary bacterial pneumonias may be preceded by an occult viral infection. Certainly many cases of *H. influenzae, Strep. pneumoniae* and *Staph. aureus* infections follow a viral infection, especially influenza. Most of the above pathogens grow readily on nutrient agar enriched with blood (blood agar) which is a standard culture medium. *H. influenzae*, like other members of this genus, require special growth factors known as X and V factors. X factor is haemin and there is no shortage of this in blood agar. Y factor (nicotinamide adenine dinucleotide, NAD) may be supplied by placing discs containing this factor on the medium or by streaking a culture of *Staph. aureus*, which liberates Y factor, on the medium. Colonies of *H. influenzæ* growing near the disc or the staphylococci will be large but those elsewhere on the medium will be very small. This phenomenon, known as satellitism, helps to identify haemophili.

Other organisms frequently observed on sputum cultures include *Staph. albus, Strep. viridans, Neisseria* species including *N. meningitidis* and various non-pathogenic corynebacteria and related genera ('diphtheroids'). These are only significant in extremely exceptional circumstances. Three other pathogens are nowadays only encountered extremely rarely in Great Britain. These are *Bacillus anthracis, Corynebacterium diphtheriae* and *Yersinia pestis*.

(b) Anaerobic cultures

Although largely neglected for many years, anaerobes are now known to be, in certain circumstances, important pathogens of the respiratory tract. They are responsible for some cases of empyaemia and lung abscesses, particularly those following aspiration of a foreign body or in association with carcinoma Anaerobes are also likely causative agents or necrotizing and aspiration pneumonias but are unlikely to be encountered in bronchitis, bronchopneumonia or lobar pneumonia. The anaerobes usually encountered are members of the genus *Bacteroides* and anaerobic or microaerophilic members of the genus *Streptococcus*. Members of the genus *Clostridium* are most unlikely to be encountered in infections of the respiratory tract. The current classification of the anaerobic bacteria is discussed by Collee in a symposium report covering many important clinical aspects of anaerobe infections [3].

Anaerobes may be cultured in the depths of a liquid medium containing a reducing agent, or more conveniently on solid media incubated in an oxygen-free environment. This is usually achieved by placing the specimens in a container which is evacuated and refilled with hydrogen. A palladium catalyst converts any remaining oxygen to water by combination with hydrogen. A commercially available system known as Gaspak (Becton-Dickenson and Co.) generates hydrogen chemically and removes oxygen catalytically, thus obviating the need for a vacuum pump and a hydrogen cylinder.

The presence of anaerobes in clinical material may be rapidly demonstrated by the detection of their volatile metabolic products by gas-liquid chromatography (see next section) but culture is required for final identification and for performing sensitivity tests.

Some aerobic organisms are also able to thrive in an anaerobic environment together with anaerobes and may contribute towards the disease process.

(c) *Mycobacteria*

The genus *Mycobacterium* consists of two subgenera which correspond to the rapid and slow growing mycobacteria. In contrast to popular belief, this is one of the best classified of all bacterial genera [4]. Even the rapid growing species grow slowly compared with most other bacteria, especially on primary isolation from clinical material. It is therefore necessary to destroy other bacteria which would otherwise overgrow the mycobacteria. Fortunately, mycobacteria are resistant to concentrations of acid or alkali which kill most other micro-organisms. In Petroff's method, for example, sputum is incubated for 30 min with an equal volume of 4% sodium hydroxide, then centrifuged and the deposit neutralized with hydrochloric acid.

Other agents used to decontaminate specimens include sulphuric acid, oxalic acid, trisodium phosphate, sodium hypochlorite, and quaternary ammonium compounds.

The most widely used medium for the culture of mycobacteria is Lowenstein Jensen medium which is one of several egg-based media. Colonies of *M. tuberculosis* usually appear on this medium after 2 to 5 weeks incubation. Only rarely is their appearance further delayed. A number of clear agar-based media for the culture of mycobacteria have been described which, although widely used by research workers, have not achieved much popularity for the primary isolation of mycobacteria from clinical material.

The first step in the identification of mycobacteria is to distinguish strains of *M. tuberculosis* from strains often referred to by the unfortunate term 'atypical mycobacteria'. This is an important distinction which should be made as soon as possible. *M. tuberculosis* is an obligate pathogen, thus each isolation is significant even if only a single colony appears on the medium (provided of course that cross-contamination of cultures does not occur in the laboratory due to poor technique). In contrast, the 'atypical' mycobacteria are environmental saprophytes which only occasionally cause overt disease. Thus their presence in clinical material need not necessarily be significant. To be considered significant, an 'atypical' mycobacterium must be isolated from sputum on at least two occasions, at least one week apart, from patients with evidence of pulmonary disease in whom other aetiologies, including *M. tuberculosis*, have been carefully excluded. This rule also applies to other opportunist organisms isolated from sputum.

The 'atypical' mycobacteria, better termed 'environmental' mycobacteria, differ in several important respects from *M. tuberculosis*. Firstly, as mentioned above, they are not obligate pathogens. Secondly, they are not transmitted from human to human except under very rare circumstances. Thirdly, the incidence of disease due to them is governed by their occurrence in the environment and the number of opportunities for infection and is thus independent of the incidence of *M. tuberculosis* infection.

It is important therefore for the clinician to be certain which entities are included within the species *M. tuberculosis*. In addition to the human type, this species contains the bovine type (*M. bovis*), the African type (*M. africanum*) and the vole type (*M. microti*) which is not virulent for humans. There is also a distinct variant originating from Asia [5].

The epithets *M. bovis*, *M. africanum* and *M. microti*, convey the false impression that these are distinct species from *M. tuberculosis*. The term 'tubercle bacillus' is also misleading because although the human, bovine and vole tubercle bacilli are members of the species *M. tuberculosis*, the avian, fish, frog and turtle tubercle bacilli, are not.

Identification of mycobacteria, other than *M. tuberculosis*, is usually undertaken by reference laboratories which may also carry out sensitivity testing.

(d) Fungi

Mycotic infections are divided into systemic, subcutaneous and cutaneous. The fungi causing systemic infections are divided into two groups – primary pathogens and opportunists.

The primary pathogenic species are *Cryptococcus neoformans, Coccidioides immitis, Histoplasma capsulatum* and *Blastomyces dermatitidis* which cause cyptococcosis, coccidioidomycosis, histoplasmosis and blastomycosis respectively. All these diseases may involve the lungs. The principal opportunistic fungi are *Candida albicans, Aspergillus* species (usually *A. fumigatus*) and the *Phycomycetes (Mucor* and *Rhizopus* species). All the above fungi may be cultivated on Sabourand's agar which is the most widely used medium in mycology. This is a simple medium containing peptone and glucose with antibiotics added to prevent bacterial contamination. Fungi are usually identified by their macroscopic and microscopic morphology and sometimes their ability to form mycelia when cultured at 37° or 22°C.

(e) Mycoplasmas

The class *Mollicutes* is composed of six genera of which only one, the genus

Mycoplasma, is known to cause disease in man. Unlike other bacteria, the mollicutes lack rigid cell walls and are thus very pleomorphic in shape and are able to pass through bacteria-retaining filters. Mycoplasmas are ubiquitous and have been isolated from patients with various rheumatic disorders and urogenital infections but they also occur in the urogenital and respiratory tracts of normal individuals, so their role as pathogens is uncertain. One species, *Mycoplasma pneumoniae*, is, without doubt, the causative agent of primary atypical pneumonia. Initially thought to be a virus, this species was originally cultured in chick embryos, subsequently in tissue cultures and eventually on an agar medium enriched with yeast extract and serum. On this medium, *M. pneumoniae* grows as minute compact granular colonies, whereas other mycoplasmas have colonies with spreading edges and heaped up centres, the so-called 'fried egg' colonies. The colonies of *M. pneumoniae* are positively identified by staining with a fluorescein – conjugated specific antiserum.

(f) *Rickettsiae and Coxiellae*

These organisms are small pleumorphic bacteria which, like the chlamydiae, are obligate intracellular parasites. The rickettsiae can only survive for very short periods of time outside a living cell and are usually spread from host to host by arthropod vectors. In contrast *Coxiella burnetti*, the causative agent of Q fever, survives in droplets and dust and is often spread by inhalation, thereby causing a pneumonia. Serum from patients with rickettsial infections agglutinate certain *Proteus* species (Weil-Felix reaction) but this reaction is not encountered in Q fever.

Coxiella burnetti infection may be diagnosed by complement fixation tests. Alternatively patients' blood may be inoculated into hamsters and guinea pigs. Infection in the animals is indicated by a rise in rectal temperature and the subsequent demonstration of the organisms in smears of splenic or peritoneal cells. Some animals show no sign of illness but are found to have a rising titre of complement fixing antibodies after several weeks which gives a reliable but retrospective diagnosis. As in the case of the chlamydiae, culture of rickettsiae and *C. burnetti* carries a high risk of infection to the laboratory staff and should therefore only be attempted in specialized centres.

(g) *Chlamydiae*

This family of organisms is more correctly known as the *Chlamydozoaceae* but in view of the difficulty in pronouncing this word (not to mention spelling it!) the abbreviated term *Chlamydia* is now in general use. These organisms were once thought to be viruses but are now recognized as minute bacteria.

They are divided into two groups, the first includes the psittacosis and lymphogranuloma venereum (LGV) agents and the second contains the causative agents of trachoma and inclusion conjunctivitis. These two groups are frequently termed the psittacosis-LGV and TRIC agents respectively.

Although bacteria, the chlamydiae are obligate intracellular parasites on account of their inability to synthesize energy-supplying phosphate esters. The principal respiratory pathogen in this family is the agent of psittacosis (parrot fever) also termed ornithosis because of its occurrence in non-psittacine birds. Infection in man is usually due to the inhalation of dried faeces from infected birds. The psittacosis agent may be isolated from sputum or, in the first few days of the illness, from blood by inoculation into the yolk sac or allantoic cavity of an embryonated egg. Characteristic particles are observed in cells on microscopy and isolated agents are identified by complement fixation or neutralization tests. Isolation procedures carry a high risk of infection and should only be attempted in specialized centres. Furthermore, specimens from patients are hazardous and should be handled with great care. Patients with the disease may shed infectious organisms for long periods of time after recovery. Rising titres of antibodies to the infecting agent may be detected by complement fixation tests.

(h) Viruses

Viruses are responsible for the great majority of respiratory tract infections, most of which are fairly mild and self-limiting. To most non-virologists, the goings-on in the virological laboratory are cloaked in a veil of mystery. Furthermore, laboratory diagnoses of viral infections cannot be expected to excite much interest when they are made, as often happens, after the patient has recovered and when there is no therapy for such infections. There are, however, changes occurring in both these respects. Techniques are becoming available for the rapid diagnosis of viral infections and antiviral chemotherapy is slowly becoming a reality. Viral infections may be diagnosed by cultural techniques, microscopy (including electron microscopy) or by the demonstration of rising titres of antibodies to the virus.

Viruses are totally dependent on living cells for the replication. In essence, a virus consists of a small unit of genetic material (either DNA or RNA but never both) within a protein container which simply serves as a vector for the genome. Viruses contain none of the organelles, enzymes or energy sources essential to living cells for their replication. Thus for the laboratory isolation of a virus, some form of living tissue is essential: either a whole animal, an egg or a tissue culture. Of these the latter is now the most widely used.

Tissues may be cultured as whole organs or as parts of them: e.g. fragments of human embryo trachea provide a sensitive system for the isolation of common cold viruses. Most virological work, however, employs dispersed cells which may be grown as a monolayer (a layer of cells one cell thick) on a glass or plastic surface. Kidney, thyroid and amniotic membrane cells may be separated by means of tryptic digestion and cultured *in vitro* as 'primary cell cultures' from which subcultures or secondary cultures may be prepared. Many cell clones may be subcultured several times but eventually they undergo changes which often include a loss of sensitivity to certain viruses. These are termed 'semicontinuous cell lines'. In other cases cells may be propagated indefinitely whilst retaining a useful range of sensitivity to viruses. Many such 'continuous cell lines' have been derived, either from normal tissues or from malignant cells. One of the best known is the *HeLa* cell line derived from a cervical carcinoma.

Monolayers of cells are cultured in media containing antibiotics to prevent contamination by bacteria present in the clinical specimens with which they are inoculated. Some viruses cause observable changes in the cell monolayer, such changes being termed cytopathic effects (CPE). Different types of CPE are encountered; thus, polio and some Coxsackie viruses cause the cells to become rounded and detached from the glass while some adenoviruses cause the cells to aggregate into colony-like clusters. Infection of the monolayer by measles, herpes or respiratory syncytial virus causes the formation of multinucleate syncytia. Viruses of the myxovirus group (influenza, parainfluenza and mumps) do not produce a visible CPE but endow the cells with the ability to absorb red cells to their surfaces (haemadsorbtion). In the case of ECHO viruses and some of the Coxsackie viruses, both CPE and haemadsorbtion occur.

Animal inoculation for the isolation of viruses has largely been superseded by the use of tissue cultures but newborn mice are still useful for the isolation of arborviruses and Coxsackie viruses causing meningitis and encephalitis. Eggs, likewise, are not used as frequently as tissue cultures although they are useful for the isolation and propagation of influenza and other myxoviruses, pox viruses, herpes viruses and, in addition, Rickettsiae and Chlamydiae.

Viruses isolated by the above three systems are identified by a variety of tests including neutralization tests, complement fixation, haemadsorbtion inhibition, haemagglutination, immunodiffusion, immunofluorescence and electron microscopy. As discussed in the section on microscopy, immunofluorescence often detects the presence of virus-infected cells before CPE is observed and may also reveal infected cells directly in clinical specimens. A very promising recent development is the use of enzyme-linked immunosorbent assay to detect viral antigen.

In general, viruses may be identified at a group level readily and rapidly but further division into serotypes is more costly and time consuming. Such additional tests, although important in epidemiological studies, do not necessarily provide useful information to the clinician.

Table 9.2 lists the viruses commonly encountered according to the nature of the illness they cause. In particular it should be noted that herpes simplex, varicella zoster, cytomegalovirus (CMV) and measles viruses are encountered as opportunist invaders of the lung in predisposed individuals.

9.6 Diagnostic use of immunological techniques

Immunological tests are used both for the diagnosis of specific infections and for the identification of pathogens isolated from clinical specimens. Under most circumstances, an infective agent elicits an immune response in its host which is manifest by a rising titre of specific antibody (humoral immune response), by the development of cell mediated immunity or by both these responses. The detection of specific antibodies to an infective agent suggests that the patient has, at some time, come into contact with that agent but does not prove that the patient is currently infected. Such proof is obtained by the

Table 9.2   The viruses responsible for respiratory infections

Infection	Virus
Common cold	Rhinovirus
	Adenovirus
	Respiratory syncytial virus
	Parainfluenzavirus
	Coxsackie A and B
Pharyngitis, laryngitis	Adenovirus
	Parainfluenzavirus
Lower respiratory tract infection	Influenzavirus A and B
	Respiratory syncytial virus
	Parainfluenzavirus
	Adenovirus
	*Measles
	*Herpes varicella zoster
	*Herpes simplex
	*Cytomegalovirus
	Enterovirus (ECHO, Coxsackie A and B)
Influenza	Influenzavirus A and B

* These viruses cause disease in immunocompromised patients.

detection of a rising level of the specific antibodies in paired sera. Antigen-antibody reactions may be detected and quantitated *in vitro* by a number of different techniques of varying sensitivity. These tests include immunodiffusion, immunofluorescence, neutralization tests, complement fixation, haemagglutination inhibition, agglutination of antigen-coated particles such as bacteria, erythrocytes and latex particles, radioimmunoassay and enzyme-linked immunosorbent assay (ELISA).

9.6.1 Immunofluorescence

This is used as a qualitative test for the presence of antibodies in serum. The appropriate antigen is fixed to a glass slide and the serum sample is poured on to the slide. After incubation to allow antibody to bind to the antigen, the slide is washed to remove all unbound immunoglobulin and is then treated with a fluorescein-labelled antihuman immunoglobulin. After further washing, the presence of fluorescence will indicate the presence of antibodies against the antigen on the slide.

9.6.2 Neutralization tests

These are used to detect antibodies which effectively prevent the pathogen from infecting its host. In practice, this class of tests is mainly limited to the study of viral infections. Neutralization tests are very sensitive and are usually very specific and have thus enabled the division of some viruses into many different serotypes. Unfortunately neutralization tests are costly and time-consuming and are therefore not usually available routinely. Depending on the virus, neutralizing antibodies may be quantitated by their ability to protect whole animals, protect tissue cultures or reduce the number of plaques forming on tissue cultures or the chorioallantoic membranes of eggs.

Neutralization tests are also used to demonstrate toxin-producing bacteria, notably *Corynebacterium diphtheriae*. Bacterial cultures are inoculated into two mice, one of which is protected by administration of antitoxin. Toxin production is indicated by death of the unprotected animal.

9.6.3 The complement fixation test (CFT) (Fig. 9.1)

CFT is one of the most widely used tests in diagnostic serology. Complement is an important effector mechanism in the immune system and, in the context of this test, is responsible for the lysis of erythrocytes in the presence of an antierythrocyte antibody. Many, but not all, humoral immune reactions cause the binding of some of the components of complement to the antigen-antibody complex. The complement is thus 'fixed' and is unable to take part in subsequent reactions. The occurrence of complement fixation is indicated by incubating an antigen with a serum which may contain specific antibodies. An indicator system consisting of erythrocytes treated with antierythrocyte serum is then added and, if unfixed complement is present, lysis occurs. If, on the other hand, the test serum contains sufficient antibody to react with the antigen, complement is 'fixed' and none remains to lyse the added erythrocytes. In practice the complement in the patient's sera is inactivated by heating the sera to 56° for 30 min and a known amount of complement added. The sensitivity of the test depends on the amount of complement added. A certain minimum amount of complement is required to cause lyses of the erythrocytes: this amount is known as the minimum haemolytic dose (MHD). If a large excess of complement is added, then a considerable amount of complement will have to be fixed in order to reduce the concentration below the MHD, thus preventing haemolysis. It is therefore necessary to standardize all reagents for the test including the antigen, the complement, the erythrocytes and the haemolytic antiserum.

CFT is used to detect antibodies to a wide range of viruses and also to chlamydiae, rickettsiae, *Coxiella burnetii* (Q fever) and mycoplasmas. In general, complement fixation tests are, unlike neutralization tests, not strain-specific because strains within a group usually share one or more antigens. It is usual to screen a single dilution of the patient's serum against many antigens, usually the second specimen of a pair of sera is examined. If

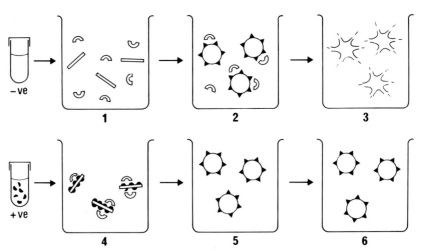

Fig. 9.1 The complement fixation test. 1. In the absence of specific antibodies complement is not consumed; 2. the complement is free to bind to sensitized red cells; 3. complement-mediated lysis occurs; 4. in the presence of specific antibodies complement is consumed; 5. no complement remains free to bind to sensitized red cells; 6. no lysis occurs.

any positive reactions are observed the antibody titres in both sera are estimated in order to detect rising titres of antibody to the relevant antigen.

9.6.4 Haemagglutination-inhibition tests

These provide a relatively simple and sensitive system for detecting antibodies to viruses that agglutinate red cells by adhering to them. These viruses include the myxoviruses (influenza, parainfluenza, measles and respiratory syncytial viruses), adenoviruses, arborviruses, ECHO and pox viruses. The test is performed by adding dilutions of the serum to suspensions of fowl erythrocytes followed by a standardized amount of the virus. The antibody titre is measured as the highest dilution of serum that inhibits the virus-induced haemagglutination. This test gives a better measure of protective antibodies and a greater degree of strain specificity than CFT and is more sensitive.

9.6.5 Agglutination reactions

These may be performed using a particulate antigen such as a bacterium or a soluble antigen bound to suitable particles such as erythrocytes, kaolin, bentonite or latex particles. Bacterial agglutination tests are of little value in the diagnosis of respiratory infection, their main applications being in the diagnosis of brucellosis, typhoid (Widal tests) and rickettsial infections (Weil-Felix text). Serum from some patients with *Mycoplasma pneumoniae* infection agglutinate an organism known as *Streptococcus* MG but there are now other more sensitive and specific tests available for the diagnosis of this infection. Two red cell agglutination tests are of particular interest in diagnostic serology: the 'cold agglutination' reaction and the Paul-Bunnell reaction.

A high proportion of infections due to *Mycoplasma pneumoniae* are associated with the ability of the serum to agglutinate human group O red cells at low temperatures. As the agglutinins are absorbed on to the patient's own red cells at temperatures below 20°C, it is important to maintain the blood sample at temperatures above 20°C until the serum has been separated. The test is often negative in the early stages of the disease and, as in the case of the *Streptococcus* MG agglutination test referred to above, is inferior to more direct ways of detecting antibodies to this pathogen (complement fixation, passive haemagglutination and ELISA).

The Paul-Bunnell reaction detects agglutinins for sheep red cells which appear in most cases of infectious mononucleosis (glandular fever). Dilutions of patients' sera are incubated with sheep red cells and the titre is recorded as the highest dilution of serum causing agglutination. A titre of 128 is suggestive and a titre of 256 is highly significant. Some normal sera and sera from patients who have recently had an injection of horse serum (e.g. antitetanus serum) may also agglutinate sheep red cells. However, agglutinins associated with infectious mononucleosis absorb onto ox red cells but not onto emulsions of guinea pig kidney, while those associated with serum therapy absorb to both these reagents.

Red cell agglutination is also used to detect and quantitate antibodies to specific antigens by attaching the latter to appropriately treated red cells. Other suitable particles include latex, bentonite and kaolin.

9.6.6 Radioimmunoassay

This is, in theory, an excellent way to detect antigen on antibody but has three major disadvantages: firstly, the radiolabelled reagents are expensive and have a short shelf life; secondly, the equipment required to measure the radioactivity is very costly to install and maintain and, thirdly, there are health hazards involved in handling radiolabelled reagents.

9.6.7 ELISA (Fig. 9.2)

All the disadvantages of radioimmunoassay are avoided while maintaining applicability and sensitivity by using a relatively new technique termed

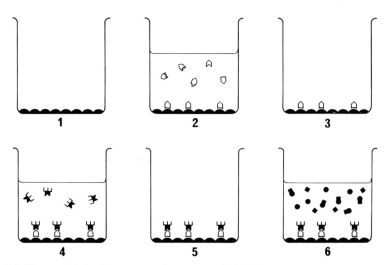

Fig. 9.2 Enzyme-linked immunosorbent assay (ELISA). 1. Wells in microtitre tray are coated with antigen; 2. specific antibodies in patient's serum combine with antigen; 3. other antibodies are removed by washing; 4. enzyme-linked antihuman globulin conbines with fixed antibodies; 5. unbound antiglobulin-enzyme conjugate is removed by washing; 6. added substrate is hydrolysed by absorbed anzyme to yield a coloured product.

Enzyme Linked Immunosorbent Assay, abbreviated to ELISA. To detect antibodies, the appropriate antigen is fixed to a solid support such as a plastic tube or the well of a microtitre tray. The patient's serum at a suitable dilution is then added to the tube and any specific antibodies bind to the fixed antigen, unfixed antibodies then being removed by washing. Next an antihuman globulin which is chemically conjugated to an enzyme is added. This binds to the antibodies which have bound to the antigen and excess conjugate is removed by washing. The amount of enzyme thus mirrors the amount of antibody in the patient's serum. A substrate is then added which is split by the enzyme to yield a coloured product which is measurable in a colorimeter. Peroxidase, alkaline phosphatase and β-galactosidase enzymes have been used. Although ELISA was only developed a few years ago, its simplicity, cheapness and versatility, have rendered it a very popular test. Certainly it is a serious rival to the CFT for the routine screening for antibodies to viruses, chlamydiae, *Coxiella* and mycoplasmas.

9.6.8 Immunodiffusion and immunoelectrophoresis

Immunodiffusion analysis has the virtue of simplicity but is relatively insensitive and requires large quantities of antigen. A more sensitive test is countercurrent immunoelectrophoresis (CIE) in which the antigen and antibody are driven into contact by the application of an electric current. This test has been used to detect viral antigens and antibodies (including smallpox antigen in pustules and hepatitis B antibodies and antigen (Australia antigen).

Much work has been performed on the detection of precipitating antibodies, sometimes termed precipitins, in bacterial chest infections. Precipitins to *Haemophilus influenzae* may be detected in many patients with chronic bronchitis and precipitins to *Pseudomonas aeruginosa* are detectable in the serum of patients with cystic fibrosis infected with this organism. The presence of such precipitins suggest that those organisms are pathogens in these diseases rather than merely commensals. Detection of these precipitins is of very dubious value in the diagnosis of infection in patients but provides a somewhat crude test for demonstrating the integrity of the humoral immune system in patients with chronic chest infections.

9.7 Non-cultural detection of pathogens

9.7.1 Detection of antigens by immunological techniques

The use of countercurrent immunoelectrophoresis (CIE) to detect smallpox virus and Australia antigen have been referred to above. CIE is also used to detect bacterial antigens in sputum. Techniques for the detection of *Strep. pneumoniae* and *H. influenzae* have been described and the method should be applicable to other microbial antigens [6]. Viruses may be detected by the use of fluorescein-conjugated antisera. Cells infected with virus may likewise be detected by the use of such sera. These cells may either be those in the original specimen or in a tissue culture infected with the virus. Immunofluorescence may reveal and identify viruses in tissue cultures much more rapidly than the observation of cytopathic effect. Immunofluorescence is also used to detect certain bacteria in sputum and tissues as well as to identify cultured organisms. Fluorescent-labelled antisera are used to identify colonies of mycoplasma and *Legionella pneumophilia*.

9.7.2 Detection of micro-organisms or their metabolites by chemical techniques

In general, micro-organisms are present in too small amounts to be detectable by chemical methods. An exception is the use of gas-liquid chromatography (GLC) to detect volatile aromatic acids produced by anaerobic bacteria. By this technique the presence of anaerobes in pus aspirated from lung abscesses or from the pleural cavity may be directly, reliably, rapidly and relatively simply confirmed.

9.8 Diagnostic use of skin tests

Serological tests are based on the ability of micro-organisms to elicit a humoral immune response in the infected host. Skin testing, on the other hand, is principally used to detect cell mediated immunity (CMI). Reagents used for skin testing are known as sensitins and are named after the organism from which they are prepared followed by the suffix -in, e.g. tuberculin, blastomycin, coccidiodin and histoplasmin.

Tuberculin is the best known skin test reagent. Koch's original Old Tuberculin is produced from old culture filtrates which contain extracellular metabolites as well as cellular components released by autolysis. Purified protein derivative (PPD) is prepared from the former by precipitating protein (and other substances) from heat-sterilized filtrates by means of acetone or ammonium sulphate. This concoction, referred to by an eminent immunologist as a 'rotted, boiled and pickled antigen', is used extensively to demonstrate delayed type hypersensitivity to the tubercle bacillus. This reagent is not specific as *M. tuberculosis* shares antigenic determinants with other mycobacteria. Thus a positive response to a tuberculin test may indicate:

1. active infection;
2. previous overt or subclinical infection;
3. previous vaccination with BCG or
4. contact with, or infection by, environmental ('atypical') mycobacteria.

The lack of specificity and the inability to distinguish between active disease and past contact severely limit the usefulness of tuberculin testing. The problem of specificity has been largely overcome by the use of 'New Tuberculins' prepared from the cytoplasm of sonically disrupted mycobacteria [7] and there is some evidence that active disease may be distinguishable from previous contact by the use of a small peptide isolated from the tubercle bacillus [8]. At the time of writing these reagents are not generally available.

The tuberculin test elicits the type of response known as delayed type, or type IV, hypersensitivity. To what extent this response correlates with immunity is still debatable [9–11].

Infection with *M. tuberculosis* leads to a development of tuberculin positivity but in some cases, especially severe infections, the skin test and other correlates of cell mediated immunity, may become negative. This is due to a trapping of the responsive lymphocytes in lymph nodes. The tuberculin test may be performed in three main ways – the Mantoux, Heaf and Tine tests.

In the Mantoux test, a known quantity (usually 0.1 ml) of the reagent is injected intradermally, a technique which requires a certain degree of expertise. Such expertise is not required for the Heaf test in which the tuberculin is driven into the dermis by means of a spring-loaded gun which fires six needles into the skin to a depth of 2 mm. Both the Mantoux and Heaf tests require the use of a solution of the tuberculin. This is rather wasteful if only one test is being performed. Thus the Tine test was introduced. This consists of four metal spikes coated with a standard dose of dried PPD and mounted on a plastic handle. When using this test it is important to allow the spikes to remain in the skin for several seconds to allow the dried PPD to dissolve otherwise an insufficient amount will enter the skin.

Skin tests reagents for fungal infections are similar in principle to tuberculin and, like the latter reagent, may indicate previous contact as well as present infection. Thus, for example, many adults in the USA react to histoplasmin, especially those living in the Mississippi valley where *H. capsulatum* is common in the environment.

9.9 Other investigations

9.9.1 Radiological investigations

Radiology plays an important role in the diagnosis of infectious diseases of the chest and also assists the management of the infection by indicating whether the disease is resolving or progressing. These investigations are discussed in Chapter 6.

9.9.2 Histological studies of biopsies

In some cases, infective agents are detected and identified by histological examination of biopsies of the lung or associated lymph nodes. Such infections include tuberculosis, fungal infections and opportunist organisms including *Pneumocystis carinii*. Tissues should be examined by haematoxylin and eosin staining and also by one of the histological modifications of the Ziehl–Neelsen method for mycobacteria and by the Grocott silver stain for fungi and *Pneumocystis carinii*. Whenever possible, biopsy material should be sent for both culture and histology but great care should be taken to avoid sending specimens placed in formalin to the microbiology department. It is surprising how often this fault occurs!

Tuberculosis is one cause of enlarged groups of lymph nodes. When surgical exploration of such nodes is performed it is not necessarily the largest node that is most suitable for histological examination as such nodes may be very necrotic.

9.9.3 Haematological studies

A total and differential leucocyte count can be performed easily and rapidly. Pneumonia of bacterial aetiology is visually accompanied by a raised leucocyte count with a predominance of granulocytes whereas the count in viral pneumonia is often normal with a relative monocytosis. The presence of characteristic mononuclear cells assists the diagnosis of glandular fever. Underlying disorders such as agranulocytosis or leukaemina may also be revealed by an examination of a blood film.

9.9.4 Immunological studies

The use of immunological techniques to diagnose infections and to detect and identify pathogens has been described above. In addition, the function of the immune system of the patient may be investigated. This involves an examination of the integrity of the humoral and cell mediated immune response and the function of the effector mechanisms of the system, namely complement and phagocytic systems. Some causes of immunodeficiency may become apparent during routine studies, namely agranulocytosis, agammaglobulinaemia, leukaemia and other malignancies. Further investigations require the use of many tests of varying cost and complexity and cannot therefore be used indiscriminately. Such investigations should be considered in cases of recurrent infection especially in children but should always be planned in consultation with the microbiologist or immunologist. Techniques for the assessment of immune function have been outlined [12].

In recent years it has become apparent that many host-parasite relationships show a spectrum of immune response. At one end of the spectrum a brisk and effective immune reaction eliminates the pathogen while at the other end the virtual absence of a response leads to a rapidly progressing and often fatal disease. Such a spectrum is most obvious in leprosy but also occurs in tuberculosis [13] and in other infections. It has also been found that the position of the patients in the spectrum determines the outcome of chemotherapy; thus there is likely to be a growing interest in immunological assessments.

9.10 Sensitivity testing – its uses and limitations

9.10.1 Principles of sensitivity testing

The purpose of sensitivity testing is to determine whether the causative organism of an infection is sensitive or resistant to therapeutic concentrations of antibacterial agents. This can be achieved by the use of simple tests to determine whether an organism is likely to be sensitive to the concentrations of antibiotic achieved by 'routine' chemotherapy. Alternatively, more formal tests may be used to establish the minimum concentration of antibiotic that will merely inhibit the organism's growth (minimum inhibitory concentration, MIC) or kill the organism (minimum bactericidal concentration, MBC). Most of the screening tests for antibiotic sensitivity/resistance involve the use of paper discs on to which a known amount of antibiotic has been dried. These discs are applied to agar surfaces which have been inoculated with the organism and, after incubation, the presence and size of zones of inhibition are recorded. This sounds simple but in practice there are numerous pitfalls for the unwary in both technique and interpretation [14]. Many errors due to faulty media and discs may be avoided by incorporating control organisms of known sensitivity into each test.

In some cases, a more exact determination of the concentration of antibiotic necessary to inhibit or destroy a bacterium is required. These determinations are performed in cases where it is essential to achieve a bactericidal concentration of antibiotic(s) in the serum, e.g. in subacute bacterial endocarditis, and also in cases where it is important to achieve a bactericidal concentration but not to exceed this greatly on account of drug toxicity. The MIC of an antibiotic for a given organism is determined by inoculating two-fold dilutions of the antibiotic in broth with a suspension of the organism and incubating overnight. The MIC is the lowest concentration permitting no visible growth. To determine whether the lack of visible growth is due to bacterial death or merely to growth inhibition, loopfuls from each tube are spread on antibiotic-free media and incubated. Growth appearing on media inoculated from the clear tubes indicates bacteriostatic activity only. The lowest concentration of antibiotic leading to no growth when thus subcultured is the MBC.

The tube dilution test may also be used to investigate the bactericidal action of a combination of two antibiotics by setting up a chequer board arrangement of tubes with various possible combinations of the antibiotics. This test is of value when unusual combinations of drugs are to be used on account of either bacterial drug resistance or untoward reactions in the patient. It is necessary to test both drugs together as in some cases one drug may antagonize the action of the other, e.g. penicillins with tetracycline; whereas in other cases a beneficial synergism may be observed, e.g. penicillins, cephalosporins or erythromycin together with an aminoglycoside such as gentamicin or streptomycin.

Despite the fact that sensitivity testing involves testing the organism under conditions quite unlike those found in the host, such testing is of value and converts antibacterial chemotherapy from mere guesswork into a rational procedure [15]. Only a small minority of bacteria encountered in hospital practice have such dependable drug sensitivity patterns as to obviate the need for sensitivity testing. It must, however, be realized that the tests outlined above are only of value if the bacterium under test is in fact the cause of the patient's disease. Many are the occasions when an infection due to a 'resistant' organism has resolved on apparently inappropriate chemotherapy when, in fact, the infection was viral in origin!

9.10.2 Sensitivity testing of *Mycobacterium tuberculosis*

It is well known that inadequate drug regimens may lead to the emergence of strains of *M. tuberculosis* which are resistant to one or more antituberculous agents. This is due to the fact that such resistance arises in this organism by mutation at a low and constant frequency, about 10^{-8} per cell division. Tsukamura [16] has emphasized that a population of *M. tuberculosis* contains many different phenotypes of resistance. Thus sensitivity testing only shows that a high proportion of the organisms is sensitive to a given antituberculous agent. This is achieved either by the proportion method, in which the exact proportion of resistant cells in a culture is measured by comparing colony counts on media with and without the antituberculous agent, or by the resistance-ratio method.

In the latter method, which is more widely used, the sensitivity of a clinical isolate is compared with that of a known sensitive strain and the difference is expressed as a ratio. Thus, for example, a resistance ratio of 4 implies that a four-fold increase in the concentration of the drug is required to destroy the same proportion of bacteria in the test strains as in the standard strain. It must be emphasized that a culture reported as being sensitive to a particular drug may nevertheless contain a few resistant organisms.

As *M. tuberculosis* is a slow growing organism, the results of sensitivity testings are not available for many weeks. Opinions vary as to the usefulness of 'routine' sensitivity testing. In the author's opinion such testing is only justifiable if it is carried out to a very high standard of accuracy, which unfortunately is not always the case. In areas where the incidence of resistance is low, more harm may be done by prescribing more toxic and less effective drugs on the basis of false reports of drug resistance than by treating cases 'blind' and modifying therapy on the grounds of clinical features and sputum microscopy.

9.11 Monitoring antimicrobial therapy

Antimicrobial agents may be detected and measured in serum, other biological fluids and tissues by chemical analysis or by bioassay. Chemical analysis usually has the advantage of rapidity whereas bioassay gives a measure of the activity of an agent which does not necessarily correlate with its concentration.

Assay of antimicrobial agents is used to determine whether sufficient serum levels are being achieved to eliminate the organism while ensuring that dangerously high levels do not occur. Such monitoring is not necessary in many cases of acute infection in otherwise healthy individuals. It is of principal value in chronic infection in patients with depressed immune responses or when the organism is physically isolated from the immune system, as occurs, for example, in subacute bacterial endocarditis. In such cases it is imperative to achieve a cidal concentration of antibiotic. Assays are also of value in cases of impaired renal function in which delayed excretion of the drug may occur.

When requesting antibiotic assays, several important points must be borne in mind. Firstly, the interval between administration of the antibiotic and taking the blood sample is of great importance. Following administration of an antibiotic the serum level increases to a peak level, the time taken depending on the route of administration, and then drops to a trough level before the next administration. Peak levels are much more variable than trough levels and give much less information about the excretion rate. Secondly, it is not necessary in all cases for the serum antibiotic level to remain constantly above the MBC of the organism. Indeed, pulsed therapy may be of more benefit than continuous high dosage. Thirdly, full details of the patient's antibiotic therapy must be given. This is of the utmost importance when more than one antibiotic is being administered as special precautions will then have to be taken to prevent the presence of one antibiotic interfering in the assay of another.

Antibiotic assays are usually performed by a tube dilution or an agar diffusion method. In the tube dilution method, the bactericidal action of serial dilutions of the serum is compared with similar dilutions of a standardized solution of the antibiotic. The agar diffusion method is based on the fact that the diameter of a zone of inhibition of a bacterial lawn on agar is proportional to the logarithm of the concentration of the antibiotic diffusing from a well in the agar, other factors being equivalent. Thus the concentration or, more properly, the activity of the antibiotic may be calculated by comparing the zone size with those produced by known concentrations of the antibiotic.

When the patient is receiving more than one antibiotic the concentration of a single antibiotic may be assayed after inactivating the other antibiotic(s). Examples include the inactivation of penicillins by lactamases and sulphonamides and trimethoprim by thymidine. Alternatively, indicator organisms which are sensitive to the required antibiotic but resistant to the other antibiotics present in the patient's serum may be selected.

The limiting factor in bioassays of antibiotics is the time taken for the test organisms to grow. However, the use of heavy inocula of rapidly growing organisms permits the results to be read after 3–5 h incubation which means that the results are available the same day if the specimen is delivered to the laboratories early enough.

Chemical methods for antibiotic assays are not widely available often because special facilities and equipment is required. Thus gentamicin may be rapidly and accurately assayed by use of radiolabelled reagents [17] providing that facilities for handling and counting radioactive materials are available. Noone *et al.* [18] assayed aminoglycosides by measuring the inhibition of urease activity in a strain of *Proteus*. Although producing a result in under two hours, the method is technically time-consuming.

An immunological technique for the assay of aminoglycoside antibiotics and several other drugs, e.g. theophylline, has recently been introduced by Syva Diagnostics Ltd., under the trade name EMIT (Enzyme Mediated Immunoassay Technique). This system is readily automated and will, hopefully, become widely used for the assay of several antibiotics as well as other drugs.

Other chemical techniques, for example the use of high pressure liquid chromatography for the assay of antituberculous drugs, are available in specialized centres.

9.12 Principles of chemotherapy

The aim of chemotherapy is to eliminate an invading pathogen by means of antimicrobial agents. Within an extremely short period of human history chemotherapy has become a very complicated medical discipline. This complication is due partially to the large number of antimicrobial substances now available and partially to the very complex interactions between the host, the pathogen, the commensal organisms and the administered agent. Although the laboratory can offer valuable assistance, it must be realized that any investigations are, by necessity, carried out in a very artificial system which bears little resemblance to the clinical situation.

Figure 9.3 illustrates some of the interactions. The host and pathogens interact, the outcome of the interaction being determined by the

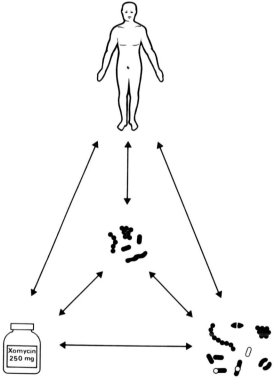

Fig. 9.3 Schematic representation of the interactions between the patient, the pathogens, commensal organisms and antibiotics (for details see text).

effectiveness of the immune response. As outlined above, the response to chemotherapy is very dependent on the nature of the immune reaction. The antimicrobial agents will hopefully destroy the pathogens but in some cases pathogens destroy the antibiotic by producing lactamases and other anti-biotic-destroying enzymes. In addition, host–antimicrobial agent interactions must be considered. The host affects the agent by variations in the rate of absorption, metabolic inactivation and excretion and by binding to proteins. Conversely, antimicrobial agents affect the host by causing various toxic side effects. Furthermore, antimicrobial agents modify the delicate balance between the host and his population of commensal organisms which themselves affect invading pathogens and may produce antibiotic-inactivating enzymes.

It is against this complicated biological background that a course of antimicrobial chemotherapy must be planned.

Space does not permit a full discussion of such therapy as this would require a whole textbook, and indeed such textbooks are available [14]. It must always be remembered that the administration of an antibiotic to a patient upsets a carefully balanced-microenvironment, sometimes with unfortunate consequences. Furthermore, indiscriminate use of broad-spectrum antibiotics leads to the selection of multiresistant organisms. The golden rule in antibiotic therapy is: if in doubt, ask the microbiologist. That is why he is there!

9.13 The future

Microbiology differs from all other branches of medicine in that it is concerned with the interaction between man and other elements of the living biosphere. Thus attention must be paid to both the 'seed' (the micro-organisms) and the 'soil' (the host) both of which are subject for continual change. Micro-organisms vary in their virulence and in their distribution. Some diseases such as diphtheria are virtually unknown in Europe while others, Legionnaire's disease for instance, make their appearance while yet others, including tuberculosis, rear their ugly heads as soon as attention is diverted away from them. New techniques will be developed adding to the range, complexity (and cost) of laboratory investigations while, hopefully, computerization will simplify the reporting and interpretation of results. New antibiotics will enable life-threatening infections to be treated more easily but will demand a greater skill and understanding from the medical profession in their use. At the same time, invasive and immunosuppressive techniques are bound to increase thereby affording more opportunites for infection by organisms normally regarded as being environmental saprophytes.

No amount of vaccines or antibiotics can erect a barrier between man and the other occupants of the biosphere. The task of the clinical microbiologist is to ensure that in all ecological battles man emerges the victor.

9.14 Summary

Clinical microbiology, in common with other medical disciplines, is a subject of ever increasing complexity. This is in part due to the changing nature of infectious processes encountered, particularly in hospital practice. As the classical pathogens decrease in incidence, the number of unusual opportunist infections are increasing. In order to be able to perform the numerous and complex investigations now available for studying infectious processes, the microbiological services consist not only of local and regional laboratories but also of specialized reference centres.

Following the clinical examination, the next step is the collection of the necessary specimens and their transport to the relevant laboratory. This step is the most crucial of the investigation as the validity and usefulness of all laboratory studies are dependent on the quality of the specimens.

Micro-organisms causing disease vary enormously in their biological properties and thus require a wide range of microscopical and cultural techniques for their detection, isolation and identification. Pathogenic micro-organisms include aerobic and anaerobic bacteria, mycobacteria, mycoplasmas, chlamydiae, rickettsiae, coxiellae, fungi, protozoa and viruses. An understanding of the biological properties of these organisms is essential if the pitfalls and limitations of the techniques used for their isolation are to be appreciated.

In addition to microscopical and cultural techniques, the detection of antibodies and, more usefully, rising titres of antibodies to known pathogens is often of considerable clinical usefulness. Many techniques have been developed for detecting and quantitating specific antibodies. These include agglutination of bacteria or antigen-coated particles, immunodiffusion, neutralization, complement fixation, radioimmunoassay and enzyme-lined immunosorbent assay (ELISA). Immunological techniques are also used to detect the presence of pathogens in clinical specimens either microscopically using fluorescein-conjugated antisera (immunofluorescence) or by countercurrent immunoelectrophoresis (CIE). Delayed hypersensitivity, particularly to mycobacteria and fungi causing systemic mycoses, is detectable by the use of skin testing reagents, although reagents currently available do not distinguish between sensitization and active disease.

The laboratory assists in the management of patients by determining the sensitivity or resistance of organisms to antimicrobial agents. In most cases a simple screening test for resistance is sufficient but in some circumstances an estimation of the minimal inhibitory or bactericidal concentrations of antibiotics to a bacterium is required. Levels of antibiotics in the patient's serum are determined either by bioassays or by chemical or immunological techniques (enzyme medicated immunoassay technique, EMIT) or by radioimmunoassay.

In conclusion, the microbiological services are able to provide a wide range of investigations to aid the diagnosis and management of infectious diseases. It is the role of the clinical microbiologist to assist the clinician to make the best possible use of these services.

References

1. Speller, D. C. E. and MacIver, A. G. (1971), Endocarditis caused by a *Coprinus* species: a fungus of the toadstool group. *J. Med. Microbiol.,* **4**, 370.
2. Cruickshank, R., Duguid, J. P. and Swain, R. H. A. (1968), *Medical Microbiology,* E. & S. Livingstone Ltd.
3. Williams, J. D. and Smith, H. (1979), Anaerobic infections – current problems and therapeutic approach. *J. Infection,* **1**, Supplement no. 1.
4. Stanford, J. L. and Grange, J. M. (1974), The meaning and structure of species as applied to mycobacteria. *Tubercle,* **55**, 143.
5. Grange, J. M. *et al.* (1978), The correlation of bacteriophage types of *Mycobacterium tuberculosis* with guinea-pig virulence and in-vitro indicators of virulence. *J. gen. Microbiol.,* **108**, 1.
6. McIntyre, M. (1978), Detection of capsulated *Haemophilus influenzae* in chest infections by counter current electrophoresis. *J. clin. path.,* **31**, 31.
7. Stanford, J. L., Revill, W. D. L., Gunthorpe, W. J. and Grange, J. M. (1975), The production and preliminary investigation of Burulin, a new skin test reagent for *Mycobaterium ulcerans* infection. *J. Hyg., Camb.,* **74**, 7.
8. Wilhelm, G. and Römer, C. (1977), An investigation of a newly isolated oligopeptide from *Mycobacterium tuberculosis* with antigenic properties specific for the diagnosis of tuberculosis. *Zbl. Bakt. Hyg., I. Abt. Orig. A.,* **239**, 379.
9. Grange, J. M. (1980), *Mycobacterial Diseases.* Edward Arnold, London.
10. Rook, G. A. W. (1978), Three forms of delayed skin-test reponse evoked by mycobacteria. *Nature,* **271**, 64.
11. Youmans, G. P. (1975), Relation between delayed hypersensitivity and immunity in tuberculosis. *Am. Rev. resp. Dis.* **111**, 109.
12. Urbaniak, S. J. *et al.* (1978), Tests of immune function. In: *Handbook of Experimental Immunology,* (ed. D. M. Weir) 3rd edn, Ch. 47.
13. Lenzini, L., Rottoli, P. and Rottoli, L. (1977), The spectrum of human tuberculosis. *Clin. exp. Immunol.,* **27**, 230.
14. Garrod, L. P., Lambert, H. P. and O'Grady, F. (1973), *Antibiotics and Chemotherapy.* 4th edn, Churchill Livingstone.
15. Howie, J. W. (1962), Recent developments in chemotherapy. *Lancet,* **i**, 1137.
16. Tsukamura, M. (1961), Variation and heredity of mycobacteria with special reference to drug resistance. *Jap. J. Tuberc.,* **9**, 43.
17. Smith, D. H., van Otto, B. and Smith, A. L. (1972), A rapid chemical assay for gentamicin. *New Engl. J. Med.,* **286**, 583.
18. Noone, P., Pattison, J. R. and Samson, D. (1971), Simple, rapid method for assay of aminoglycoside and antibiotics. *Lancet,* **ii**, 16.

CHAPTER TEN

Immunology

M. E. H. Turner-Warwick and P. L. Haslam

The object of this chapter is to summarize the current place of immunological tests in the investigation of lung diseases. Only the principles of the tests will be mentioned and the details regarding the concepts as well as the actual techniques should be obtained from standard immunological references [1–5]. The purpose of immunological investigation in a clinical context is either to define causes of disease in man or to obtain further evidence regarding pathogenesis. The research aspects of immunological investigation will not be discussed except insofar as they may have practical implications in the near future.

One of the great difficulties in any discussion upon immunology is to impose limits to the subject. Immunology merges into mechanisms of inflammation and inflammation is the basis of the majority of diseases. The present discussion will be limited to the following subjects:

1. Measurement of total immunoglobulins.
2. Specific antibodies to extrinsic antigens.
3. Autoantibodies in disease.
4. Circulating immune complexes.
5. Tissue immune complexes.
6. Complement.
7. Lymphocytes.
8. Macrophages and lung lavage.
9. Immunological mediators.

Three major groups of immunological systems are used in clinical practice.

(a) *In vitro* measurement of immunological factors can be used to assess the situation *in vivo* without antigenic challenge, e.g. measurement of total immunoglobulins, lymphocyte populations, the detection of circulating or tissue-bound immune complexes, complement conversion products or activation of alveolar macrophages.

(b) Immunological tests can be performed to assess responses to antigenic challenge *in vivo*, e.g. prick or intradermal skin tests, nasal and bronchial challenge tests.

(c) *In vitro* antigenic challenge tests can be undertaken to detect specific interactions with antibodies or cells obtained from the patient.

10.1 Antigens

Clearly all tests involved in (b) or (c) listed above depend for their reliability upon standard potent antigens and currently these are rarely available. This single fact has been and continues to be a major drawback to the application of immunological techniques in clinical practice.

There are many explanations for the lack of standardization of antigens used. On many occasions a crude product, for example *Dermatophagoides pteronyssinus* is known to provoke respiratory symptoms but contains a large number of potential antigens, many of which are likely to be relevant. Indeed the exact nature of the specific antigen or antigens within crude extracts is often unknown and cannot therefore be standardized. Attempts have, of course, been made to do this. Such an example is the standardization of the total protein or polysaccharide components of pollens and fungi. Different batches of soluble antigens can be reacted with a standard and potent antiserum using methods such as crossed electrophoresis (Fig. 10.1). In this the soluble antigens are first electrophoresced in agar in one dimension to separate the components, the strip of agar is cut out and placed against an agar strip containing antiserum and electrophoresis performed at right angles to the original; the antigens spread into the antiserum containing agar and react to create a series of precipitin peaks. In this way the uniformity of antigen content of different batches can be checked. The method is not, however, suitable for particulate antigens. Some antigens are extremely difficult to handle *in vitro* and complexed products have been developed for clinical tests. For example, platinum salts have been attached to albumin-coated Sepharose beads to enable their use in a radioallergosorbent test (RAST) to measure specific IgE antibodies in sensitized workers [6].

Particulate antigens such as extracts of whole organisms are usually standardized crudely on a weight/volume basis.

The purpose of this discussion is to emphasize that with current limitations on standardization of antigenic preparations, results from different centres are likely to vary widely and understanding of these laboratory limitations is essential if the physician is not to be misled. A good example of this problem is the wide difference in results obtained from many parts of the world on the frequency of bronchopulmonary aspergillosis based on identifying precipitating antibody in the serum of patients under investigation.

10.2 Measurement of total immunoglobulins

The standard method for measuring the well recognized classes of IgG, IgM,

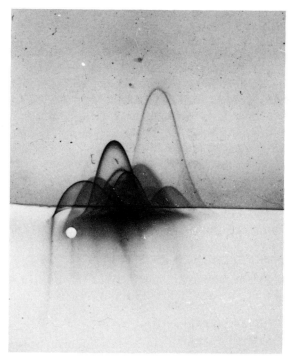

Fig. 10.1 Multiple immunoprecipitation arc indicating spectrum of antigens in an *Aspergillus fumigatus* serodiagnostic extract (Bencard Allergy Division, Beecham's) after cross-electrophoresis against a standard pool of Aspergilloma sera containing multiple antibodies.

IgA and IgD is by the single radial immunodiffusion Mancini method. Test serum is added to wells cut in agar containing antibodies directed against individual immunoglobulins. Precipitin rings develop, the sizes of which are related to the amount of immunoglobulin present; the ring size is referred to a standard curve relating ring sizes to known amounts of immunoglobulin.

Measurement of the total levels of individual classes of immunoglobulins in the serum is particularly important to detect hypogammaglobulinaemia which may affect one or all classes in patients with repeated infection often of the upper or lower respiratory tracts. Correct diagnosis is exceedingly important because of the opportunities for introducing replacement therapy. There are many varied combinations of immunoglobulin defects [7]. The clinical significance of reduced total IgA is much debated. On the one hand subjects with absent IgA may remain entirely healthy and on the other it is the only defect detectable in a number of patients with recurrent chest infections. Under the latter circumstances it is difficult to avoid the conclusion that the two are related. Some patients with a low serum IgA respond to fresh, frozen plasma perhaps because of an as yet unidentified but associated defect [8].

Total levels of IgA can also be measured in the saliva or sputum by using dialysed, lyophilysed and reconstituted samples on special Mancini plates containing adjusted amounts of antibody to precipitate optimally with the small amounts of IgA found in the secretions. In general, measurements of the total IgA in secretions has not proved to be of great clinical value. When serum IgA is very low it is usually also absent in the secretions. Only very rarely has absent IgA in the secretions been found in association with normal serum levels and vice versa.

Increased amounts of total immunoglobulin classes have provided only limited information. Elevation of IgG, IgM and IgA are frequently found in chronic bacterial infections of the lung. Selective increases are found in some of the connective tissue disorders and in cryptogenic fibrosing alveolitis but there is no consistent pattern. In sarcoidosis IgM and IgA are particularly raised in the more active stages and tend to fall with spontaneous remission but the association is not close enough to be a useful indication of activity in assessment of the individual case. High levels of IgM have been found in patients with cryptogenic fibrosing alveolitis and digital vasculitis but the explanation is unknown.

Measurement of the total serum IgE is more difficult because it occurs in such very small amounts (i.e. less than 500 ng/dl). Several methods are available including the radioimmunosorbent test (RIST) the stages of which are illustrated in Fig. 10.2. Other methods have been evolved which avoid using radiolabelled material such as the enzyme-linked immunosorbent test (ELISA). In this the antibody to IgE is linked not to a radiolabel but to a suitable enzyme which can then be measured quantitatively after exposure to the relevant substrates (see Chapter 9). A modified Mancini method has also been developed where the ring developed between antigen and antibody can be identified by layering it with a radiolabelled antibody to IgE which can subsequently be developed by autoradiography and measured.

Total IgE increases moderately up to about 600–1500 IU/ml in about 60% of atopic asthmatics and especially those with eczema and bronchopulmonary aspergillosis. It probably has little value in the routine management of individual atopic patients. It is however valuable in the differential diagnosis of pulmonary eosinophilia. In bronchopulmonary aspergillosis the total IgE is in general higher than in extrinsic asthma (often around 2000–5000 IU/ml) where the blood eosinophilia is around 1.00/nl. By contrast in cryptogenic pulmonary eosinophilia the bood eosinophil count is higher (2–10/nl) but the the total IgE relatively less, usually less than 1000 IU/ml. In florid helminth infestations the total IgE count is exceedingly high (up to 10 000 IU/ml) and the eosinophil count is also greatly raised. Thus the relative response

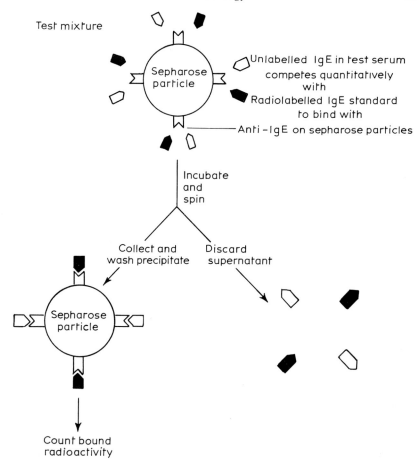

Fig. 10.2 Stages of the radioimmunosorbent test (RIST) for the measurement of total serum IgE. The counts of radioactivity vary quantitatively according to the amounts of unlabelled IgE in test sera. These are expressed as International Units of IgE by reference to the inhibition produced by reference standards containing known amounts of unlabelled IgE.

between IgE and blood eosinophil counts can be of considerable diagnostic importance in cases presenting wtih eosinophilia and pulmonary infiltrates.

10.3 Specific antibodies to extrinsic antigens in serum

Measurement of specific antibodies of different classes requires different techniques depending on the amount and character of antibody present. Probably the easiest method of measuring IgG (and IgM) specific antibody is by precipitation and in clinical practice the double diffusion method of Ouchterlony is standard. In this, serum containing test antibody is placed in a well cut in agar with antigen in a neighbouring well. As the reactants diffuse outwards from the respective wells, precipitation occurs at the line of equivalence which can be easily demonstrated using a protein stain, such as Coomassie blue. While the principle of this test is straightforward, the exact size and distance between the rings and the concentrations of antigen are all critical to produce the best result. Even under carefully controlled circumstances, the precipitin line may be delicate and quite difficult to see. Care has to be taken about the specificity of the reaction because C-reactive protein which is a non-immunoglobulin constituent of serum which tends to increase in acute or chronic inflammation can interact to form non-specific precipitates with C-polysaccharide substance present in fungal and bacterial antigens and with various antigens having a high negative charge. Interaction with C-substance can be prevented by the addition of citric acid to the agar. Another elegant way of ensuring specificity in the case of IgG antibodies and highly anionic antigens such as DNA is to combine the double diffusion principle with countercurrent electrophoresis. The antibody is placed in the anodal well and electrophoresis performed to cause negative drift migration of the IgG antibodies towards the cathode. The antigen is placed in the cathodal well and electrophoresis continued to cause its anodal migration to meet the IgG antibody. The specific precipitation occurs between antigen and antibody which has been thus separated from other serum components (Fig. 10.3). Antibody has to be present in substantial

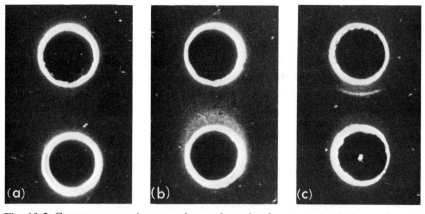

Fig. 10.3 Countercurrent immunoelectrophoresis of test sera in the lower (anodal wells) against DNA (20 µg/ml) in the upper (cathodal) wells showing: (a) a negative appearance, (b) non-specific precipitation only, (c) an additional distinct specific immunoprecipitation line due to DNA antibodies in test serum.

amounts to form precipitates and it is therefore a fairly insensitive test. Further, not all antibodies form good precipitates with antigen and in this case other tests have to be used.

The detection of specific precipitating antibodies is particularly useful in suggesting possible causes of disease in patients with suspected extrinsic allergic alveolitis due to a variety of organic dusts, especially due to fungi and animal proteins. However, detection of precipitins is usually an indication of exposure and not necessarily of disease. For instance, 20% of farmers are reported to have precipitins to mouldy hay without evidence of disease and 40% of healthy pigeon breeders are also found to have precipitins. A much closer correlation between precipitins and disease has, however, been reported amongst budgerigar fanciers developing disease and precipitins are rarely found in healthy exposed individuals.

Detection of precipitins is valuable in the diagnosis of bronchopulmonary aspergillosis although the precipitin lines using standard antigens are few in number and can be difficult to detect. This contrasts with the much greater number of easily identifiable precipitin lines seen in patients with aspergillomas. For this reason it is useful in clinical practice to report the number of lines visible as well as their presence. Serial precipitin tests can be useful after exposure to antigen has apparently been withdrawn or following resection of aspergillomas. However, disappearance of precipitin lines is a crude method of quantitation and is therefore of limited value.

Agglutination tests involve attaching antigen to the surface of a visible particle such as latex, bentonite or a suitable erythrocyte and reacting this with test serum. These tests are simple and more sensitive than precipitation and are quantitative. They also can be used when antibody is not precipitating in type. Agglutination tests have been developed and used for quantitative studies in patients with avian protein hypersensitivity and for detecting bacterial antibodies. Study of the latter is occasionally of value in certain patients with recurrent infections where the total amounts of immunoglobulin classes are normal but where there is a qualitative defect and specific antibodies to infecting agents are not made. Thus patients have been identified with repeated staphylococcal infections with normal total immunoglobulins and immunoglobulin classes but in whom antistaphylococcal antibodies are absent. Analogous tests have been employed to study patients following test immunization with tetanus toxoid. Agglutination tests have also been developed to detect IgM antibodies to tuberculosis as a diagnostic test of active disease. Unfortunately, the application of this test is not straightforward and there are too many false positive and false negative results to make the test reliable. The reason for this limitation is probably due to the preparation of antigen and developmental work continues in many laboratories.

A modification of the agglutination test has been developed as a haemagglutination inhibition (HIA) test which is of value in clinical virology. Selected viruses have the property to agglutinate erythrocytes directly. This reaction can be inhibited by specific antibody if this is present in test sera as in the case of HIA test for influenza and rubella antibody. Fourfold or greater rises in HIA titre between acute and convalescent sera are indicative of recent infection or vaccination.

Complement fixation tests depend on the principle that many antigens when combining with antibody also fix complement. If this is added in a standard dose the amount of free complement is reduced and less is available to cause lysis of subsequently added antibody-coated red cells. This is a sensitive and quantitative test provided that the antibody is complement-fixing in type, and that other substances such as immune complexes are not present in the serum which fix added complement in the absence of the test antigen and which render the test unusable. Such sera are termed anticomplementary.

Complement fixation tests are used routinely to detect recent viral infection. They are also used to identify fungal disease, such as coccidioidomycosis, histoplasmosis and cryptococcosis because such antibodies are only present in active disease. Complement fixing antibodies are also useful in detecting living helminth infestation, such as *Echinococcus* and *Toxocara canis*.

Solid phase radioimmunoassay has been developed as a special method when antigens may be inappropriate for conventional tests and where a very sensitive test is required. However, this is not usually the case in clinical practice and the test system is still mainly used as a research procedure. It has potential, for example, if specific antibody in secretions needs to be measured.

Specific IgE antibodies can also be measured but again special methods have to be used because of the minute quantities present. The RAST method has been used but other analogous methods not involving radio labels have now been developed. The best known of these is the ELISA method.

Tests for specific IgE correlate very closely with prick skin test results so that when the latter are feasible there is little practical advantage of measuring specific IgE. If skin test material is not available as in the case of some of the special chemical agents relating to occupational asthmas, e.g. platinum salts and isothiocyanates, then these methods have important clinical value in diagnosis (see Chapter 17).

10.3.1 Skin tests

Recent interpretation of early studies has now demonstrated that immediate skin test responses to antigens introduced by prick testing in the human skin represent an IgE-mediated reaction [9, 10] and the tests correlate very closely with the amount of specific IgE in the serum [11]. In clinical investigation of allergy, skin tests provide an extremely simple and rapid method of demonstrating *in vivo* sensitization. Positive responses to a range of common environmental allergens, including house dust, pollens, animal danders, food and fungi, suggest that the individual has an increased propensity to develop IgE antibodies (i.e. he is an 'atopic subject'). This information is useful in the diagnosis of less typical cases of airflow obstruction, because in some phases of asthma, airflow obstruction is not reversible with β-agonists and the identification of atopy increases the likelihood (but does not prove) that asthma may be the underlying condition and that with more intensive treatment reversibility may be achieved. Routine skin testing in known asthmatics is useful because it may suggest agents to which the patient is sensitive and prompt further questioning. Skin tests *per se* do *not* indicate the cause of respiratory symptoms and this distinction should always be made to the patient. Demonstrable positive reactions are often useful at an educational level having obtained, in addition, a positive history. Under these circumstances, the patient may be encouraged to undertake better environmental control of their bedding, for instance, or by removal of pets.

Where there is a history of seasonal asthma and/or hayfever, together with an isolated response to pollen, results of specific desensitization may be particularly good [12]. However, blunderbuss desensitization to all positive reactants is of no proven value and in the authors' view should not be undertaken.

Late skin reactions occurring after 4–8 h may be mediated by more than one mechanism. Pepys *et al.* [13] demonstrated a close relationship between positive late 6–8 h skin tests using certain antigens especially *A. fumigatus* and avian proteins and specific IgG precipitating antibodies. Upon this basis he suggested that these reactions might represent an IgG-mediated Arthus response. More recent evidence suggests that IgE responses alone may induce a late reaction under certain circumstances [14] and injection of certain immunopharmacological mediators such as kallikreins will also induce a response having the same characteristics. Thus pharmacological mediators liberated both from mast cells and possibly from other cells of inflammation, e.g. platelets and granulocytes, may also be responsible. Late skin reactions (whatever the pathogenesis) may nevertheless be of considerable clinical value in diagnosis of organic dust and fungal hypersensitivity disease where prick tests are negative and precipitins not demonstrable. Late skin tests are mainly seen on intradermal testing. Prick tests should always be done first. If the positive reaction is less than about 3 mm induration, it is safe to proceed to an intradermal injection of 1/10 of the strength used in the prick test. If the test is negative it may be repeated using increasing strengths. In the authors' experience, late skin reactions have been useful in suggesting a possible aetiology for cases showing chronic, especially upper zone, shadowing, with or without evidence of bronchial wall thickening, in which a diagnosis of bronchopulmonary aspergillosis or extrinsic allergic alveolitis is suspected but where precipitins and prick tests are negative.

10.3.2 Bronchial challenge tests (See Chapter 11)

In an immunological context, these tests demonstrate that an agent is able to cause changes in the bronchi but it does not necessarily demonstrate pathogenetic mechanisms. An immediate reaction may closely parallel the immediate skin test and it is for this reason bronchial challenge tests are rarely indicated when the prick test is positive; under these circumstances a mast cell mediated pathogenesis may be presumed. However, an immediate bronchoconstriction also occurs in individuals exposed to irritants of many types and an immunological event cannot be necessarily presumed. There is much greater controversy over the pathogenesis of the late airways obstruction and the same issues are under current discussion as were mentioned above in Section 10.3.1.

Inhalation challenge tests are particularly valuable in the demonstration of specific causes in relation to occupational asthma, where appropriate skin test solutions are not available. By reproducing the job undertaken at work, challenge tests may be devised where exposure involves fumes, aerosolized droplets or chemicals, none of which can readily be prepared as specific skin test agents. The nature of these agents also makes demonstration of specific antibody in the serum difficult or impossible. Examples of agents identified by inhalation which cause respiratory symptoms in the absence of suitable skin or serological tests include colophony, formalin, various hardwood, flux, ethanolamine and isothiocyanate (see Chapter 17).

Late restrictive defects can also be demonstrated by inhalation challenge and this may also confirm the cause of respiratory symptoms in occupational exposures where skin or serological tests are not feasible. A recent example of such a case is the identification of humidifier lung [15].

10.4 Autoantibodies in disease

Antibodies to cell nuclei (antinuclear antibodies (ANA)) and to altered gammaglobulin (rheumatoid factors (RF)) are the principal autoantibodies studied in relation to lung disease but antibodies to collagen will also be mentioned.

10.4.1 Antinuclear antibody (ANA)

ANA is usually detected using an immunofluorescent technique where test serum is layered on to a suitable substrate of nucleated cells such as a frozen section of rat or mouse liver, and a fluorescent labelled antibody to human globulin is subsequently applied. When viewed under ultraviolet light the nuclei fluoresce at the sites of attached antibody. Thus a number of distinct patterns can be identified as illustrated (Fig. 10.4). Dilutions of serum can be applied in the same test so that a semiquantitative estimate is made.

ANA often in high titre is found in a number of connective tissue disorders involving the lungs, especially systemic lupus erythematosus (SLE). Lower titres are found in about 45% of cases of cryptogenic fibrosing alveolitis reported in some series [16] but not in others [17]. ANA in very low titre of around 1/10 is found in some cases of asbestosis (about 23%) and coal miner's pneumoconiosis, and higher titres in some cases of accelerated silicosis, in the latter two instances relating to the radiographic extent of disease. ANA is, however, much less frequently present in certain other forms of pulmonary fibrosis such as sarcoidosis, extrinsic allergic alveolitis and radiation pneumonitis, so that it has some general diagnostic value in distinguishing the more likely causes of pulmonary fibrosis. Nuclei contain a number of distinct antigens, and antibodies appear to be directed against different antigenic components in different disorders. For instance, antibodies to double stranded DNA demonstrated either by countercurrent electrophoresis or by radiolabelled DNA binding tests are found especially in SLE but are much less frequent in other types of connective tissue disorders in which ANA by immunofluorescence is present. Antibodies to single stranded DNA (detected by the same basic methods) are, however, also found in the latter conditions. In SLE, antibodies to deoxyribonucleoprotein are found (these can be demonstrated by immunofluorescence using deoxyribonucleoprotein smears) and these correspond to the presence of LE cells. Such antibodies are not usually seen in other connective tissue disorders of the lung and neither are LE cells found. Apart from these general statements it must be emphasized that a number of cases have been seen having clinical criteria for SLE including the presence of LE cells in which the double stranded DNA binding test has been negative. It appears that the DNA binding tests are more specific for some forms of SLE especially when the kidneys are involved but may be absent when other organs are predominantly affected. In our experience many patients with predominant thoracic involvement have negative DNA binding and it cannot therefore be used as a pathognomonic test in pleuro-pulmonary SLE. Titres however tend to fluctuate with activity of the disease.

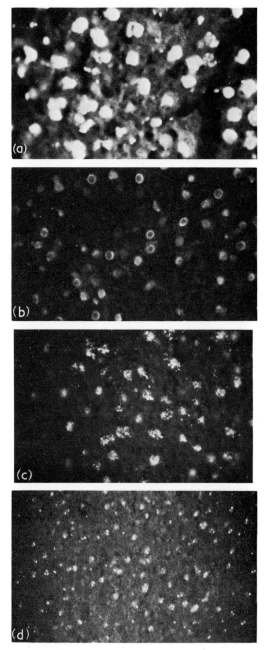

Fig. 10.4 Patterns of immunofluorescent staining attributable to attachment of antinuclear antibodies from test sera to the nuclei of rat liver cells using indirect immunofluorescent staining: (a) diffuse (b) membrane (c) speckled (d) nucleolar staining patterns.

ANA having a speckled pattern on immunofluorescence and representing a soluble nuclear antigen has been identified in a high proportion of cases with systemic sclerosis [18] and this is also the case when the lungs are involved. However, speckled antibody is found in other cases including cryptogenic fibrosing alveolitis (CFA) and Sjögren's syndrome, so that it cannot be regarded as pathognomonic of systemic sclerosis.

The presence of autoantibodies in CFA has no detectable influence on prognosis or steroid responsiveness [19] and is only helpful as a general diagnostic pointer in the clinical context.

10.4.2 IgM rheumatoid factor (RF)

IgM RF measured by an agglutination test with sheep cells coated with rabbit gammaglobulin as antigen (Fig. 10.5) or by agglutination of gammaglobulin coated latex particles is found particularly in cases when diffuse lung shadowing is associated with polyarthritis and is also found in about 15% of lone CFA [16].

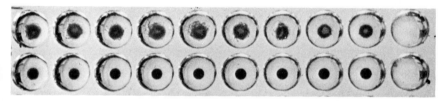

Fig. 10.5 Rose-Waaler sheep cell agglutination test demonstrating: in the upper row, positive agglutination of sheep red cells coated with rabbit gamma globulin which indicates the presence of rheumatoid factor in a patient's serum to a dilution (titre) of 1/256 (the wells contain doubling dilutions of the patient's serum from left to right). The lower row shows absence of agglutination using a test serum without rheumatoid factor.

It is also found in coal miner's pneumoconiosis especially those with typical and atypical Caplan's syndrome. RF in CFA is closely associated with the presence of circulating immune complexes measured by a C_1q binding method (see below) and this is also found in bronchiectasis.

The detection of RF is, like ANA, more common in some forms of interstitial lung disease (e.g. CFA, SLE, and Sjögren's syndrome) than others (e.g. sarcoidosis and extrinsic allergic alveolitis) and is thus of some diagnostic value. However, cases with overlapping immunological features exist so that the distinction is not a highly reliable one.

Antibodies to collagen were identified many years ago by Burrell and his associates [20]. While they have been detected in a wide range of lung diseases using a complicated and difficult test of antiglobulin consumption their practical clinical value is to detect a glomerular basement membrane antibody (GBMA) (possibly type IV collagen) as a diagnostic feature of Goodpasture's syndrome. The test for circulating GBMA is not yet available for general use but good results have now been reported from at least two centres using a radioimmunoassay [21].

10.5 Circulating immune complexes

More than thirty different tests have been developed in an attempt to measure immune complexes in the circulation. Unfortunately so far a good correlation between the various tests does not exist. This may in part be due to technical factors and in part because they vary in the fundamental principles employed, and in sensitivity and measure complexes of different type and size. A widely used test which has been explored in a preliminary way in lung disease is the C_1q binding test. In this, radiolabelled C_1q is added to test serum and any complexed globulins precipitated by polyethylene glycol; after washing, the amount of radiolabelled C_1q bound within the globulin precipitate is counted and expressed as a percentage binding (Fig. 10.6).

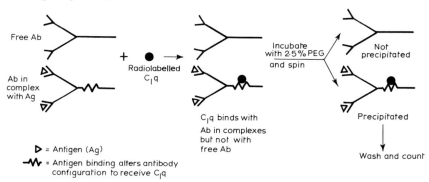

Fig. 10.6 Principle of the polyethylene glycol (PEG) C_1q binding test for measurement of circulating immune complexes.

Circulating immune complexes have been demonstrated in a number of lung disorders. These include particularly the connective tissue diseases SLE, rheumatoid arthritis and Sjögren's syndrome and also in more than 50% of patients with CFA. The C_1q binding test has proved negative in our own studies of hypersensitivity pneumonitis and sarcoidosis and if this is confirmed then it may be of some general diagnostic value, although other tests have indicated that circulating immune complexes of some type may occur in sarcoidosis [22]. Of greater potential interest are the possible therapeutic implications in an attempt to treat these cases with plasmaphoresis but this, so far, remains a suggestion for the future.

The immune complexes demonstrated in bronchiectasis may reflect spill-over of antigen into the circulation but the clinical significance of this is unknown; it may however explain the association of bronchiectasis with rheumatoid arthritis. Circulating immune complexes have also occasionally been found in patients with ulcerative colitis and bronchiectasis and it has been suggested that antigen may reach the circulation through disorganized bowel mucosa.

10.6 Tissue immune complexes

Studies of lung biopsies using immunofluorescent techniques or electron microscopy enable the sites of deposition of antibody, complement or both to be identified. So far such evidence of immune complexes in the lung has been demonstrated in CFA [23–25], SLE [26], rheumatoid arthritis [27, 28], and one case of veno-occlusive disease [29]. A linear staining pattern of IgG deposit on pulmonary basement membrane has been demonstrated in Goodpasture's syndrome by Bierne *et al.* [30], and identification of such a pattern in biopsy material would be helpful in diagnosis, especially in view of the currently limited facilities for routine serological tests.

Dreisin *et al.* [24] have further suggested that cases in which they were able to identify complex deposition responded well to corticosteroids; these results, however, have not been confirmed by other workers. There have been one or two reports of deposits of complement in the lung in patients with acute extrinsic allergic alveolitis but these results too have not been confirmed. Moreover it is likely that biopsy material has to be obtained within a very short time from exposure to obtain such results so that their practical clinical value must remain in doubt.

When biopsy material is obtained for diagnostic purposes in patients with diffuse interstitial lung disease the opportunity should be taken for the sample to be studied for possible immune complexes using both immunofluorescence and electron microscopy. However, it has to be recognized at the present time that the results are very frequently negative.

10.7 Complement

Complement is a compound term which covers a group of proteins found in serum which interact in a series of enzymatic steps (the complement cascade), triggered often by the interaction of antigen with antibody (the classical pathway of complement activation) and also by certain agents including endotoxin and aggregated gammaglobulin which cause its activation through the alternative pathway. Complement plays several very important roles in inflammation. Completion of the cascade may result in cytotoxic effects through membrane damage to cells. If the target cell is an invading micro-organism this mechanism of action is protective; activation of complement components (especially C_3 and C_5) results in the generation of fragments which are anaphylotoxic and also highly chemotactic for neutrophils and eosinophils which in turn liberate enzymes promoting tissue damage. In this way complement is involved in amplification of inflammation and recruitment to the damaged area of cells with phagocytic properties. Complement products can also interact with complement receptors on the surface of certain cells, especially phagocytes, promoting cell functional activities.

Quantitative tests for total complement function using a standard haemolytic system, and quantitation of the major complement components (C_3 and C_4) using single radial immunodiffusion Mancini technique are within the capacity of most routine pathology laboratories. However, they have at present little practical value in diagnosis and staging of pulmonary disease or indicating prognosis. Reduced amounts of circulating complement have been shown to correlate with renal involvement (and prognosis) in SLE but in cases with pulmonary involvement kidneys are often not affected and complement levels of C_3 and CH_{50} are usually normal or elevated. Studies of other groups of lung disease in which circulating immune complexes have been suspected or demonstrated have also failed to show depleted levels, and it is possible that soluble complexes of this type contain relatively little complement. Complement levels have been shown to be low in pleural fluids in rheumatoid arthritis and in secondary carcinoma suggesting consumption of complement but these are not yet routine diagnostic tests and of course are not specific.

Detailed studies of complement components are usually limited to specialist laboratories and may be valuable in elucidating certain types of progressive chest infection where immune deficiency is suspected but in which immunoglobulin, lymphocyte and granulocyte defects cannot be identified. Cases with genetic defects in C_2 have been reported amongst patients with recurrent chest infections but are exceedingly rare.

10.8 Lymphocytes

Lymphocyte function is of central importance to normal defences and subtle defects of function are being identified in many types of lung disease, including recurrent infections, malnutrition, sarcoidosis [31], neoplasm [32] and some stages of hypersensitivity pneumonitis [33] and pneumoconiosis [34, 35]. Defects have also been implicated in the induction of atopy [36].

Many of the *in vitro* tests are difficult and time-consuming to perform accurately and their use is still mainly limited to research laboratories (see Chapter 12). Blood lymphocytes can be divided on the basis of a relatively simple rosetting technique which demonstrates different types of receptor sites on the cell membrane, into T (thymus-dependent cells) characterized by rosettes forming spontaneously with sheep erythrocytes (Fig. 10.7) and B (bursa equivalent cells) characterized by C_3b receptor sites on their surface demonstrated by red cells coated with antibody and complement or by surface immunoglobulins demonstrated by immunofluorescence. Of the total lymphocytes in peripheral blood about 60% are T cells and 20% B cells; 20% have no characteristic membrane marker and are termed null cells. Total lymphocyte numbers are reduced in a number of immune deficiency states, especially those affecting T cells; lymphocytes are also reduced by immunosuppressants and this effect predisposes to the range of opportunist lung infections occurring in these patients. T cells are also reduced in sarcoidosis [37]. The simplest *in vivo* test for T cell function is the performance of delayed skin tests to antigens to which most adults are normally sensitized. Several antigens should be used because it cannot be assumed all normal individuals have been exposed to all such agents. Those frequently used include purified protein derivative (PPD), *C. albicans*, trichophyton, mumps antigen and streptokinase. Unfortunately, all have their limitations. With control of tuberculosis in the

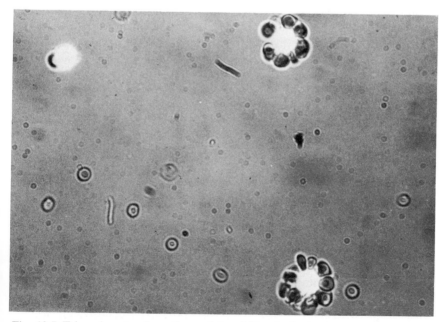

Fig. 10.7 T lymphocytes from the peripheral blood of a healthy donor volunteer distinguished from other lymphocytes by rosettes of attached sheep erythrocytes.

community there are increasing numbers of adults who have never been exposed to this micro-organism and negative reactions to PPD are becoming increasingly common. *C. albicans* induces an Arthus reaction (6 h response) in many patients and therefore a mixed late and delayed skin reaction can result with overlapping time features so that a positive reaction at 48 h does not necessarily reflect pure T cell activity. Mumps and streptokinase antigen are not always available. Further difficulties in interpretation have to be remembered. The size of reaction depends on the dose so that a full range of doses must be given if anergy is to be diagnosed reliably. In practice we have found that if three antigens are used, namely PPD 100 TU, 10 TU and 1 TU, *C. albicans* (whole cell preparation) w/v 1/1000 and 1/100, trichophyton w/v 1/1000, 98% of a series of hospital patients not suspected of having an immune deficiency showed a positive response of 4 mm or greater induration to at least one antigen. However, in order to complete such a battery of tests, properly observing each response over at least 48 hours, takes a minimum of six days.

In vitro tests of lymphocyte function are also time-consuming and often lack reproducibility. Lymphocyte transformation to a non-specific mitogen such as phytohaemagglutin (PHA) is probably the easiest to handle but only fairly gross defects will be detected. Demonstration of antigen-specific lymphocyte sensitization as a diagnostic aid remains a research tool. It has been suggested that such sensitization is a more specific diagnostic test in hypersensitivity pneumonitis than the detection of antibodies which are present also in many exposed healthy subjects. Such tests are limited to certain non-cytotoxic agents such as avian protein and are not in routine use. *In vitro* lymphocyte tests are also used in research to detect serum inhibitors of lymphocyte function (e.g. immune complexes and other agents). A PHA test on lymphocytes cultured in the presence of autologous or normal human serum is one example. Some apparent lymphocyte defects are shown in fact to be due to serum inhibitors when autologous and heterologous serum is used for cell culture. Such inhibitors have been shown in patients with bronchiectasis, lung infections and some tumours and may well in fact represent circulating immune complexes (see Chapter 12).

10.9 Macrophages and lung lavage

With the introduction of lung lavage, alveolar macrophages and other inflammatory cells can be obtained and studied in a number of ways. Thus differential cell counts may be performed using light microscopy (Fig. 10.8) and cell morphology may also be studied by electron and scanning electron microscopy; their phagocytic and secretory potential can be examined; their heterogeneity may also be studied using special histochemical stains, and their interaction with micro-organisms or particles examined, as well as their

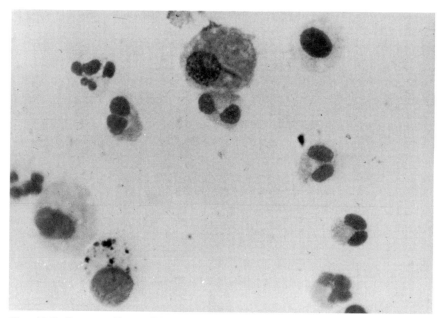

Fig. 10.8 Cytocentrifuge slide preparation of lung lavage cells from a patient with cryptogenic fibrosing alveolitis stained with May-Grünwald stain demonstrating the presence of macrophages, neutrophils and eosinophils (x 345.6).

interaction with other cells, such as macrophage/lymphocyte interactions. These studies are providing unique information about mechanisms of pathogenesis of lung disease and it may well be that simple tests will be developed which will select patients for specific treatment. Indeed preliminary findings in CFA suggest that lavage lymphocyte increases may predict corticosteroid responders while lavage eosinophil and/or neutrophil increases unaccompanied by increases in lymphocytes may predict nonresponders [38].

It is certain that the opportunity to obtain living tissue macrophages and inflammatory cells using a simple procedure on repeated occasions may well form the basis of entirely new practical tests for the future but currently these have not been defined. The research potential directed towards understanding pathogenesis is enormous and this is reflected in the explosion of publications over the last two years on this subject.

10.10 Immunological mediators

The development of radioimmune assay as well as other techniques now enables accurate measurement of minute amounts of inflammatory mediators. These include histamine, slow reacting substance of anaphylaxis (SRS-A), serotonin, eosinophil chemotactic factor of anaphylaxis (ECF-A), platelet aggregating factor (PAF) and prostaglandins. Further, with sputum and bronchoalveolar lavage available, inflammatory sites in the lung can now be sampled and the non-cellular components of lung injury can be analysed and monitored. The potential for developing tests upon which drug treatment may be planned and titrated is obviously exciting and offers clear therapeutic applications, as well as the theoretical but major interest in enabling us to understand the nature of pathogenesis in a way that is not yet available in most other fields of medicine.

10.11 Conclusions

While a number of simple tests (especially those detecting specific antibody) are of diagnostic value, and others reveal defects in normal immunological defence mechanisms which suggest the explanation for proneness to infection, it has to be admitted that much of the value of immunological studies to date has been in their contribution to the understanding of the nature of disease; thus their main value is often as a research tool. However, the logical link between understanding pathogenesis and designing therapy is such that understanding the immunological implications of disease in the individual remains of central importance.

References

1. Roitt, I. (1977), *Essential Immunology*, 3rd edn, Blackwell Scientific Publications Ltd., Oxford.
2. Hobart, M. J. and McConnell, I. (1976), *The Immune System: a Course on the Molecular and Cellular Basis of Immunity*, Blackwell Scientific Publications Ltd., Oxford.
3. Weir, D. M. (1978), *Handbook of Experimental Immunology*, 3rd edn, Blackwell Scientific Publications Ltd., Oxford.
4. Humphrey, J. H. and White, R. G. (1970), *Immunology for Students of Medicine*, 3rd edn, Blackwell Scientific Publications Ltd., Oxford.
5. Thompson, R. A. (1977), *Techniques in Clinical Immunology*, Blackwell Scientific Publications Ltd., Oxford.
6. Cromwell, O., Pepys, J., Parish, W. E. and Hughes, E. G. (1979), Specific IgE antibodies to platinum salts in sensitized workers. *Clin. Allergy*, **9**, 109–17.
7. Hobbs, J. R. (1970), Immunoglobulins in some diseases. *Br. J. hosp. Med.*, **3**, 669.
8. Cole, P. J. (1979), Unpublished observation.
9. Ishizaka, K. and Ishizaka, T. (1971), Mechanisms of reaginic hypersensitivity: a review. *Clin. Allergy*, **1**, 9–24.
10. Johansson, S. G. O. (1976), IgE antibodies in diagnosis of human allergy. In:

The Role of Immunological Factors in Infections, Allergic and Autoimmune Processes. (Eds R. F. Beers Jr. and E. G. Bassett), Raven Press, New York.

11. Stenius, B. and Wide, L. (1969), Reaginic antibody (IgE), skin, and provocation tests to *Dermatophagoides culinae* and house dust in respiratory allergy. *Lancet*, **ii**, 455.

12. McAllen, M. K. (1961), Bronchial sensitivity testing in asthma: an assessment of the effect of hyposensitization in house dust and pollen sensitive asthmatic subjects. *Thorax*, **16**, 30.

13. Pepys, J., Turner-Warwick, M., Dawson, P. and Hinson, K. W. F. (1968), Arthus (Type III) skin test reactions in man. Clinical and immunopathological features. In: *Allergology*. Excerpta Medica International Congress Series, 162. (Eds B. Rose, M. Richter, A. Sehon and A. W. Frankland), Excerpta Medica, Amsterdam, p. 221.

14. Dolovich, J. *et al.* (1973), Late cutaneous allergic responses in isolated IgE dependent reactions. *J. Allergy clin. Immunol.* **52**, 38.

15. Banaszak, E. F., Thiede, W. H. and Fink, J. N. (1970), Hypersensitivity pneumonitis due to contamination of an air conditioner. *New Engl. J. Med.* **283**, 271.

16. Turner-Warwick, M., Burrows, B. and Johnson, A. (1980), Cryptogenic fibrosing alveolitis: Part I. Clinical features and their influence on survival. *Thorax*, **35**, 171.

17. Crystal, R. G. *et al.* (1976), Idiopathic pulmonary fibrosis: clinical, histologic, radiographic, physiologic, scintigraphic, cytologic and biochemical aspects. *Ann. Intern. Med.* **85**, 769–88.

18. Rothfield, N. F. and Rodnan, G. P. (1968), Serum antinuclear antibodies in progressive systemic sclerosis (scleroderma). *Arthritis Rheum.* **11**, 607.

19. Turner-Warwick, M. Burrows, B. and Johnson, A. (1979b), Cryptogenic fibrosing alveolitis: Part II. Response to corticosteroid treatment and its effect on survival. *Thorax*, **35**, 593.

20. Burrell, R. G., Esber, H. J., Hagadorn, J. E., and Andrews, C. E. (1966). Specificity of lung reactive antibodies in human serum. *Am. Rev. resp. Dis.*, **94**, 743.

21. Lockwood, C. M., *et al.* (1976), Immunosuppression and plasma-exchange in the treatment of Goodpasture's syndrome. *Lancet*, **i**, 711–15.

22. Daniele, R. P., McMillan, L. J. Dauber, J. H. and Rossman, M. D. (1978), Immune complexes in sarcoidosis. *Chest*, **74**, 261–4.

23. Nagaya, H., Elmore, M. and Ford, C. D. (1973), Idiopathic interstitial pulmonary fibrosis. An immune complex disease? *Am. Rev. resp. Dis.*, **107**, 826.

24. Dreisin, R. B., Schwarz, M. I., Theofilopoulos, A. N. and Stanford, R. E. (1978), Circulating immune complexes in the idopathic interstitial pneumonias. *New Engl. J. Med.*, **298**, 353.

25. Turner-Warwick, M., Haslam, P. L. and Weeks, J. (1971), Antibodies in some chronic fibrosing lung diseases. 11. Immunofluorescent studies. *Clin. Allergy*, **1**, 209.

26. Turner-Warwick, M. (1974), Autoantibodies in allergic respiratory disease. In: *Progress in Immunology*, 11, Vol. 4., Clinical Aspects 1. (Eds L. Brent and J. Holborow), North Holland, Amsterdam, p. 283.

27. de Horatius, R. J., Abruzzo, J. L. and Williams, R. C. Jr. (1972), Immunofluorescent and immunologic studies of rheumatoid lung. *Arch. intern. Med.*, **129**, 441.

28. Turner-Warwick, M. (1969), Rheumatoid arthritis, rheumatoid factors, and lung disease. *Br. J. hosp. Med.*, **2**, 507.

29. Corrin, B. *et al.* (1974), Pulmonary veno-occlusion – an immune complex disease? *Virchows Arch. path. Anat. Histol.*, **364**, 81.

30. Beirne, G. J., Octaviano, G. N., Kopp, W. L. and Burns, R. O. (1968), Immunohistology of the lung in Goodpasture's syndrome. *Ann. intern. Med.*, **69**, 1207.

31. Mitchell, D. N. and Scadding, J. G. (1974), Sarcoidosis. State of the Art. *Am. Rev. resp. Dis.*, **110**, 774.

32. Holmes, E. C. and Golub, S. H. (1976), Immunologic defects in lung cancer patients. *J. thorac. cardiovasc. Surg.*, **71**, 161.

33. Haslam, P. L. *et al.* (1979), An immunological profile of patients with acute extrinsic allergic alveolitis: skin responses, lymphocyte studies, serology and bronchoalveolar lavage findings. In preparation.

34. Haslam, P. L., Lukoszek, A., Merchant, J. A. and Turner-Warwick, M. (1978), Lymphocyte responses to phytohaemagglutinin in patients with asbestosis and pleural mesothelioma. *Clin. exp. Immunol.*, **31**, 178–88.

35. Campbell, M. J., Wagner, M. M. F., Scott, M. P. and Brown, D. G. (1980), Sequential immunological studies in an asbestos exposed population. 11. Factors affecting lymphocyte function. *Clin . exp. Immunol.*, **39**, 176.

36. Soothill, J. F. *et al.* (1976), Predisposing factors and the development of reaginic allergy in infancy. *Clin. Allergy*, **6**, 305.

37. Daniele, R. P. and Rowlands, D. T. Jr. (1976), Lymphocyte subpopulations in sarcoidosis: correlation with disease activity and duration. *Ann. intern. Med.*, **85**, 593.

38. Haslam, P. L. *et al.* (1980), Broncho-alveolar lavage in pulmonary fibrosis: comparison of cells obtained with lung biopsy and clinical features. *Thorax*, **35**.

CHAPTER ELEVEN

Bronchial Challenge

M. C. F. Pain

11.1 Introduction

11.1.1 Scope and definition

As an investigative procedure, non-specific bronchial challenge is used to demonstrate that a particular subject at a particular time has heightened bronchial reactivity. Bronchial reactivity can be defined as the ability of the bronchial tree to alter acutely its effective airway diameter in response to some normal or abnormal stimulus. Since the intact bronchial tree in man normally exhibits some degree of bronchial reactivity, the importance of non-specific bronchial challenge tests arises from subjects who exhibit a marked degree of reactivity. In contrast to bronchial challenge with specific allergens, usually no conclusions can be made about causative relationships between the provoking agent and the production of clinical symptoms. Because many pulmonary conditions associated with reversible airways obstruction are aggravated in a non-specific way by many inhaled substances, non-specific bronchial challenge tests may actually have more clinical relevance and are certainly less prone to spontaneous fluctuations.

The aim of this chapter is to provide the practical information for setting up non-specific bronchial challenge testing, to indicate the dangers and precautions and to discuss the clinical implications of the results of testing. It is not intended as a review of the whole field of bronchial reactivity, an area with a rapidly increasing literature. Fortunately several excellent reviews of the general topic have recently appeared and the reader is referred to these for a more detailed discussion [1, 2, 4].

11.1.2 Background

The concept of an oversensitive bronchial tree as part of the pathogenesis of bronchial asthma is an old one and a history of asthmatic attacks in response to a variety of inhaled stimuli has been used as evidence of the asthmatic state. Deliberate provocation of wheezy attacks by challenge seems to have developed from experimental pharmacology and the study of respiratory changes in man in response to parasympathomimetic aerosols was well studied by Dautrebande [3] and other European workers by the early 1940s. The suggestion that a non-specific reaction to a cholinergic agent might be a useful index of asthma was made regularly in the non-English literature but it certainly was not taken up with any enthusiasm and World War II probably postponed any familiarity with this prewar work. Although the original observation that derivatives of acetylcholine could cause acute asthma was first noted in the American literature in 1932, by the end of 1945, references were starting to appear noting the effect of histamine administration on patients with asthma and suggesting that procedure as a useful one for studying the relative efficiency of the newly available antihistamines. In English speaking centres, the publications of Itkin and Parker did much to reawaken interest in methacholine as a satisfactory provoking agent and since that time the number of articles dealing with bronchial challenge has increased very significantly. A considerable experience has developed with histamine and methacholine aerosols and more recently with exercise stress testing. Exercise testing and its role in bronchial hyper-reactivity assessment is discussed in Chapter 4.

11.2 Provoking agents

The inhalation of many substances has been found to cause an acute increase in airways resistance and some of these have been used to study airway dynamics in animals and man (Table 11.1). They broadly divide into non-specific agents whose action is presumed to be mainly an irritative one and non-specific agents with known pharmacological actions on the bronchial tree. Dust particles, smoke, extremes of temperature, citric acid, urea, hypertonic saline are examples of the former and histamine, 5-hydroxytryptamine, acetylcholine and its stable derivatives, carbachol and methacholine are examples of the latter. In practical terms, by far the commonest agents used for non-specific bronchial provocation tests are histamine and methacholine.

11.2.1 Histamine

Its wide distribution in plants and animals, its potent pharmacology and actions on many organs, its central role as a mediator in the allergic reaction makes histamine aerosol inhalation a most interesting phenomenon. The action of histamine inhalation on the bronchial tree is thought to result from a combined effect on capillaries allowing endo-bronchial oedema formation, contraction of smooth bronchial muscle and a direct irritant action stimulating vagal reflex bronchoconstriction. This is dose-related and given

Table 11.1 Non-specific bronchoprovoking agents

	Reference
Inert	
Charcoal, calcium carbonate, India ink, aluminium dust	Dubois, A. and Dautrebande, L. (1958), *J. clin. Invest.*, **37**, 1746–55.
4 M urea	Pain, M. and Denborough, M. (1967), *Med. J. Aust.*, **2**, 68–9.
Ultrasonic nebulization	Pflug, A. *et al.* (1970), *Am. Rev. resp. Dis.*, **101**, 710–14.
Pharmacologically active	
Histamine	Bouhuys, A. (1969), *Am. Rev. resp. Dis.*, **95**, 89–93.
Acetylcholine, methacholine	Itkin, I. (1967), *J. Allergy*, **40**, 245–56.
5-Hydroxytryptamine	Herxheimer, H. (1933), *J. Physiol.*, **122**, 49.
Prostaglandin $PGF_2\alpha$	Mathe, A. *et al.* (1973), *Br. med. J.*, **1**, 193–6.
Carbaminoyl choline	Orehek, J. *et al.* (1977), *Am. Rev. resp. Dis.*, **115**, 937–43.

sufficient aerosol, all subjects will show endobronchial oedema but in lesser amounts, the smooth muscle contraction seems to be the predominant action. The effects are virtually immediate and, provided care is taken not to use excessive dosage, the action is transient, passing off spontaneously in 2–5 min. Delayed reactions occurring some 4–6 h after administration have been reported but are not severe or common.

11.2.2 Cholinergic agents

(a) *Acetylmethylcholine – methacholine*

This substance has been used therapeutically since 1933. It is slowly destroyed by cholinesterase and hence is more stable than acetylcholine and it also has little of the ganglionic and skeletal muscle actions of acetylcholine. The actions of methacholine are thought to be on the receptor cells of the cholinergic fibres. Thus it stimulates the vagus, the cholinergic vasodilator fibres of the sympathetic system and the smooth muscle of the bronchial tree, intestines, bladder and uterus through their parasympathetic innervation.

(b) Carbachol

Unlike methacholine, this substance does stimulate autonomic ganglia and skeletal muscle. It is more potent and of longer action and although some workers have used carbachol aerosol as a provoking agent there seems little to recommend it over methacholine. Similar remarks apply to urecholine.

Pilocarpine and related derivatives have not been used extensively as provoking agents presumably because of their other actions although as aerosols they have a similar action to acetylcholine.

11.2.3 Mechanism of action

It is fortunate that the complete understanding of their site and mode of action is not a prerequisite to the use in clinical medicine of various substances used in therapeutics or diagnosis. This is particularly true in the field of agents altering bronchial airway calibre and much research continues into the nature of airway receptors, the neural connections between the various airways structures and between them and the central nervous system, the role of naturally occurring mediators and the regulations of bronchial muscle tone and the links between the upper airways and lower airways [5].

Any schema attempting to explain the sites of action of different provoking agents must at least take into account the well established anatomical facts and the factors known to influence the effects of these agents. It seems clear that not all inhaled substances acting as bronchoprovoking agents act at the same receptor site or in the same part of the bronchial tree. For example, the differences between histamine and methacholine response and histamine and hemp dust and their different modifications by substances such as corticosteroids, antihistamines and sodium cromoglycate make it necessary to postulate more than one pathway of action.

(a) Vagal integrity

Early concepts of bronchial asthma as a state of increased vagotonia point to the recognition of the importance of the vagus innervation in the regulation of bronchial calibre. The ease with which atropine can abolish laboratory induced asthma or block the anticipated response to bronchoprovoking inhalations and recent experimental work in dogs on vagal blockade using differential cooling certainly supports this. That the vagus is not the sole or even a very important modulator of bronchial tone in man, however, is suggested by the disappointing results of vagal blockade in clinical asthma. Vagal connections do provide a mechanism whereby irritant receptors in the upper airways may induce bronchial narrowing in lower airways.

(b) Local reflexes

An isolated perfused lung preserves a degree of bronchial tone and can be induced to increase airways resistance in response to inhaled irritants and chemicals so that there exists some local response system which may be cholinergic in its synapse operating between bronchial mucosa and bronchial muscle.

(c) Mediator release

Inhaled provoking agents may themselves interfere with mast cell function and induce mediator release which then acts directly on bronchial smooth muscle or the mast cell may be under the influence of vagal efferent signals.

(d) Vascular reactivity

It is still uncertain how much of the acute airways response is due to acute endobronchial oedema secondary to capillary dilatation. The action of histamine on systemic capillary leakage is easy to imagine as translated into the bronchial tree although the sudden onset and transient action of histamine in small doses would suggest that oedema formation and resolution is unlikely to be the major mechanism.

(e) Direct action

Both histamine and methacholine have a direct action on isolated smooth muscle and it remains possible that the inhalation of these soluble substances results in sufficient local concentration across the mucosa to directly stimulate the smooth muscle. If this is the major mechanism of action then the quantitative and qualitative differences between histamine and methacholine aerosol challenge in certain individuals are unexplained.

   It seems most likely that an inhaled bronchoprovoking agent acts by more than one pathway and stimulation at one portion of the bronchial tree may induce acute changes there as well as acute changes in another site. Fig. 11.1 attempts to illustrate these possibilities.

11.3 The challenge test procedure

A successful bronchial challenge test requires an effective means of administering the provoking agent and a means of following changes in pulmonary function so that some end-point can be recognized and measured. This also should provide some index which can be used for between- and within-subject comparisons. The test must be performed with as little discomfort to the subject as possible and with adequate precautions and measures to deal with alarming symptoms should they occur.

11.3.1 Administration of the agent

Techniques for delivering the aerosol to the patient have varied from a fully enclosed environmental chamber, a closed spirometer system containing the aerosol, nebulization into a face mask during quiet breathing to repeated single inhalations from an aerosol generator. Recently electronically timed pulses of aerosol from an intermittently pressurized aerosol generator have been used [6].

Whilst all these methods of delivery are effective in the sense that they can all produce satisfactory responses to inhaled aerosols, any attempt at quantitation combined with objective assessment and early cessation of delivery once an end-point has been reached, demands an intermittent controlled exposure rather than a continuous one. Most protocols, therefore, advocate a delivery system of repeated single inhalations of an aerosol with increasing concentrations rather than continuous exposure to a single concentration.

To ensure reasonable penetration of the bronchial tree and deposition, most of the nebulizers used for administration of sympathomimetic bron-

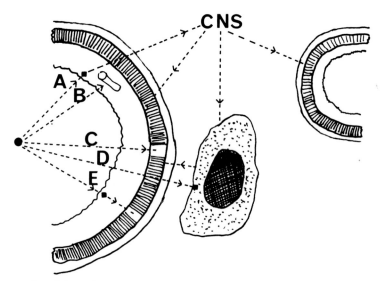

Fig. 11.1 Possible actions of non-specific inhaled bronchoprovoking agents. (a) Stimulation of irritant receptors with afferent and efferent central nervous system connections to bronchial smooth muscle and for mast cell; (b) direct alteration of vascular permeability; (c) direct action on smooth muscle; (d) direct action on mast cell; (e) direct action on receptor with local reflex action on smooth muscle.

chodilator aerosols are suitable, especially if they are able to nebulize very small volumes of liquid. The Bennett 'Vaponephrin' Type 0634 driven by an oxygen flow rate of 5 l/min has been found particularly useful and has been used in my laboratory for the last decade for challenge testing. It delivers approximately 0.02 ml of aerosolized liquid over 3 s which is the average time of an inspiratory manoeuvre and can operate with only 0.5 ml of liquid.

Inhalations are given with the mouth open, nose clip in place and from functional residual capacity rather than residual volume to provide a better distribution of the aerosol. With some co-ordination, the aerosol generation is commenced and the nebulizer brought close to the mouth as the subject commences to inspire slowly to total lung capacity. On reaching this point, the nebulizer is switched off and the subject breath-holds for 5 s. Control of aerosol generation is conveniently obtained by rapidly connecting and disconnecting the compressed gas supply to the nebulizer.

An alternative method of delivery involves tidal breathing of the aerosol for a set period – commonly two minutes. Single breath manoeuvres and tidal breathing may result in different patterns of aerosol deposition but whichever technique is used, careful development of a standard procedure (e.g. inspiratory flow rate, breath-holding time) is important if comparisons between subjects using the same technique are to be made.

11.3.2 Measurement of airway function

Many pulmonary function tests have been used in association with bronchial challenge testing. Thus, the spirometric vital capacity and Tiffeneau test have been used since the original work but have been complemented by measurements of maximal mid-expiratory flow rate, airways resistance or conductance, lung volumes determined by a closed circuit or plethysmographic techniques, single breath nitrogen plateau, flow volume curves with helium/oxygen and air breathing, and compliance and closing volume measurements. Admittedly, some of these studies have been primarily concerned with 'testing the tests' or determining the site of change of airway calibre rather than simply determining whether or not a state of bronchial hyper-reactivity exists. Since spirometry provides the simplest, most convenient and most readily available technique to use in bronchial provocation testing, it is necessary to consider its disadvantages and whether these are of sufficient importance to justify, in a context of clinical practice, recommending any other procedure.

(a) Sensitivity

Any abnormality demonstrated by spirometric testing can be demonstrated more sensitively by some other procedure but the question arises as to what extent abnormalities which could be detected by some other procedure would be missed by spirometry. It seems clear that changes in small airway function, unless very gross, will be underestimated by vital capacity, timed expired volume and maximum mid-expiratory flow rate measurements, although the maximum mid-expiratory flow rate may not be as insensitive as the former. It also seems that the first detectable changes induced by inhaled bronchodilator or bronchoconstrictor agents and the interval disability in asymptomatic patients with asthma occurs in the small airways. Using spirometric indices in conjunction with bronchial provocation testing with thus overestimate the degree of airway normality initially and not detect the earliest or smallest change. On the other hand, symptomatic disability is associated with spirometric abnormality in asthma and even mild induced asthma attacks are invariably associated with a fall in either time expired volume or slow vital capacity or usually both [7]. If vital capacity, forced expired volume and maximal mid-expiratory flow rate are unchanged after bronchial challenge, then the response to the challenge has been slight, asymptomatic and perhaps confined to small airways. Since normal subjects will show some impairment of small airway function to bronchial challenge, increasing the sensitivity of testing does not necessarily make separation of 'abnormal' from 'normal' easier; this point is taken up in Section 11.6.1.

(*b*) *Manoeuvre-induced bronchoconstriction*

In some subjects with heightened bronchial reactivity, forced respiratory manoeuvres such as are required for performance of vital capacity and forced expiration can themselves produce transient airways narrowing [8, 9]. This has been used as support for tests which employ submaximal effort or tests carried out during quiet respiration. Whilst this induced broncho-constriction may blur the bronchoconstrictive action of the inhaled agent and make quantitation difficult, the influence of maximal respiratory manoeuvres on airway calibre in susceptible individuals is much less than that of bronchoactive aerosols and in any case is additive. If the objective of the test is to demonstrate bronchial reactivity then to some extent any additive augmentation is an advantage.

The arguments against simple spirometry as an appropriate monitor of airway function in bronchial provocation testing do not, to me, provide sufficient weight to negate its advantages in terms of simplicity, convenience, ease of access to the subject and ready availability. Peak flow measurements are of less value because they are dominated by the effort-dependent stage of forced expiration, do not detect changes in vital capacity and usually do not provide any tracing or written record.

(c) The end-point

There are two end-points for consideration. Firstly, a decision as to when to cease administration of the bronchoprovoking agent is required since excessive administration of these active substances may induce very profound bronchial obstruction. One approach is to allow the subject to breathe the aerosol until symptoms are produced. At this point, administration is ceased and measurements of the response commenced or continued. Whilst there may be some value in some subjects in producing symptomatic attacks and relating this to pulmonary dysfunction, there remains a considerable group of subjects who are consistently poor at perceiving their state of airway patency and who can tolerate quite considerable obstruction without symptoms. This group and others with an abnormal perceptive ability are at risk from excessive administration of potent bronchoactive agents. Another method provides a standard delivered dose with measurement of the response to that dose regardless of symptoms although the dose sequence may be abridged or extended depending on the response. A further approach is to deliver the aerosol in increasing concentrations or accumulative doses of the same concentration until some predecided degree of deviation from the initial airway function has been reached.

Secondly, an end-point measurement must be chosen. This will usually be the measurement which shows the maximal change from the baseline value and to obtain this point, several measurements during onset and offset of the usually transient induced episode will be necessary. If dose response curves are to be constructed, then some precise timing in relation to the delivered dose is required.

(d) Protocol for a semi-qualitative test using methacholine

This test is a modification of an earlier test [10] and has been used satisfactorily without catastrophe in my laboratory for five years in over 1500 subjects. Without constructing a full dose response curve it provides a reasonable measurement of bronchial reactivity in a test taking about fifteen minutes.

Baseline measurements of slow vital capacity and forced timed expiration are made usually requiring three or four manoeuvres before full co-operation is obtained. The highest value for vital capacity, forced expired volume at one second (FEV_1) and maximum mid-expiratory flow rate are taken as the baseline value. Some brief explanation as to the test procedure and the chance that the various sprays may cause some altered sensation of breathing is given combined with reassurance that any symptoms will be mild and transient. Using a Bennett 'Vaponephrin' nebulizer with an oxygen flow rate of 5 l/min, the subject is allowed one maximal inspiration from functional residual capacity during which an aerosol from a solution of methacholine (2.5 mg/ml in normal saline) is delivered into the open mouth. The subject is encouraged to breath-hold for about five seconds at total lung capacity and is then allowed to exhale normally. After 1 min, a forced expirogram is recorded and the subject questioned about symptoms. Some coughing is not uncommon during this time but does not necessarily harbinger significant airways obstruction. If there is no change in the expirogram, the measurements are repeated at 2 and 3 min after the delivery. No change at 3 min makes it very unlikely that the initial dose will produce any further change and a second single inspiration and delivery from another nebulizer containing 25 mg/ml of methacholine in saline is then given. Measurements are made at 1, 2 and 3 min following that dose. In the absence of any significant change to that dose over 3 min, a second single dose of aerosol from 25 mg/ml solution is given. Measurements are made again at 1, 2 and 3 min and no further methacholine is given. To reverse any induced airway narrowing, 30 s of inhalation of an aerosol of 1% isoprenaline is given as a routine and measurements made 1 min later. If there is not a substantial return towards baseline values the subject is observed for an hour in the laboratory and a further dose of isoprenaline given at that time.

The initial dose of methacholine aerosol usually does not cause any dramatic change and most information is gained by the response to the larger concentration. Carefully selected normal subjects (no past or current history of asthma or other respiratory illness or atopy) will show less than a 5% fall in vital capacity and less than a 10% fall in FEV_1 in response to two delivered doses of 25 mg/ml methacholine aerosol. Many normal subjects will show no change at all.

In contrast, all subjects with current or interval asthma will show changes of greater than 10% in vital capacity, 15% in FEV_1 and 25% maximal mid-expiratory flow rate. In some subjects, the change is very considerable and in these, the response to the 2.5 mg/ml aerosol is sufficient to preclude the need for the more concentrated aerosol. Thus a positive test by this technique would require as the minimum at least a change in vital capacity ($> 10\%$), FEV_1 ($> 15\%$) or maximum mid-expiratory flow rate ($> 25\%$) to two single inspiratory doses of aerosol from 25 mg/ml methacholine solution. Greater changes in ventilatory capacity or achieving these changes to either the 2.5 mg/ml aerosol or a single dose of 25 mg/ml aerosol are taken as indicating a greater degree of bronchial reactivity.

Fig. 11.2 illustrates some responses using this protocol. These have been chosen because they make a number of points about bronchial hyper-reactivity. Thus patient A shows a response which is barely significant at the 25 mg/ml dose but the subsequent response to bronchodilator suggests that the change with methacholine was a genuine one. Patient B had a sufficiently significant change with 2.5 mg/ml not to require any further administration. The response to inhaled bronchodilator was satisfactory. Patient C had a larger response to 2.5 mg/ml aerosol only. Patients D and E did not change significantly with 2.5 mg/ml but the large concentration induced very significant falls in FEV_1 which in patient E was not immediately responsive to bronchodilator aerosol. A subsequent dose and the passage of time reversed the induced episode satisfactorily.

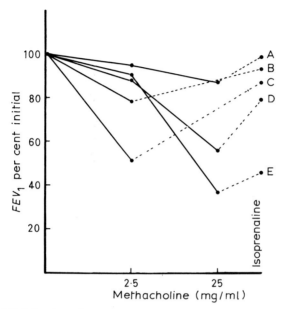

Fig. 11.2 Selection of responses to methacholine aerosol (see text).

(e) Quantitative testing

This test, although simple and quick, is rather crude in the sense that it delivers a relatively enormous dose of methacholine. Many subjects with bronchial hyper-reactivity would show measurable changes to doses much less than 25 mg/ml bolus. It is possible, then, that this approach would fail to separate two subjects who both reached a similar significant degree of induced airways obstruction to a large amount of methacholine by different time courses as a result of a different degree of reactivity. A more quantitative procedure would seem desirable and several attempts to achieve this have been made.

The refinements have been related to timing and incremental increases in aerosol dosage delivered and dose-response curve construction has been undertaken. A limiting factor in these attempts is the variable and uncertain dosage of aerosol delivered and retained in the bronchial tree. Thus there will always be some uncertainty about the points in a dose-response curve in relation to the dose axis. Refining the technique of measuring the response or the time of the response will not alter this uncertainty. Nevertheless there is some advantage in standardization of techniques if an examination of differences in bronchial reactivity is being made. The technique of Chai and others provides serial increases of methacholine dosage (5 breaths at each dose) and seeks to determine the concentration required to produce a 20% fall in FEV_1 from the control value. This protocol, recommended by the United States National Institute of Health, suggests nine concentrations of methacholine from 0.075 mg/ml up to 25 mg/ml and would take up to 45 min to perform [11].

(f) Protocols using histamine

Histamine diphosphate aerosol has a history as long as methacholine as a bronchoprovoking agent, and like it, protocols have developed from a fairly simple qualitative test to more recent attempts to refine and standardize a histamine provocation test. Thus an example of a simple protocol is that described by Stanescu and Brasseur [12] in which a nebulized solution of histamine of 1 mg/ml concentration is delivered for 1 min and symptomatic response assessed. If the subject is asymptomatic, further nebulizaton or a higher concentration is given until breathlessness or wheeze is noted.

A refinement of this protocol is used by Bryant and Burns [13] who commenced with a 1–2 min period of aerosol delivery of 0.01 mg/ml solution and recorded FEV_1 over the next 13 min. Absence of a significant change (<20%) in FEV_1 is followed by a further period of nebulization. The sequence is repeated for 20 min of nebulization and if still there is no response, the histamine solution concentration is increased to 0.1 mg/ml and the sequence continued until a significant change in ventilatory capacity is recorded. The test result is expressed as the total nebulized amount of histamine delivered to produce the 20% significant change in FEV_1. They show that the mean dose required for normal subjects was about 2 mg and for subjects with asthma it was of the order of 0.2 mg.

A more quantitative protocol was used by De Vries and others [14] by administering aerosols over 30-s periods from concentrations of 0.0625, 1.0, 4.0, 16 and 32 mg/ml. A lack of change in vital capacity or FEV_1, resulted in the next highest concentration being delivered. The administration was stopped when the change in vital capacity and/or FEV_1 of >10% was produced and the lowest histamine concentration causing this change was termed the histamine threshold. Recommendations by Chai et al. [11] to standardize the histamine provocation test suggest 5 inhalations of an aerosol of a low concentration (0.03 mg/ml) of histamine solution and recording the forced expired volume measurement immediately afterwards and at 3 min. A negative response ($<20\%$ change in FEV_1) is followed by 5 breaths of the next highest concentration and the procedure continued until a fall of 20% or greater is sustained over a 3-min period. Concentrations of histamine recommended are 0.03, 0.06, 0.12, 0.25, 1.0, 2.5, 5.0 and 10.0 mg/ml.

Details of various techniques currently in use for non-specific bronchial challenge are provided in the articles listed in the references.

11.4 Precautions

To avoid alarming episodes of airways obstruction, the following points are constantly kept in mind.

1. Provocation in patients with severe airways obstruction is potentially risky and usually unnecessary since the subsequent response to bronchodilator and a course of corticosteroids will indicate diagnosis and to some extent the degree of bronchial reactivity. Patients with acute bronchoconstriction will show a significant response to inhaled bronchodilator. Rarely, one might require an immediate assessment of bronchial reactivity in obstructed patients but as a routine, my laboratory staff now never provoke a subject whose FEV_1 is <1 l.
2. Before proceeding to a higher concentration of provoking aerosol, sufficient time must have elapsed to ensure that any change induced by the low concentration has occurred. This means at least three minutes between inhalations and final measurements at any particular concentration. Shortening the time interval increases the risk of a sudden large response due to cumulative effects of previous doses.
3. Decisions about response or lack of response should be based on changes in measured indices rather than the symptoms of the patient. Many subjects will not make comments even in the presence of a large drop in ventilatory capacity.
4. Medical supervision and resuscitative measures must be quickly available. Given technical staff of considerable experience, I do not think a medical officer must actually give the agents but one must be in the laboratory during the test to make decisions concerning the advisability of the test, the possible need to abort the test and to provide resuscitative help if necessary.
5. An episode of induced airways obstruction should be terminated, as distinct from allowing it to subside spontaneously over a few minutes, if the subject becomes so distressed that he cannot perform any useful measurements of pulmonary function. This situation may be associated with sweating, central cyanosis and a sensation of 'having the air completely cut off' and demands prompt intervention in the form of oxygen

by face mask at high concentrations, aerosol bronchodilator administration (I prefer 1% isoprenaline for 30 s because of its rapid action) and an intravenous injection of atropine sulphate at a dose of 1.2 mg for an adult. Intermittent positive pressure ventilation may be necessary if rapid improvement does not occur.

Less severe episodes do not prevent obtaining a valid measurement but having obtained that, oxygen and bronchodilator aerosol can be given immediately and the response measured. Partial recovery is further encouraged by a second period of bronchodilator aerosol in 1 h. In an experience of over 3000 provocation tests using methacholine, swift termination using atropine has been required twice and rapid reversal with oxygen and bronchodilator on twelve occasions. No fatalities have occurred and no long-term consequences of an induced attack have become apparent.

11.5 Expression of results

The majority of studies involving bronchial provocation express the results as percentage change of an index from the initial value and up until this point, no other approach has been mentioned. The reactivity can be expressed as the dose of an agent to produce a certain percentage change in an index or the percentage change in that index to a standard dose of provoking agent. The question immediately arises as to whether a 20% fall in FEV_1, for example, from an initial value of 4 l is more significant, less significant or of the same significance as a 20% fall from an initial value of 1.5 l.

Because of the dominance of radial changes in relationships expressing changes in resistance in a tube, it is apparent that smaller absolute radial changes will be required to produce the same percentage fall in flow rate if the initial radius is already abnormally reduced. The problem would be resolved if all subjects started with the same initial value but since studies are done on subjects with an initial ventilatory capacity varying from normal though to moderate impairment, the influence of the initial status on reactivity and its quantitation needs some consideration.

It has been postulated that on the analogy of the *in vitro* dose-response curve for smooth muscle, increasing tone of bronchial smooth muscle will be associated with a larger response to the same dose of agent over the steep portion of the dose-response curve. Bronchial reactivity thus would be determined to a large extent by the resting tone [1]. However, that using the percentage change from initial value irrespective of the degree of initial impairment may have some respectability is suggested by the exponential relationship that is found between airways conductance and methacholine dose in an individual subject given relatively high concentrations of methacholine aerosol. This means that if the slope of the line expressing airways conductance with methacholine dose is taken as the index of bronchial reactivity, then expressing the change as a percentage change from the initial value will produce the same gradient if reactivity is unchanged [17].

That a distinction should be made between the dose-response gradient and the final change in ventilatory capacity induced by bronchoprovocation has been argued by Charpin and his group [18]. They point out that there is no correlation between the dose of carbachol to cause a 25% decrease in airways conductance (which they term bronchial sensitivity) and the slope of the dose-response curve (bronchial reactivity) in a small group of normal and asthmatic subjects. Subsequent changes in ventilatory function following further doses of carbachol after the 25% change point has been achieved are widely divergent in normals and asthmatics, suggesting that different mechanisms may be operating and making it likely that both indices (reactivity and sensitivity) are characteristics of an individual bronchial response. Some normal subjects seem to have a sensitivity in the asthmatic range but normal reactivity. The practical significance of this is that a response curve can only be interpreted with some confidence if the dose given has been large with no response or if the change has been considerably greater than 25%. A 3 point test, i.e. baseline value and changes at two concentrations, would seem the minimal desirable for an acceptable test. Expressing results as a percentage change from initial value seems as good as any, at least in our present state of ignorance.

11.6 Clinical implications of non-specific bronchial challenge

As stated in the introduction, the purpose of non-specific bronchial challenge is to demonstrate the degree of bronchial hyper-reactivity in an individual. It remains to consider the reasons why this may be helpful in the investigation of patients with respiratory diseases and to summarize the present state of knowledge concerning hyper-reactivity in man.

11.6.1 Normal or abnormal?

Since many normal subjects will show no evidence of bronchial reactivity using the techniques and agents discussed, it could be argued that any degree of reactivity demonstrated using these techniques is a deviation from normal. To do so would be to place a label of abnormality on a large proportion of the healthy population. No large surveys of bronchial reactivity measurements in a random sample of the population have been performed but experience with small samples suggests that there is a continuum of reactivity with most of the population showing very little reactivity but merging continuously into a tail with very bronchoreactive members

[10]. Rather than attempting to decide if an individual response to a bron-chial challenge is normal or abnormal, it is more useful to think of the subject as being a member of the population and his response places him somewhere between a complete non-response and an obviously large response. Using sensitive tests of airway dynamics, it is probable that all persons can be made to show a degree of bronchial reactivity but still differences between them will be present. It seems that about 10% of a random sample of the popula-tion will show a degree of bronchial hyper-reactivity significantly greater than a selected normal population. From within that 10%, patients with clinical lung disease, usually asthma or bronchitis, or a past history of asthma will account for about half but the remainder will appear to have bronchial reactivity as great as many patients with asthma and yet be symptom-free, have no past history of asthma and have normal pulmonary function. This latter group is a very important group for further study.

11.6.2 Bronchial asthma

Whilst not all persons exhibiting heightened bronchial reactivity will have asthma, all persons with bronchial asthma will show bronchial hyper-reactivity. This rather sweeping statement needs some qualifications in the light of experience gained from responses in asthma subjects to various provoking agents and their modification. Thus a number of studies have shown that the reactivity to methacholine is more constant and more univer-sal amongst asthma subjects than the response to inhaled allergens or histamine [19]. Furthermore, whereas antihistamines, corticosteroids and sodium cromoglycate will reduce the reactivity to histamine, these agents do not greatly alter the response to methacholine. In general, however, re-sponses to histamine and methacholine agree quite well [16]. Bronchial hyper-reactivity is abolished for a variable time after the inhalation of sympathomimetic aerosols or iprotropium or the intravenous administra-tion of atropine in patients with asthma. Therefore these agents should be withheld for at least two hours before any bronchial challenge. Bronchial hyper-reactivity continues after clinical remission in asthma. Removal of a subject with asthma induced by some specific agent from that environment, may be followed by a gratifying improvement or complete disappearance of wheezy attacks but hyper-reactivity can remain for years. There is currently some dispute concerning the relationships between the degree of hyper-reactivity and the severity of clinical asthma [15, 17, 18]. Some studies show a good agreement between the histamine response and the bronchodilator requirements of patients with asthma [15] whilst others show no correlation between clinical severity, initial airways obstruction and response to methacholine [17]. Part of this contradiction may be due to differences in technique or differences in expression of response [18]. Thus bronchial hyper-reactivity seems to be an essential component of bronchial asthma. It is a remarkably constant property of patients with overt asthma, patients in an interval phase or in long term remission and the reactivity to methacholine in particular seems to be largely independent of corticosteroids or sodium cromoglycate treatment [21].

11.6.3 Obstructive bronchitis

The majority of patients with chronic obstructive bronchitis show no evidence of bronchial hyper-reactivity on non-specific bronchial challenge (Fig. 11.3). There are many, however, who show a degree of reactivity as great as patients with asthma or who are in an intermediate situation. Whether the former are really patients with chronic bronchial asthma or asthmatic bronchitis is of interest physiologically and epidemiologically. Therapeutically, what is important is that some significant clinical improvement can be anticipated using antiasthma therapy.

The inter-relationships between cigarette smoking, chronic bronchitis and bronchial reactivity are of interest. As a non-specific bronchial irritant, inhaled tobacco smoke would be expected to aggravate patients with bronchial asthma and worsen the situation of patients with chronic bronchitis

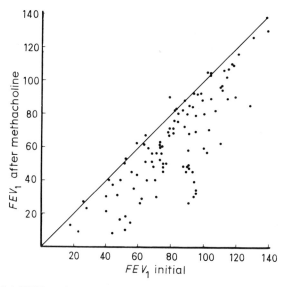

Fig. 11.3 Initial FEV_1 and postmethacholine FEV_1 in 104 unselected patients with suspected asthma. Points lying on the line of identity indicate no change with provocation. Note the spectrum of responses at all levels of initial FEV_1 and the lack of response in some patients despite considerable obstruction initially.

who exhibit bronchial hyper-reactivity. It is possible that chronic cigarette smoke inhalation may induce bronchial hyper-reactivity. Much work is in progress on these questions but at the moment, there seems no evidence to suggest that cigarette smoking can induce bronchial hyper-reactivity although it is possible that a previous state of asymptomatic heightened bronchial reactivity may be associated with a more rapid reduction in FEV_1 with time in smokers. The acute inhalation of tobacco smoke causes an increase in airways resistance in subjects with heightened bronchial reactivity. Recent studies showing evidence for cigarette smoking in asthmatic populations are therefore surprising [23]. There is some evidence that the presence of hyper-reactivity in subjects with chronic bronchitis may adversely influence long-term prognosis.

11.6.4 Miscellaneous conditions

Despite many studies examining the question, there is no well-established relationship between atopic status and non-specific bronchial reactivity. This is in contrast to a reasonable agreement between bronchial challenge to inhaled allergens and immunological evidence such as positive skin hypersensitivity or elevated immunoglobulin levels. Thus many subjects with clinical asthma and non-specifice bronchial hyper-reactivity will not show atopic features and many patients with allergic diseases such as rhinitis will show normal non-specific bronchial reactivity. Some studies have suggested that patients with allergic rhinitis have a degree of reactivity which is not clearly asthmatic but still greater than normal [20, 24]. Patients with asthma with a clearly allergic component have been found to vary in their bronchial response to allergen and histamine but not to methacholine.

Bronchial reactivity has been shown transiently to increase in some normal subjects following upper respiratory tract viral infections and various vaccinations and presumably a similar enhancement of reactivity may explain some exacerbations of clinical asthma in relation to viral infections but the question has been little studied. A high proportion of patients with cystic fibrosis will show an increase in bronchial reactivity.

Some diurnal variation in reactivity has been demonstrated and this may be the explanation for the marked diurnal variation in ventilatory capacity demonstrated in some patients with bronchial asthma. Administration of β-blocking agents does not usually induce a state of non-specific bronchial hyper-reactivity in normal subjects although episodes of asthma may be induced in subjects with unsuspected asthma and the degree of control in established asthmatics may be upset.

11.6.5 Implications of bronchial hyper-reactivity

The demonstration of the presence of bronchial hyper-reactivity is most useful in the context of confirming a clinical suspicion of bronchial asthma. Many patients give a very atypical history and in the absence of airways obstruction, the diagnosis may remain speculative. Bronchial hyper-reactivity is strongly supportive of the diagnosis and a negative response is strongly against the diagnosis.

Other lung conditions with associated bronchial hyper-reactivity (obstructive bronchitis, cystic fibrosis) should be considered as having an asthmatic component and treated accordingly.

The apparently healthy subject with hyper-reactivity remains an enigma (Fig. 11.4). One could speculate that this subject is at greater risk of developing asthma or intrinsic airway disease and that he should be protected from occupations that provide a known inhalational hazard. There are large areas of ignorance concerning bronchial hyper-reactivity. What determines it? Is it acquired in response to external factors? What is the distinction between a non-asthmatic and an asthmatic individual with identical bronchial reactivity? What is the long-term influence of bronchial hyper-reactivity on the incidence and rate of progression of chronic lung disease? Some of these questions will be answered by research being undertaken on cell mediators, receptor function and in the field of neurophysiology but very useful clinical information will be provided by a more widespread use of simple non-specific bronchial challenge testing.

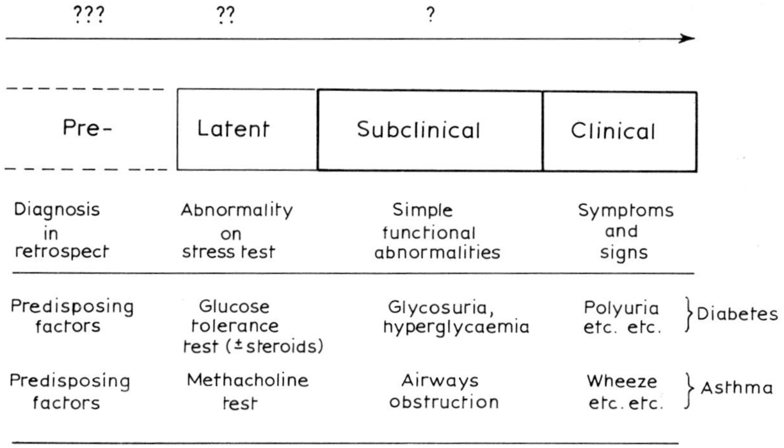

???	??	?	
Pre-	Latent	Subclinical	Clinical
Diagnosis in retrospect	Abnormality on stress test	Simple functional abnormalities	Symptoms and signs
Predisposing factors	Glucose tolerance test (±steroids)	Glycosuria, hyperglycaemia	Polyuria etc. etc. } Diabetes
Predisposing factors	Methacholine test	Airways obstruction	Wheeze etc. etc. } Asthma

Fig. 11.4 A parallel between non-specific bronchial hyperreactivity in relation to asthma and abnormal glucose metabolism and diabetes mellitus. (Reproduced with permission from *Aust. N.Z. J. Med.* (1971), **1**, 22–25.)

11.7 Summary

Accurate determination of bronchial hyper-reactivity using non-specific bronchial challenge tests in man is limited by uncertainties about dose delivered and deposition, distribution differences between subjects, sites and mode of actions of provoking agents and the most appropriate method of measuring the response and expressing the result. Despite these limitations, a simple bronchial challenge using a non-specific provoking agent has proved to be a quick, safe and useful addition to the repertoire of pulmonary function laboratories. Its most useful role is in studying the patient with possible bronchial asthma but who has normal ventilatory function. It also offers a means of study of the natural history of asthma, chronic bronchitis and their modification by external factors and treatment.

References

1. Benson, M. K. (1975), *Br. J. Dis. Chest.*, **69**, 227–39.
2. Charpin, J., Orehek, J. and Gayrard, P. (1977), *Therapie*, **32**, 9–17.
3. Dautrebande, L. (1962), *Microaerosols*, Academic Press, New York.
4. Mueller, R. A. (1977), In: *Anesthesia and Respiratory Function* (ed E. Kafer) In: *Int. Anesthesiol. Clin.*, **15**, 137–67.
5. Widdicombe, J. G. (1974), Reflex control of breathing. In: *Respiratory Physiology*, Physiology Series One, Volume 2, Butterworths, London.
6. Rosenthal, R., Norman, P. and Summer, W. (1975), *J. Allergy clin. Immunol.*, **56**, 338–46.
7. Rubinfeld, A. R. and Pain, M. C. F. (1977), *Thorax*, **32**, 177–81.
8. Gimeno, F., Berg, W. C., Sluiter, H. J. and Tammeling, G. J. (1972), *Am. Rev. resp. Dis.*, **105**, 68–74.
9. Orehek, J., Gayrard, P., Grimaud, C. and Charpin, J. (1975), *Br. Med. J.*, **1**, 123–5.
10. Cade, J. F. and Pain, M. C. F. (1971), *Aust. N.Z. J. Med.*, **1**, 22–25.
11. Chai, H. *et al.* (1975), *J. Allergy clin. Immunol.*, **56**, 323–7.
12. Stanescu, D. and Biasseur, L. (1973), *Scand. J. resp. Dis.*, **54**, 333–40.
13. Bryant, D. H. and Burns, M. W. (1976), *Clin. Allergy*, **6**, 373–81.
14. de Vries, K., Goei, J., Booy-Noord, H. and Orie, N. (1962), *Int. Archs Allerg.*, **20**, 93–101.
15. Cockroft, D. W., Killian, D. N., Mellon, J. J. A. and Hargreave, F. E. (1977), *Clin. Allergy*, **7**, 235–43.
16. Juniper, E. F. *et al.* (1978), *Thorax*, **33**, 705–10.
17. Rubinfeld, A. R. and Pain, M. C. F. (1977), *Am. Rev. resp. Dis.*, **115**, 381–7.
18. Orehek, J. *et al.* (1977), *Am. Rev. resp. Dis.*, **115**, 937–44.
19. Townley, R. G., Ryo, U. Y., Kolotkin, B. M. and Kang, B. (1975), *J. Allergy. clin. Immunol.*, **56**, 429–42.
20. Fish, J. *et al.* (1976), *Am. Rev. resp. Dis.*, **113**, 579–86.
21. Cade, J. F. and Pain, M. C. F. (1971), *Lancet*, **2**, 186–8.

22. Lichtenstein, L. M. and Austen, K. F. (1977), *Asthma, Physiology, Immunopharmacology and Treatment*, Academic Press, New York.
23. Higenbottam, T. W., Feyeraband, C. and Clark, T. J. H. (1980), *Br. J. Dis. Chest*, **74**, 279–84.
24. Felarca, A. B. and Itkin, I. (1966), *J. Allergy*, **37**, 223–5.

CHAPTER TWELVE

Host Defences

P. J. Cole

This chapter will attempt to apply the general theory of immunological responsiveness and non-responsiveness of the host to respiratory syndromes seen by the clinician in both general and specialist environments. Application of such theory can result in recognition of particular syndromes with common pathogenetic mechanisms, greater understanding of their pathogenesis (and in some cases aetiology), rationale for treatment feasible at present, and directions for research which may yield improved treatment in the immediate future.

Normal mechanisms of defence against invasion of the host via the respiratory route will be described. Clinical syndromes arising from malfunction of these mechanisms will be discussed, and classification of these will be attempted in a manner allowing logical clinical investigation in order to define a cause or pathogenetic mechanism. Finally, treatment for the conditions will be described with a brief consideration of the lines in which research is developing in pursuing better treatment for such conditions.

12.1 Concept of elimination or persistence of antigen

Environmental pressure during evolution has forced man to accept a number of changes in anatomy and physiology to befit him for survival. One of these is acquisition of an air-breathing mechanism, the lung; another is ability to walk upright. Both of these advantages outweigh the penalties incurred by such evolution, but simultaneously man has had to evolve defences against those disadvantages which endanger him. Thus, with evolution of the lung came the disadvantage of exposure to pollution in respired air which demanded evolution of mechanisms to defend the host against noxious agents using the respiratory tract as portal of entry to the body. Similarly, with acquisition of upright posture came the task of clearing secretions within the respiratory tract against gravity and development of more sophisticated active clearance mechanisms.

Generally, the response of the body to foreign, potentially injurious matter is an attempt to eliminate it. Local responses have been developed to achieve this in the lung and such host response, if successful, eliminates the agent concerned. An unsuccessful host response may have one of two results. Dysfunction of defences against a highly invasive agent will allow the host to be rapidly overwhelmed and to die. However, should elimination of noxious matter (whether it is invasive or not) be slow or incomplete, host mechanisms inevitably continue to attempt to eliminate it and in doing so may actually cause damage to host as well as invader (Fig. 12.1).

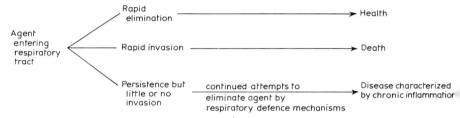

Fig. 12.1 Concept of elimination or persistence of antigen.

Host response to this persistent foreign material forms the basic pathogenesis for a number of diseases seen in the respiratory tract. The importance of this concept lies in the understanding it gives to mechanisms of diseases and, therefore, to potential treatment of them.

12.2 Normal defence mechanisms available to the respiratory tract

These are summarized in Table 12.1 where it can be seen that there are 'first line' local defences but, should these be hard pressed, circulating 'back up' defences can move to the environs of the lung to form a second line of defence. Some defences depend on immunological mechanisms which are specific but there are also important ones which are non-immunological.

12.2.1 Non-specific local defence mechanisms

(a) 'Explosive' clearance mechanisms

A number of respiratory manoeuvres use respired gas as a hydraulic fluid to transmit energy from the respiratory muscles to other sites in the respiratory tract – these can result not only in ventilation and sound production but also in clearance of material from within the system. Thus, coughing and 'huffing' clear the central airways and larynx; throat clearing, hawking and spitting expel material from the pharynx and mouth; sneezing, 'snuffling' and nose blowing expel material from the upper respiratory tract or upper airways. A number of these are reflexes which are largely involuntary, but

Table 12.1 Defence mechanisms available to the respiratory tract

---

(a) **Local** (First line)
    1. Non-specific
        reflexes (e.g. 'explosive', nervous)
        anatomical (e.g. air–blood barrier, cilia)
        lining materials (e.g. mucus, surfactant)
        antimicrobial agents (e.g. lysozyme, interferon, lactoferrin, transferrin)
        phagocytes (e.g. alveolar macrophage, airways macrophage, interstitial
            macrophage)
    2. Specific
        antibody (mainly IgG and sIgA)
        lymphocytes (BALT and luminal cells)

(b) **Systemic** (Second line recruitment)
    1. Non-specific
        serum factors (e.g. complement)
        phagocytes (e.g. PMN, PB monocyte)
    2. Specific
        antibody (mainly IgG and IgM)
        lymphocytes (T and B cells)

Ig = immunoglobulin; sIgA = secretory IgA; BALT = bronchus-associated lymphoid tissue; PMN = polymorphonuclear leukocyte; PB = peripheral blood.

both voluntary and involuntary build-up of pressure against a closed glottis allows expulsion of air through upper airways at speeds which shear secretions of suitable viscoelastic properties from the walls and propel them into the pharynx.

(b) Nervous reflexes

Two general advantageous characteristics of nervous reflexes, prompt response and ability to recruit rapidly much of the body's physiology, lend invaluable defence to the respiratory tract. These properties allow prompt response to less than life-threatening situations which would otherwise require slower humoral control systems.

Such reflexes may protect by initiating sneeze or cough (mentioned above), laryngo- and bronchospasm and mucus secretion, etc.

(c) Lining material of the respiratory tract

'Mucus' is widely used to designate the fluid material lining the respiratory tract. It is heterogeneous and differs in constitution in different regions within the tract. In 1934 it was realized that it was a bilayered system – a lower layer of periciliary fluid which is thin and serous in which the cilia beat, and viscid material secreted by goblet cells which lies in discontinuous drops and plaques on the surface of the periciliary layer. Mucous glands may contribute secretion to both layers. The lower layer is fairly uniform in depth and continuous whereas the viscid layer varies a great deal throughout the respiratory tract.

Surfactant, probably produced by the type II pneumocyte, is a substance present in the alveolar region which reduces alveolar and perhaps bronchiolar surface tension. Such forces may cause flow of this substance towards bronchioles and this may be assisted by cilia in respiratory bronchioles. Relatively little is known about clearance mechanisms in peripheral airways.

(d) Cilia

Ciliated epithelial cells are known to occur in all parts of the respiratory tract except the alveolar sacs and anterior nares. Cilia themselves are approximately 5 μm cellular projections displaying intense motility by virtue of cytoplasmic fibrils whose active motion causes changes in shape of the cilium resulting in a beating cycle. Cilia contain claw-like processes at their tips which project into the more viscid upper layer of respiratory tract lining fluid and propel it onwards as the cilium beats. Eventually the mucus plaques and any contained particles reach the glottis and can be swallowed or coughed out.

(e) Pulmonary alveolar macrophage

This cell is one of three, possibly four, types of mononuclear phagocyte in the respiratory tract: the free alveolar macrophage, the airway macrophage (probably an alveolar macrophage which has been transported from the alveolus through the bronchiole into the airways, although it could have migrated through the bronchial epithelium), the interstitial macrophage, and the macrophage in the pleural space.

These are scavenger cells which protect the host against respired particles small enough to enter alveoli. Their complex functions are discussed later.

It is important to remember that bronchoalveolar lavage samples the first two types of cell (alveolar and airway macrophage), and these may not be representative of the type of macrophage (interstitial) believed to be implicated in the cause of a variety of pulmonary diseases (e.g. fibrosis). Much work is required to define the derivation of alveolar macrophages, their stages of maturation and their subpopulations.

Present knowledge of the origin and maturation of these cells suggests that they are ultimately derived from haematopoietic tissue. Bone marrow promonocytes can divide and give rise to circulating monocytes which leave the blood at a rapid exponential rate (after about 8.5 h in man). Such monocytes can enter the pulmonary interstitium. There, a population of mononuclear cells is known to be capable of mitosis, and such cells have been seen to arrive at the alveolar surface. That these interstitial cells are of monocyte origin is likely, but an intrapulmonary origin has not been completely excluded. Some macrophages have been seen to divide in the alveolus.

The fate of these cells is either death in the alveolus with subsequent ingestion by other macrophages, transport by the alveolobronchiolar route (which could be direct, via the interstitium of the alveolar walls or via lymphatics), or, much less likely, transport into the circulation. This fate is not purely academic because these cells are capable of transporting non-degradable, often toxic, agents. Their route and final resting place is therefore of practical significance to the host.

(f) Antimicrobial substances

The respiratory secretions contain a number of substances with recognized antimicrobial activity but relatively little work has been done in this area. However, it is known that the enzyme lysozyme has bactericidal activity and that alveolar lining material enhances intracellular bactericidal activity of alveolar macrophages. The latter, as well as other cells in the respiratory tract, are capable of producing interferon which has antiviral properties.

Lactoferrin and transferrin are found in bronchial secretion and by binding iron ensure that bacteria are not supplied with too abundant a source of free iron which might increase their pathogenicity. Complement components have been found in bronchial lavage fluid but the significance of this in terms of local protection of the respiratory tract is unclear.

(g) Lymphatics

Pulmonary lymphatic endothelial cells engulf large molecules and particulate molecules from the interstitium where they may arrive having crossed bronchial and alveolar walls from the lumen of the respiratory tract.

(h) Air-blood barrier

The delicate alveolocapillary barrier is adapted to rapid gas exchange in an efficient manner. It also functions as an important anatomical barrier against penetration of airborne noxious agents. Although this function is poorly understood, it is recognized that three properties of the alveolar epithelium are protective. First, the epithelium is selectively permeable to lipid-insoluble macromolecular diffusion. Second, pinocytosis (droplet transport) by type I pneumocytes delivers bacteriostatic substances from blood to alveoli and there is similar transport of fluid from alveoli to the interstitial space. Third, type I pneumocytes can phagocytose and thereby remove some inhaled particulate material from the alveolar space.

12.2.2 Specific local defence mechanisms

(a) Antibody

In 1927 it was suggested that a local mucosal immune response might exist independent of serum-derived immunity. Later it was shown that antibody in respiratory tract secretions was locally produced, and in the 1960s Tomasi and his colleagues clearly established that a distinct secretory immune system existed. Three observations led to this concept: first, that immunoglobulin (Ig) A predominated in mucosal secretions despite scanty presence in serum; second, that the IgA in secretions (secretory IgA, sIgA) had a different structure; and third, that sIgA components were locally synthesized.

IgA in serum is mainly monomeric (7sIgA), whereas most IgA in secretions is dimeric, consisting of two 7sIgA monomers linked to a non-Ig secretory component and a 'J' chain. The whole molecule is 11sIgA and secretory component is responsible for its unique chemical and antigenic properties and its resistance to proteolysis. 'J' chain is a low molecular weight polypeptide which links Ig molecules in polymeric configurations.

Synthesis of sIgA, as a 10sIgA dimer, occurs in plasma cells in the lamina propria of the respiratory mucous membrane. It passes into intercellular spaces after crossing the basement membrane but is diverted into epithelial cells by the tight junctions at the apical end of these cells. It combines with secretory component (secreted from the epithelial cell) either in the intercellular space, in the epithelial cell itself or on its luminal surface.

Determining the derivation and quantitating Ig found in the respiratory tract raises problems. First, there is difficulty in distinguishing serum-derived Ig from that locally produced and second, there is danger of a considerable dilution artefact when one considers that respiratory secretions are both serous and mucous – probably with separately controlled secretion rates. However, in the case of sIgA the structure gives clue to its derivation, although in nasal secretions it has been shown that up to 20% IgA may be in monomeric form indistinguishable from serum IgA, and therefore may be serum-derived or represent dissociated sIgA. A similar finding occurs in bronchial lavage fluid where up to 10% IgA may be monomeric. Unbound secretory component is often found in lavage fluid from the lower respiratory tract, but IgM is rarely found. IgG is present in lower respiratory secretions in larger amounts in smokers than non-smokers (although there appears to be dose-relation), whereas smoking does not appear to affect the amount of sIgA present.

Beside being thought to act as an antitoxin neutralizing viral infectivity and to inhibit bacterial adherence to mucosal surfaces – obvious protective roles – sIgA appears to block transport of enterochelin from bacteria. Enterochelin is an iron-chelating substance synthesized by bacteria which can remove iron from unsaturated transferrin or lactoferrin and provide it for metabolism (and increased pathogenicity) in the bacterial cell. Although it has been proposed that sIgA has a major opsonizing role, evidence for this in the case of human alveolar macrophage function is poor.

Some bacteria produce IgA proteases in an attempt to overcome the protective effects of this Ig on mucosal surfaces.

(b) Lymphocytes

In 1958 Humphrey and his colleagues showed the importance of lung tissue as a major source of antibody production following intravenous immunization. In 1973, Bienenstock and his colleagues noted subepithelial follicular lymphoid aggregates in several species and named them *bronchus-associated lymphoid tissue* (BALT) although allusion to such tissue had been made in the literature as far back as 1868. They are analogous to gut-associated lymphoid tissue (GALT) including Peyers patches, and may be part of a wider mucosal immunological system. The discovery of this lymphoid system, peculiar to the airways but similar to that of the gut, is important because both these organs are subjected to a constant stream of potential pathogens, both possess a local secretory IgA system and both are derived from endoderm. BALT, lying as it does in sentinel positions at bifurcations of the bronchial tree below mucosa modified by its possession of microvilli but not cilia, would therefore be an excellent recognition and priming system. Antigen could specifically stimulate proliferation of sensitized cells which could then be directed to other mucosal sites where they might protect against invasion by that antigen. There is support for this hypothesis in that although BALT develops in germ-free animals it proliferates far more in conventionally reared or wild animals. Absence of plasma cells, despite presence of lymphocytes, strongly suggests that BALT differs from other peripheral lymphoid tissue and could be a site of B and T cell differentiation. Cell transfer studies have suggested that BALT cells can repopulate lung and gut lamina propria with IgA-producing cells. If the analogy holds good the T cells in BALT help IgA production but suppress IgG and IgM production.

This may be important not only in terms of protection of the lung but also in terms of pathogenesis of atopy, if this is due to hypothesized overstimulation of B cells. This is postulated to occur because of increased permeability of gut and, perhaps, bronchial mucosa to antigen molecules at the time of relative IgA deficiency in infancy. The immunogenicity of such molecules may be reduced by combination with IgA in or at the mucosal surface, or by suppression of the immune response to them in GALT by suppressor T cells. Perhaps a similar situation exists with respect to BALT.

12.2.3 Systemic defence mechanisms

Just as an army requires reinforcements when hard pressed, so the respiratory tract relies on 'back-up' defences from the circulation to aid the 'front-line' local defences when these are stressed. These reinforcements can be classified similarly to local defence mechanisms (Table 12.1).

(a) Antibody

IgG and IgM antibodies are found predominantly in the intravascular compartment but are available to local tissue sites when inflammatory response to a pathogen increases vascular permeability. Obviously IgM, being a large molecule, is less able to penetrate such tissue sites but protects the adjacent vascular compartment to prevent spread by this route.

(d) Phagocytes

Traffic of polymorphonuclear (PMN) leucocytes to sites of invasion in the respiratory tract occurs rapidly and forms the 'advance guard' of reinforcement. These cells are extremely active in phagocytosis and intracellular killing of microbes, the mechanisms of which are fairly well understood.

Circulating mononuclear phagocytes are mobilized to invasion sites less quickly but, as in the case of the PMN, the bone marrow increases production to keep pace with traffic to the invasion site. If such stimulus continues indefinitely immature precursor cells enter the blood and, like scantily trained troops, are less effective in their functions.

(c) Lymphocytes

Lymphocytes, themselves mononuclear cells, are seen to enter the area of invasion at about the time of mononuclear phagocytes. They are of two lineages: thymus-processed (T cells) capable of exhibiting delayed hypersensitivity (DH) cellular reactions, and bursa-derived (B cells) capable of exhibiting humoral functions such as maturation into plasma cells secreting antibody of the various classes. T cells, if already sensitized to invading antigens, will be stimulated to make a response which can be termed cell mediated immunity (CMI) if it is protective. If the antigen is novel, sensitization is necessary, usually helped by presentation of the antigen via the macrophage ('macrophage processing'), so that a CMI response can be mounted in the immediate or distant future. Such T cell sensitization also results in co-operation with B cells to enable a more efficient antibody response by the latter than could be achieved by antigen presentation to the B cell alone.

(d) Serum factors

Factors, such as complement, gain access to the lung in larger quantity when an inflammatory reaction occurs there. They assist in direct and indirect antimicrobial reactions. In addition, a number of chemotactic substances appear in local tissues and enter the serum when inflammation occurs. These mobilize and direct circulating cells to the site where they are required as described below.

12.3 Mobilization of defences

Unless local defences can 'home in' on invading agents with speed and accuracy these first line defences will totally fail in their function. Even if they achieve this, it is important that they be able to rapidly and efficiently communicate with other local defences and with distant back-up defence mechanisms in the circulation to disseminate knowledge of the state of invasion and its extent. Only in this way can local defence be amplified. The signals emitted to produce directional movement of phagocyte cells are chemical (chemotaxins, chemoattractants) and the process of attraction named chemotaxis or chemoattraction.

Similar substances are involved in attracting polymorphonuclear leuko-cytes (PMN) and alveolar macrophages (AM) but some only act on one cell type, although it must be said that there is little information about this aspect of the AM. With respect to PMN, bacterial products, classical pathway complement components and materials derived from the alternative path-way of complement are strong attractants. PMN and AM lysis-products attract mononuclear cells and PMN themselves. In this way the traffic inflammatory cells to the site of invasion is amplified. Several of these substances also affect other aspects of cell function such as microtubule assembly, lysosomal enzyme release and cell metabolism. However, inhibit-ing factors occur in several diseases, including systemic infections, and can oppose the action of chemotactic agents.

12.4 Phagocyte function

Because the AM occupies such a sentinel position in the defences of the respiratory tract, and because circulating PMN form such an efficient 'flying hit squad' once invasion has occurred, it is important to understand the known functions of these cells. This is particularly important because of the clinical relevance of this information to treatment, as will be discussed later.

Broadly, the function of phagocytes is to phagocytose invading agents, kill them (if living) and degrade them. In the case of living and non-living organic agents this is relatively straightforward, but in the case of inorganic particles and fibres the functional situation is complex and may cause distress to the host.

Phagocytosis of a particle can be dissected into a series of steps – attraction of the cell to the particle (discussed above), movement of the cell towards the attractant, adherence to the particle and, finally, ingestion of the particle. Killing involves activation of metabolic processes, and degradation involves activation of lysosomal enzymes.

It is important to recognize the essentially 'one hit' nature of PMN function which contrasts with the capacity of the macrophage to modulate its response in the light of information derived by it from the environment through a process of sampling extracellular fluid (pinocytosis). An example of this is the recent demonstration that AM adapt to changes in oxygen tension by altering their level of an enzyme superoxide dimutase which is mentioned later. This is particularly important in the case of the foetal lung adapting to hyperoxia.

12.4.1 Motility

(a) Locomotory apparatus

Phagocytosis involves both movement of the cell in its environment and movement of subcellular structures, such as lysosomes, within the cell itself. These, in turn, depend upon contractile mechanisms acting on intrinsically rigid intracellular features. Electron microscopy has revealed contractile microfilaments which insert into the cell membrane and mechanically supportive microtubules, the latter also orientating flow of the cell. The contractile proteins, together with cyclic nucleotides, also regulate mobility of receptors in the cell membrane.

(b) Energetics

The energy required for motility is supplied by adenosinetriphosphate (ATP) in the presence of divalent cations. In AM, motility can be inhibited by inhibitors of oxidative phosphorylation and by hypoxia, but PMN can sustain motility by anaerobic glycolysis. However, only a very small proportion of oxygen consumption by AM is expended in movement and ingestion so the balance (well over 95%) must be used for other functions including production of microbicidal metabolites of oxygen.

12.4.2 Attachment

It appears that in AM, attachment of the cell to an artificial surface involves cyanide-sensitive metabolism, even at 4°C. However, once attachment has occurred neither cyanide nor cytochalasin B (a microfilament poison) affect it, therefore non-energy requiring forces, such as ionic ones, may be important in maintaining adhesion.

Particle adherence to phagocytes probably involves such mechanisms but there are, in addition, substances (opsonins) which promote both adherence and ingestion and these play a major role in this phase of phagocytosis. Opsonins include heat-stable serum factors including Fc and Fab fragments of IgG_1 and IgG_3 sub-class molecules (which can be increased by immunization) and heat-labile complement-derived factors from both classical and alternative pathways of the latter's activation.

All these promotors of adherence have an influence in the process through which a phagocyte goes in order to select a particle for ingestion. But receptors on the cell surface augment the selection procedure. Fc receptors on AM, estimated at about two million per cell, bind IgG antibody (particularly in the presence of polyvalent and divalent haptens) and, even more avidly, immune complexes of antigen and antibody. In different phagocytes, some opsonins promote either attachment or ingestion, or both (e.g. C3b promotes only attachment of immune complexes to AM and IgG is required by the AM to ingest immune complexes after adherence, whereas both attachment and ingestion is promoted by C3b-coated bacteria in the case of PMN).

12.4.3 Ingestion

This step involves formation of a phagocytic plasma membrane-lined vacuole which is transported within the cell and fuses with vesicles containing degradative enzymes (lysosomes) which then become activated. Although the triggering mechanism for ingestion is unknown a number of essentials for the process to occur in different phagocytes is known. Examples are suitable extracellular fluid osmolality and pH, and presence of divalent cations.

12.4.4 Plasma membrane resynthesis

Formation of a phagocytic vacuole involves loss of a significant amount of plasma membrane from the cell surface to the interior. It is known that peritoneal macrophages and blood monocytes replace this by resynthesis within 6–12 h. The situation in PMN and AM is not certain, although in the former it appears that little resynthesis occurs – again reflecting its 'one off' nature.

12.4.5 Intracellular killing

Inside the phagocytic vacuole is a chemical world of its own. A variety of reactions occur which serve both killing and degradation of micro-organisms. The cellular metabolic changes entailed are triggered by the membrane perturbations of phagocytosis. Energy is produced, microbicidal oxidizing substances are generated and lysosomal enzymes are activated. The important area of oxygen metabolism is now mentioned.

(a) Hydrogen peroxide (H_2O_2)

It was first shown in the PMN that oxygen was not required for ingestion but was required for optimal killing, and that phagocytosis triggered cyanide-sensitive oxygen consumption, formation of H_2O_2 and stimulation of conversion of glucose to carbon dioxide via the hexosemonophosphate (HMP) shunt. H_2O_2 can, of course, be extremely toxic to the cell itself so the PMN has two pathways for removal of excess – catalase and glutathione systems. H_2O_2 is part of the myeloperoxidase–halide system of bacterial killing which operates by one of three mechanisms: directly on the bacteria, by fixation of halide to the protein of the bacteria, or by formation of aldehydes (from amino acids) which are toxic to bacteria.

In AM, H_2O_2 formation, oxygen consumption and glucose conversion occur, but to a less extent. The mechanism of the bactericidal action of H_2O_2 in the cell is unclear. Although histochemical and several biochemical assays have failed to detect myeloperoxidase activity in AM, peroxidase activity has been shown more recently using different substrate and conditions. This activity kills only with iodide and not chloride anions (in PMN it occurs with both anions). Also, iodide radicals, H_2O_2 and a granular fraction of homogenized AM are strongly bactericidal, but no formation of active aldehydes seems to occur in this fraction of the cell.

(b) Superoxide anion (O_2^-)

In 1975 the superoxide anion's importance in cells was shown. This anion is a one electron reduction of oxygen (O_2) and is thus a free radical having an unpaired electron. It is a vigorous oxidizing agent but spontaneously dismutes to H_2O_2 and O_2, a process which is catalysed by superoxide dismutase (SOD) enzyme in cells. This anion is only one of a number of highly reactive oxygen reduction products. PMN release the anion when phagocytosing and, for several reasons, it is thought to be a bactericidal agent in its own right, although it may co-operate with the H_2O_2 system as well by supplying H_2O_2 on dismutation. It is also possible that O_2^- and H_2O_2 react to form the unstable, very reactive free hydroxy radical (OH$^.$). In AM little is known except that O_2^- generation occurs at rest and during phagocytosis, and that SOD is found in the cytoplasm.

(c) Singlet excited oxygen ($^1O_2^*$)

This is formed by shift of one electron from a ground energy state orbit to a higher energy state orbit within the oxygen molecule. It was found in PMN using carotenoid pigment, an acceptor of $^1O_2^*$, but whether it is present in AM in uncertain.

The relative importance in bactericidal killing of the various products of oxygen reduction found in phagocytes is not yet determined.

(d) Subcellular localization

It is important to recognize that localization of chemical processes within the complex confines of the cell plasma membrane may be critical in determining whether they are helpful or harmful to the host cell. For instance, reactive oxygen reduction products and H_2O_2 may be efficient in killing micro-organisms within plasma membrane-lined phagocytic vacuoles ('islands of the exterior' within the cell) but can kill the cell itself if liberated into the cytosol without a suitable disposal mechanism.

Localization of chemical processes is also important in determining function itself. In AM, oxygen reduction in the mitochondrial location provides energy for the cell whereas the same process in the phagocytic vacuole promotes the function of microbial killing which defends the host. Elsewhere in the cell such processes may be responsible for other functions, such as tumour cell killing by oxygen metabolites.

12.4.6 Degradation

Lysosomal enzymes are stored inactive within phagocytes as lysosomal granules. Solubilization and activation of the enzymes occurs as lysosomes fuse with phagocytic vacuoles. The regulation of this process is briefly discussed.

(a) Lysosomal degranulation

It is probable that contact between plasma membrane constituents of the wall of the phagocytic vacuole (altered by the act of phagocytosis) and lysosomes triggers degranulation and activation of the enzymes. The phagocytic vacuole is directed towards the lysosomes by microtubules.

That which is known about the sequence of such enzyme release is derived from study to PMN – little being known about it in AM. PMN contain azurophil and specific granules, each containing different enzymes (peroxidase and proteases in azurophil granules; alkaline phosphatase, collagenase and most of the lysozyme in specific granules). The specific granules release their enzymes in the first minute of phagocytosis, but by 10 minutes the phagocytic vacuole contains enzymes from both types of granule.

(b) Lysosomal enzyme release

In PMN it appears that release of lysosomal enzymes is regulated by levels of the cyclic nucleotides cAMP and cGMP via their effects on the polymerization of tubulin (specific dimeric proteins, thirteen of which comprise a microtubule) to form organized microtubules. Neurohumoral agents tending to increase intracellular cAMP diminish release, and vice versa (β-adrenergic drugs diminish release while cholinergic drugs stimulate it; atropine blocks the latter effect). Unfortunately little is known about the regulation of enzyme release in AM and there is considerable conflict in the data available.

(c) Release of lysosomal enzymes independent of phagocytosis

Although it is usual to consider lysosomal enzyme release to occur during phagocytosis, it has been possible to detect release of lysosomal enzymes from phagocytes which have been activated by a C5a-like serum factor and by non-phagocytosable antigen–antibody complexes bound to millipore filters. In addition cytochalasin D, a microfilament 'poison', selectively depresses particle ingestion but not attachment. Its use has allowed demonstration of selective lysosomal enzyme release independent of the ingestion phase of phagocytosis. Lysozyme (muramidase), found mainly in the specific granules of PMN and in high specific activity in human AM, is secreted by such cells in culture and is very little, if at all, influenced by induced phagocytosis. This enzyme is, therefore, used as a marker for measurement of the 'pool' of PMN and/or macrophages in clinical situations.

(*d*) *Neutral proteinases*

Recently, it has been demonstrated that AM contain a variety of biologically important enzymes that PMN have been known to possess for some years. Examples are collagenase and elastase.

(*e*) *Disease*

It is obvious that such complex cells as phagocytes could harm instead of protect the host by a number of mechanisms. It is almost an axiom that deficiency of protective function, particularly phagocytosis and intracellular killing, allows invasion of the respiratory tract by noxious agents. But in a more subtle way the complex machinery of the cell may cause tissue damage by continuous attempts to eliminate 'indigestible' agents. For example, repeated priming of AM by endotoxin during infection could activate a number of synthetic cell processes which then 'back-fire' by releasing tissue-damaging enzymes when attempting to digest, for instance, cigarette smoke-derived inert particles.

Recent work has suggested that the macrophage may have an important role to play in fibrogenesis. Although controlled fibrogenesis is important as a defence or healing mechanism (e.g. walling off an abscess), uncontrolled fibrogenesis undoubtedly causes disease (e.g. cryptogenic fibrosing alveolitis).

12.4.7 Activation of phagocytes

There are a number of non-specific and immunologically specific ways in which macrophages can be 'activated', although relatively little is known about these processes in AM. Two important points require emphasis. First, use of the term 'activation' should always be qualified by exactly what it is that is being activated (e.g. microbicidal mechanisms, adherence, etc.) and how it is being achieved. This will help to amend confusion which has occurred in the literature because of loose usage of the term. Second, 'activation' of any kind is a property of macrophages not PMN which, as has been mentioned before, are essentially 'one-off hit cells' having little 'cross-talk' with the environment.

Lymphokines, those soluble factors produced by lymphocytes which can regulate macrophage behaviour, are an important field of their own with potential clinical importance.

12.5 Clinical syndromes arising out of dysfunction of respiratory defence mechanisms

Although there are a variety of diseases whose pathogenesis is known to depend, or may depend, upon failure to eliminate antigen or noxious agents from the respiratory tract (e.g. extrinsic alveolitis, silicosis, asbestosis, etc.), the main syndromes discussed here will be those due to failure to eliminate infective agents.

Eighteenth century literature describes a syndrome of frequent respiratory infections, and in the 19th century Walshe [1] and also Van Zeimssen [2] wrote about rapid recurrence of respiratory infection after apparently perfect recovery and about the similarity of such episodes to chronic bronchitis except for more rapid development of mucopurulent sputum. Dobell [3] tried to identify those at risk from 'colds going to the chest' and in doing so developed an excellent questionnaire which is the forerunner of several current ones used to identify asthmatic and chronic bronchitic populations.

12.5.1 Recurrent acute infections

The principal syndromes in adults fall into two clinical and radiographic groups which occur principally in non-smokers of a mean age of approximately 25 years.

(a) Without radiographic signs

Recurrent acute, usually upper, respiratory tract infections may occur with varying frequency but all hallmarked by the fact that they rapidly affect the lower respiratory tract provoking expectoration of purulent sputum. In the interval between such infections the patient enjoys normal health. Many such upper respiratory tract (URT) infections are viral and the periods between them vary enormously in length in different patients. It is difficult to define when frequency exceeds the 'normal' incidence because of seasonal variation in exposure to viruses, environmental factors, etc. However, a useful clinical rule is to consider the frequency to be abnormal if it affects the patient's social or working life sufficiently to bring him or her to the doctor. It is surprising in many cases how rapidly the lower respiratory tract is affected (within hours rather than days) and how frequent such episodes can be at the severe end of the spectrum (one episode every two weeks with little intervening sputum-free interval). Such episodes may tend to linger longer than might be expected in the case of a normal adult suffering the average cold, and do not appear to be related to cigarette smoking. There is a definite association of this syndrome with recurrent sinusitis.

(b) With radiographic signs of pneumonia

This syndrome may consist of recurrent URT infections affecting the chest, but is most commonly seen as pneumonia arising *de novo* in the chest at the same or different sites. When the same site is involved each time there is somewhat more likelihood of a local mechanical cause than immunological abnormality.

12.5.2 Chronic purulent sputum production

A third syndrome exists, usually in non-smokers of a slightly greater mean age (45 years), where daily expectoration of purulent sputum occurs and which is often found to be due to bronchiectasis when a bronchogram is performed.

Although in about 20% of these patients there is a good history of a preceding serious respiratory infection in infancy, childhood or shortly before development of the syndrome, it arises 'out of the blue' in the majority of patients. This syndrome is found in association with rheumatoid disease, inflammatory bowel disease and several other conditions loosely classified as 'auto-allergic', e.g. thyroiditis, pernicious anaemia. There is an association of this syndrome with chronic sinusitis.

All three syndromes are associated with a high incidence of wheezing during sputum production and, although antibiotic usage is greatest in patients with daily sputum production, there is a higher incidence of antibiotic (and other drug) allergy in those with recurrent acute infections – perhaps reflecting altered immunological control in this group.

12.5.3 Non-infective syndromes

Inability to eliminate known non-living organic and inorganic particles and fibres from the lung results in a variety of pathological situations including granuloma formation and fibrogenesis. It is hypothesized that other conditions (e.g. emphysema) may be due to inappropriate release of tissue-damaging proteolytic and lysosomal enzymes from phagocytes within the lung – perhaps in situations, as already suggested, where active cells are subjected to the effects of tobacco smoke and other toxins. Such conditions have been reviewed [4, 5] (see Chapter 8).

12.6 Investigation of patients with infective syndromes due to possible dysfunction of respiratory defence mechanisms

Whenever a patient presents with recurrent infections it is imperative to exclude allergy first as sole cause of apparent 'infections'. Once infection is truly established the indication to investigate the patient is interference with normal social or working life by such illnesses. Experience derived from investigating over 400 patients with these three infective syndromes [6] has taught that there are certain routine tests (Table 12.2) which should be done

Table 12.2 Routine schedule for investigation and treatment of patients with a possible respiratory defence mechanism defect

Test	Result, diagnosis and further tests	Treatment
1. History	Defines the syndrome to be evaluated in case non-routine tests necessary	
2. Prick skin tests ± serum IgE Blood for eosinophils Sputum for eosinophils Provocation tests	Diagnoses **allergy** and suspect 'intrinsic' asthma and rhinitis	Hyposensitization Block result of allergic reaction (DSCG) Treat result of inflammatory mediator release (bronchodilators, corticosteroids, etc.)
3. *Aspergillus* prick skin tests Blood for *Aspergillus* precipitins	Diagnoses **allergic bronchopulmonary aspergillosis** ± Bronchogram	Corticosteroids, bronchodilators, etc.
4. Examination of URT Sinus radiographs	Diagnoses **recurrent/chronic sinusitis perennial rhinitis post nasal discharge**	Antimicrobial agent, local corticosteroid spray, drainage, surgery, etc.
5. Serum immunoglobulins	Diagnoses **selective Ig deficiency hypogammaglobulinaemia** → haemopoietic tests gut function tests *Giardia lamblia* infestation Detects raised Igs in response to infection	Non-routine tests required (Table 12.3, 12.5) Gammaglobulin replacement Supplements for malabsorption Metronidazole Non-routine tests required (Tables 12.3, 12.4, 12.5)

Test	Result, diagnosis and further tests	Treatment
6. Sputum microscopy Sputum and blood culture and and sensitivity including AAFB CIE of serum and blood (in serious acute infections)	} Diagnoses **acute pneumonia** with a classical pathogen	Antimicrobial agent
7. Clinical tests of CMI (Mantoux, etc.)	Detects non-exposure or possible defect in CMI	Requires non-routine tests (Table 12.4)
8. Diary card completion daily until next clinic visit	Obtains more objective picture of frequency and severity of syndrome	
9. Non-routine tests (Tables 12.3, 12.4, 12.5)		

Ig = immunoglobulin; URT = upper respiratory tract; AAFB = acid and alcohol-fast bacillus; DSCG = disodium cromoglycate; CIE = counter immunoelectrophoresis; CMI = cell mediated immunity.

on every patient. These can be done in any routine laboratory attached to a chest clinic and will reveal any major deficiencies in respiratory defence mechanisms. Should such screening be negative, the patient will require more sophisticated investigation (Tables 12.3–12.5), which may not be immediately available and which may require referral to a suitably equipped centre.

The flow chart in Table 12.2 shows one sequence of routine investigations which is satisfactory in practice. It attempts to exclude allergy as sole cause of the syndrome, detect and treat any wheezing and rhinitis secondary to infection, provide a more objective record of the patient's illness than can be obtained solely by questions at intermittent clinic visits, assess the upper respiratory tract for parallel infective problems and finally, exclude serum immunoglobulin deficiencies.

The importance of such investigations lies in the fact that almost all dysfunction of defences detected by routine tests is treatable. But prognosis will inevitably depend on how soon before irreversible damage occurs diagnosis is made. It is sad that at present most cases of hypogammaglobulinaemia presenting to chest clinics have severe bronchial destruction which, despite replacement of the deficient immunoglobulin, continues to cause problems for the patient and may lead to death despite such treatment. The clinical lesson to be learned is 'when in doubt, test for immunoglobulin deficiency' – the penalty for missing such deficiency is too great to risk.

Although further non-routine tests may reveal conditions for which no treatment exists at present, nevertheless, it is of importance to delineate groups of patients with such deficiencies so that research can be directed towards understanding them better and possibly designing treatment to rectify them.

The tests referred to in the flow charts in Tables 12.2–12.5 are detailed slightly more fully in Tables 12.7–12.9.

12.7 Conditions revealed by investigation

Once allergy and mechanical causes have been excluded as sole cause of a syndrome, infective conditions broadly divide into two main groups both clinically and immunologically. Recurrent infections tend to have immunological deficiencies or no detectable defect, but chronic infection often carries the stigmata of heightened immunological response and a possible vicious circle of self-destruction in the respiratory tract [6].

12.7.1 Exclusion of allergy (Table 12.2)

Episodes closely resembling recurrent upper and lower respiratory infection may be mimicked by allergic conjunctivitis, rhinitis and asthma. The latter

Table 12.3 Non-routine schedule for further investigation and treatment of patients with recurrent-acute respiratory infections including pneumonia

Test	Result, diagnosis and further tests	Treatment
1. History and clinical examination for clue to aspiration	Detects cause of **aspiration pneumonias**	Treat the cause
2. Sweat Na$^+$ excretion Pancreatic function tests (exocrine and endocrine)	Diagnoses **cystic fibrosis**	Physiotherapy, antibiotics, genetic counselling, pancreatic extracts, etc.
3. Bronchoscopy	To detect a **local mechanical cause** for recurrent pneumonia at same site foreign body postinfective bronchial stenosis bronchial tumour	Usually surgical
4. Bronchography	Detects **localized bronchiectasis**	Surgical
5. Pulmonary angiography	Detects **sequestrated segment**	Surgical
6. Immunological tests (Table 12.4)	Detect **immunity deficiencies**	Table 12.4
7. Local tests of respiratory defence mechanisms	Detect dysfunction of a variety of local defence mechanisms	Table 12.9

Table 12.4 Non-routine schedule for immunological investigation of patients with recurrent respiratory infections including pneumonia

Test	Result, diagnosis	Treatment
1. Igˢ in nasal secretions (Table 12.7)	Detects **sIgA deficiency**	
2. Antigen challenge (Table 12.7) (vaccine)	Detects **inability to mount a 1° or 2° antibody response**	Gammaglobulin
3. IgG sub-class (Table 12.7) estimation	Detects a **sub-class deficiency**	Gammaglobulin
4. Antibody affinity (Table 12.7)	Detects production of **poor affinity antibody**	Gammaglobulin
5. Serum opsonin (Table 12.8) estimation including complement	Detects **serum opsonin deficiency** and complement deficiencies relevant to opsonization	FFP
6. PB phagocyte function (Table 12.8)	Detects **blood phagocyte dysfunction**	? immunostimulation
7. Cell mediated immunity (mitogen and antigen stimulation of PB lymphocytes in autologous and normal serum)	Detects **T cell defect**	Replacement or ? immunostimulation
8. AM function (Table 12.9)	Detects **AM dysfunction**	? immunostimulation

Ig = immunoglobulin; sIgA = secretory IgA; FFP = fresh frozen plasma; PB = peripheral blood; AM = alveolar macrophage.

Table 12.5 Non-routine schedule for further investigation and treatment of patients with chronic purulent sputum production

Test	Result, diagnosis and further tests	Treatment
1. History and clinical examination for clue to aspiration	As in Table 12.3	Treat the cause
2. Sweat Na⁺ excretion Pancreatic function tests (exocrine and endocrine)	As in Table 12.3	As in Table 12.3
3. Bronchoscopy if mechanical cause suspected	As in Table 12.3	As in Table 12.3
4. Bronchography	**Bronchiectasis**	Surgery if localized
5. Serum and nasal Ig^s	Detects **hypogammaglobulinaemia** see Table 12.2	Gammaglobulin
	If raised	1. Reduce load of antigen (physiotherapy, antimicrobial agents)
6. Serum autoantibodies	If present	
7. Circulating IC^s	If raised	2. Plasmaphoresis and/or filtration of IC^s
8. Serum inhibitory factors for lymphocyte and monocyte function	If present	3. ?Anti-inflammatory drugs and/or immunosuppressants
9. Lung and nasal clearance	If impaired	
10. Cilia ultrastructure	Detects dynein arm deficiency, etc.	
11. Sperm ultrastructure	Detects dynein arm deficiency, etc.	
12. Cilia function *in vitro*		
13. Mucus viscoelasticity		
14. Mucus chemistry		

(Tests 6, 7, 8: collectively these may be pathogenetic in causing local tissue damage)

IC^s = immune complexes; Ig = immunoglobulin.

Table 12.6   Factors diminishing the efficiency of defence mechanisms available
to the respiratory tract

(a) *Factors exposing the respiratory tract to infection by affecting systemic (± local)*
defences of the host
    extremes of age
    protein calorie malnutrition
    alcoholism
    diabetes mellitus
    virus infection
    malignancy
    immunity-suppressed states (congenital and acquired)

(b) *Factors exposing the respiratory tract to infection by affecting local defence*
mechanisms
  1. Those providing abnormal quantity or quality of exposure
      highly pathogenic micro-organisms
      aspiration
      postnasal discharge
      excess or abnormally viscid mucus secretion
      pulmonary infarction
  2. Those causing abnormal clearance
      cough suppressants (e.g. analgesics, pain, unconsciousness)
      cilia depressants (e.g. congenital states, general anaesthesia)
      mucosal damage (e.g. virus infection)
      bronchial obstruction (e.g. tumour, foreign body, emphysema)
      respiratory myopathy (e.g. motor neurone disease)
      tracheostomy
  3. Dysfunction of the immunity mechanisms (Tables 12.3, 12.5)

---

can also be exacerbated by virus infection, and these symptoms (in a skin test negative 'intrinsic' form) may occur for the first time following a virus infection. It is important to recognize these pitfalls and to treat them before embarking on the more complicated, time-consuming and expensive tests of protective immunity. Suggestive history, positive immediate hypersensitivity skin prick tests to common allergens, presence of eosinophils in nasal secretions and/or sputum and blood eosinophilia are all pointers to an allergic basis for the syndrome of recurrent 'infection'.

The relationship between allergy and infection in the respiratory tract is fascinating but eludes understanding at present. It is possible that a number of allergic manifestations are the penalty which man pays for a very efficient antiparasitic defence mechanism which, unfortunately, can be hoodwinked by such agents as pollen into responding as though against parasitic invasion.

Table 12.7 Tests of local and systemic humoral immunity

Qualitative serum Ig^s (immunoelectrophoresis)
Quantitative serum Ig^s of classes G, A and M (radial immunodiffusion)
Serum antibody production in response to antigen challenge

1. to naturally occurring antigens (e.g. isohaemagglutinins, *Escherichia coli*)
2. As primary and secondary response to acute challenge (e.g. influenza virus vaccine)

Serum IgG sub-class estimation
Ig^s in nasal secretions (esp. sIgA)

Ig = immunoglobulin; sIgA = secretory IgA.

Table 12.8 Tests of opsonization and phagocyte function

Total number of neutrophils in peripheral blood
Total number of monocytes in peripheral blood
Chemotaxis *in vivo:* skin window or chamber test
            in vitro: movement through a filter
Tests of phagocytosis: particles or micro-organisms
Tests of intracellular killing of micro-organisms
Tests of metabolism (e.g. NBT test, chemiluminescence)

Use of autologous and normal serum to opsonize particles or micro-organisms
    prior to phagocytosis and killing, and analysis of any such deficiency in the
    patient's serum in terms of the intact nature of classical and alternative
    pathways of complement, immunoglobulin, etc.

NBT = nitrobluetetrazolium.

Table 12.9 Tests of respiratory tract defences

Clearance of radiolabelled particles
Ig^s in nasal and bronchial secretions
Cilia – structure (light and electron microscopy)
      – function *in vitro* (beat frequency)
Free lung cells – differential cell count
                – immunological markers
                – alveolar macrophage function
Physical and biochemistry of mucus

Ig = immunoglobulin.

12.7.2 Antibody deficiencies

(*a*) *Selective immunoglobulin deficiency* (Tables 12.2, 12.4 and 12.7)

From discussion earlier in this chapter it is easy to understand the deleterious effect on the host of absence of locally produced secretory IgA (sIgA) in the respiratory tract. This can be detected by measuring sIgA in nasal or bronchial secretion. Absence of serum IgA is usually accompanied by absent sIgA, but in some cases antibody is produced locally in the absence of serum antibody and may account for normal health in some individuals with no serum IgA. When serum IgA is low but not absent there may be enough locally produced sIgA to protect the respiratory tract against a large proportion of infections. There are documented rare cases of low sIgA with normal serum levels of IgA, so it is important to sample nasal/bronchial secretions as well as to test serum. Nevertheless, as has been discussed in the first part of this chapter, the role of sIgA in protection of the respiratory mucosa is not completely understood, and it may be that deficiency of IgA in serum or secretions needs to be accompanied by a lack of compensatory protective mechanisms (e.g. IgM production) or by other defects in order to be manifest clinically.

Treatment of selective IgA deficiency is difficult. There is insufficient IgA in replacement immunoglobulin preparations to be of use, and boosting IgG levels by such preparations in the hope of encouraging transfer of the molecule across mucous membranes to protect them has not been shown to be effective clinically [7]. Indeed, use of immunoglobulin preparations containing small quantities of IgA may result in severe adverse reactions if the patient with absent IgA possesses antibodies directed against IgA (anti-IgA antibodies). Fresh frozen plasma has apparently helped some patients with this disorder (but who do not produce anti-IgA antibodies); however, because not all patients respond, the situation is complicated and requires further study.

(*b*) *Hypogammaglobulinaemia* (Tables 12.2 and 12.7)

Although a generalized defect, this condition usually presents with respiratory infections or gastrointestinal malfunction. In many cases it does not lead to polytopic infections but manifests itself solely by respiratory tract symptoms. After diagnosis it is very important to investigate the haemopoietic and gastrointestinal symptoms in order to detect complications of this condition – in particular giardiasis which is easily treated with metronidazole.

Treatment with replacement human immunoglobulin is highly effective in reducing frequency and severity of infections, therefore it is imperative to have a high index of suspicion of the condition in order to diagnose it before irreversible lung damage, which can cause debility and death despite therapy, occurs.

(c) *Immunoglobulin G sub-class deficiencies* (Tables 12.4 and 12.7)

These are more difficult to detect and usually require specialist laboratory assistance. It is important to test for them when no other defect has been found because they usually respond to immunoglobulin replacement therapy.

(d) *Inability to mount an antibody response to antigen* (Tables 12.4 and 12.7)

Tests of antibody response to antigens 'naturally' present in the body (e.g. red blood cell isoantigens, *E. coli* antigens in the gut) will reflect gross humoral immunity deficiency but will not detect those patients who, while they can respond to such strong chronic antigen stimulation, cannot respond promptly to the type of acute antigen challenge that is so common in daily life. Such inability to respond can be detected by slowness or inability to mount an antibody response to artificial challenge with such antigens as are contained in influenza virus vaccine or tetanus toxoid. Here again one might expect such persons to be helped by normal human immunoglobulin replacement therapy.

(e) *Poor antibody affinity* (Tables 12.4 and 12.7)

Despite normal levels of immunoglobulin of the various classes it is possible for the antigen-combining ability of the contained antibodies to be poor. A small quantity of antibody with good 'grabbing' quality might be of more use to the host than much antibody with poor such function. Again, replacement normal human immunoglobulin might be of advantage to the host in such circumstances.

12.7.3 Opsonin deficiencies and phagocyte defects (Tables 12.4 and 12.8)

(a) *Opsonin deficiencies*

Immunoglobulin deficiency, principally of IgG, will cause defective phagocytosis of particles in the respiratory tract, but deficiency of other serum factors such as complement components will also cause this. Such deficiency may be specific for a given micro-organism but is usually more general in its effect. The use of chemiluminescence (light emission by virtue of active oxygen radical production by cells) is revolutionizing the diagnosis of such defects and allows serum opsonization of a variety of different particles from micro-organisms to be tested very rapidly [8]. By its use new data is emerging about various factors contributing to opsonization [9].

Replacement of such deficiencies by regular infusion of fresh frozen plasma is highly effective in rectifying such defects and this therapy can be easily and rapidly monitored by chemiluminescent techniques.

(b) Phagocyte defects

These are rare and often present to non-respiratory specialist departments of medicine (e.g. patients with chronic granulomatous disease, CGD, although suffering from respiratory infections and granulomata, being young often present to paediatricians or with skin sepsis to dermatologists). However, there are occasions when such patients with recurrent infections are seen by the respiratory physician and then they require careful investigation by a specialist centre to define the underlying defect in phagocyte function – be it in chemotaxis, motility, phagocytosis, microbial killing or particle degradation, as discussed earlier in this chapter. This is a rapidly expanding field and there is promise from several lines of research of potential therapy for such disorders by activating such cell functions with lymphocyte extracts and immunostimulant drugs. In acute situations transfusion of phagocytic cells may allow time for more definitive therapy to be planned.

12.7.4 Defects in cell mediated immunity (Table 12.4)

From experience provided by 400 patients studied in a clinic at Brompton Hospital defective lymphocyte function is rare, but often seen in association with hypogammaglobulinaemia (itself rare).

12.7.5 Defects in alveolar macrophage (AM) function (Tables 12.4 and 12.9)

A small number of patients with recurrent respiratory infection have abnormal AM phagocytosis and killing of bacteria not due to opsonin deficiency. Such defects are partially rectified *in vitro* by culture with certain immunostimulant drugs. Treatment of these patients with such drugs has been successful in the few who can tolerate such therapy. The majority of patients, however, are prevented from continuing treatment by toxic effects of the drugs available at present. Stimulated AM oxidative metabolism can be measured using lucigenin-dependent chemiluminescence [10].

12.7.6 Immunological overactivity

The immunological abnormalities described hitherto (with the notable exception of hypogammaglobulinaemia) are commonly seen in recurrent rather than chronic respiratory infection (Tables 12.10 and 12.11). Chronic

Table 12.10 Abnormalities found in the immunological defence mechanisms available to the respiratory tract in 218 patients with recurrent acute respiratory infection

	Recurrent respiratory infection (little or no radiographic signs)	*Recurrent pneumonias*
Hypogammaglobulinaemia	1	4
Selective IgA deficiency (absence)	78 (7)	6 (4)
Opsonin deficiency	21*†	7‡
Failure to mount antibody response to antigen	9*	1
One or more Ig classes raised	17	1
None	96	3
Total number of patients	200	18

* 1 with hypogammaglobulinaemia.
† 3 with absent IgA.
‡ 4 with hypogammaglobulinaemia.
Ig = immunoglobulin.

Table 12.11 Abnormalities found in the immunological defence mechanisms available to the respiratory tract in 200 patients with chronic purulent sputum production

Hypogammaglobulinaemia	9
One or more Ig classes raised	156
Lymphocyte stimulation depressed	6*
Serum inhibitory factor(s)	32
Autoantibodies present	51
Autoallergic disease	20
Opsonin deficiency	9*
None	25
Total patients studied	200

* all with hypogammaglobulinaemia.
Ig = immunoglobulin.

respiratory infection may be due to hypogammaglobulinaemia, but if this deficiency is excluded the common picture seen is exuberant humoral response with increased immunoglobulin levels (doubtless a response to bacterial antigen), production of serum factors inhibiting lymphocyte function (among them immune complexes), production of autoantibodies and prevalence of autoallergic or inflammatory bowel disease in the patient or his family. Such features, detected by tests outlined in Table 12.5, raise the possibility of a vicious circle of bronchial destruction occurring through exuberant immunological response against a bacterial load and possibly against self – directly, by cross reaction, or through complement fixation by immune complexes of antibody and bacterial antigen deposited in the wall of the respiratory tract.

It is interesting that titres of immune complexes are higher in those bronchiectatics whose disease appears to be rapidly progressing despite strict physiotherapy, postural drainage and rotating combinations of antibiotics. Although this may be a secondary effect, it is important to study this further in case such immune complexes are pathogenetic. The implication for treatment, should this be so, is almost heretical because it would involve removing the immune complexes by plasmaphoresis or filtration and suppressing their formation by immunosuppression, as well as reducing bacterial antigen load in time-honoured manner with physiotherapy and antimicrobial agents.

12.7.7 Defective clearance

Various methods [11] of measuring clearance of isotopically labelled particles from the respiratory tract have resulted in definition of a number of patients with chronic purulent sputum production who have reduced capacity to clear such particles. Further studies on such patients may reveal abnormalities which could account for their poor clearance.

(*a*) *Cilia abnormalities* (Tables 12.5 and 12.9)

Rarely, such patients show a morphological abnormality of ultrastructure of cilia such as dynein arm deficiency. This abnormality may also be manifest in the sperm tail of such patients (which has similar structure to a cilium). Such abnormality may be responsible for malfunction of ciliary activity because dynein is thought to act as a contractile protein in this process. It is one cause of the 'immotile cilia syndrome' described by Eliasson *et al.* [12]. Dynein arm deficiency is seen in Kartagener's syndrome (see Chapter 15). Bizarre abnormalities in cilium ultrastructure are found in a rapidly fatal bronchiectatic syndrome seen in Polynesians [13]. Measurement of ciliary beat frequency is now possible by a brushing technique [14].

(*b*) *Mucus abnormalities* (Tables 12.5 and 12.9)

Although much attention is being paid to control and quality of secretion of mucus in the respiratory tract, the significance of subtle changes in viscoelasticity and chemistry of such secretions to clinical disease is ill understood. This area is of considerable importance because of theoretical amenability of these properties to pharmacological intervention.

(*c*) *'Reservoir' of infection*

In a series of patients with *cystic fibrosis* it has been shown that alveolar macrophages contain live intracellular bacteria not killed by the cell's microbicidal mechanisms and able to slowly multiply despite conventional treatment with parenteral antibiotics [6]. Whether this is a property of the bacteria or AM is under study. This phenomenon could conceivably explain exacerbations of infection with the same organism seen after treatment which apparently eradicates the organism from the sputum.

(*d*) *Neglected potential pathogens*

The use of selective bacteriological media under appropriate conditions can show potential pathogens, such as *Haemophilus influenzae*, to be present in sputum from patients with chronic suppurative respiratory disease which, if cultured under usual laboratory conditions, show overgrowth of such organisms as *Pseudomonas aeruginosa* [15]. The rapid *in vitro* growth of such organisms swamps other underlying potential pathogens which grow slowly *in vitro*. The application of such bacteriological techniques to the study of chronically infected patients may lead to better antimicrobial management.

12.8 Specific treatment

Conventional treatment for infection (antimicrobial agents, physiotherapy and bronchodilators if wheeze is present) is particularly important when the host's protective clearance mechanisms are at fault. Because success of such measures may in turn depend upon the integrity of a number of the host's defences, it is important to consider specific therapy to remedy abnormalities of such defences.

12.8.1 Normal human immunoglobulin (gammaglobulin)

Situations in which replacement therapy with this material is indicated have been discussed. Therapy is usually administered by intramuscular injection. Loading doses of 50 mg/kg body weight/24 h are given for five days, followed by weekly injections of 25 mg/kg body weight. Initially, it is important to monitor the level of IgG in serum just before the weekly dose is administered to ensure that the material is not being lost abnormally rapidly by some mechanism. If it is, an increased dose weekly or twice weekly is required. In practice the volume of material is large and the injection usually painful; nevertheless patients prefer it to their infections. Reactions to the material (tachycardia, rigors, limb and back pain, abdominal colic, shock) may occur within 30 min – mainly in patients with deficiency of immunoglobulin other than congenital hypogammaglobulinaemia or secondary immunodeficiency. They may be due to aggregates of IgA in the material or to complement activation by IgG aggregates. Such reactions can often be prevented by centrifugation of the material before administration. Anti-IgA antibodies in patients with selective IgA absence may cause anaphylaxis if gammaglobulin is given in this situation. In the latter case it is important to screen for such antibodies against several IgA myeloma proteins to detect true anti-IgA antibodies (rather than an idiotypic antibody to a particular IgA myeloma) because such reactions can be fatal.

Fifty mg/kg body weight/week is significantly more effective in preventing infections than the 25 mg/kg/week mentioned above, but it is usually an unacceptably large injection for a single administration. An intravenous IgG preparation is now available in which aggregates are prevented by mild chemical manipulations. The new preparation has several advantages: its half-life is about three weeks, it contains over 80% of its original antibody activity and it can be given in large volume by intravenous infusion whereas the intramuscular preparation of gammaglobulin used at present lacks the Fc portion of the IgG molecule, which makes it subnormal in opsonizing quality and short in half-life (five or six days), because it is enzyme-digested. Side effects of the intravenous preparation (nausea, fever, flushing and cramps) are not as severe as may occur with the intramuscular preparation but occur in about 30% of primary antibody-deficient patients. They may be lessened or abolished by taking 600 mg of aspirin 30 min before infusion. Other intravenous preparations under trial are acid-treated and S-sulphonated IgG, the latter reverting to native form within 24 h of administration and persisting for an approximately three-week half-life.

12.8.2 Fresh frozen plasma (FFP)

Regular infusions of this material have successfully reduced the frequency and severity of recurrent infections in patients with opsonin deficiencies [7]. Some of these patients have lacked IgA but such infusions do not seem to benefit this condition if it is solitary – only if it is associated with an opsonin deficiency or IgG subclass deficiency. Similar precautions with regard to anti-IgA antibodies as in therapy with gammaglobulin must be taken if the recipient lacks IgA in the serum. There is a slight risk of serum hepatitis from this treatment although donor material is screened for hepatitis B antigen. Infusions every eight weeks have been found to be necessary in most patients to allow them to lead a normal life.

12.8.3 Transfer factor

In very rare cases of T-lymphocyte deficiency transfer factor may help, but usually becomes relatively less effective as time and repeated administration continue. This material is composed of informational molecules derived from disrupted leucocytes.

12.8.4 Thymus grafts

In the case of thymic dysplasia with deficient T-lymphocyte function (rarely seen in a chest clinic, unless paediatric) grafting irradiated thymus to the anterior rectus sheath can induce maturation of T-lymphocytes under the influence of thymic substances.

12.8.5 Bone marrow grafts

In cases of B-lymphocyte and stem cell deficiency histocompatible bone marrow grafts can repopulate the recipient and lead to normal immuno-logical function. The graft procedure is complicated and hazardous, involving immune suppression of the recipient so that the graft is not rejected. Graft reactions against host can occur in this situation and management of this form of therapy can be exceedingly difficult requiring specialist skills.

12.8.6 Immunostimulants

(a) Vaccines

Anti-pseudomonas vaccines, for use in patients prone to chronic respiratory infection with the organism, show signs of being helpful in management, but it is too early to be sure of their place in therapy. Pneumococcal vaccines have been more widely used, particularly in the USA, in situations where systemic host defences are compromised – with promise. But the situation with regard to chest infection in the UK requires further study.

(b) Biological and pharmacological agents

A variety of drugs and other agents (Table 12.12) possess the property to activate various parts of the immune response. An example is levamisole, first noted to have such properties when being used as an antiparasitic agent. It has no effect on normally functioning lymphocytes and phagocytes but can restore deficient function to normal *in vitro* and *in vivo*. Unfortunately, it is a toxic drug which is poorly tolerated. However, work with a variety of analogues is proceeding in an attempt to find more active, less toxic agents.

Table 12.12   Immunostimulants

Microbial	Biological	Pharmacological
BCG	Transfer factor	Levamisole
C. parvum	Thymic hormones	Isoprinosine
Mixed bacterial vaccines	Lymphokines	Muramyl dipeptide and analogues
Pseudomonas vaccine	Interferon	Interferon inducers
Pneumococcal vaccine		Copolymer pyran
		SM 1213
		Lynestran
		Bestatin

Interferon deserves special mention because it has already been shown to be effective in protection against rhinovirus infection of the upper respiratory tract when applied locally. Provision of adequate supplies from cell cultures and from 'genetically engineered' bacteria holds promise for its use in the future.

12.9 Concluding remarks

Failure to eliminate inhaled living and non-living antigenic material from the respiratory tract may cause damage to the host from invasion by such material or continued frustrated host response against it, or both. The investigation and treatment of defective respiratory defence mechanisms (whether it be to increase or decrease them) are now becoming as important to survival as has been modification of the invading material in the past.

Further Reading

Bateman, E., Emerson, R. and Cole, P. J. (1980), Mechanisms of fibrogenesis. In: *Lung Biology in Health and Disease,* Vol. II (*Occupational Lung Diseases*). (Eds M. Turner-Warwick and H. Weill) (Executive ed. Claude Lenfant), Marcel Dekker, New York and London pp. 237–90.

Green, G. M., Jakab, G. J., Low, R. B. and Davis, G. S. (1977), Defence mechanisms of the respiratory membrane. *Am. Rev. resp. Dis.*, **115**, 479–514.

Hocking, W. G. and Golde, D. W. (1979), The pulmonary-alveolar macrophage. *New Engl. J. Med.*, **301**, 580–7; 639–45.

van Furth, R. (ed.) (1980), Mononuclear phagocytes in immunity, infection and pathology. Blackwell, Oxford.

Brain, J. D., Proctor, D. F. and Reid, L. M. (eds) (1977), Respiratory defence mechanisms Part I and II. In: *Lung Biology in Health and Disease*, Vol. 5. (Executive ed. Claude Lenfant), Marcel Dekker, New York and London.

References

1. Walshe, W. H. (1871), In: *A Practical Treatise on the Disease of the Lungs*. (Ed. Smith) Elder and Company, London.

2. Van Zeimssen (1876), *Diseases of Respiratory Organs.* Cyclopaedia of the Practice of Medicine, Vol. 4. London.

3. Dobell, H. B. (1866). *On Winter Cough, Catarrh, Bronchitis, Emphysema and Asthma*, Churchill and Sons, London.

4. Allison, A. C. (1977). Mechanisms of macrophage damage in relation to the pathogenesis of some lung disease. In: *Lung Biology in Health and Disease*, Vol. 5. (Respiratory Defence Mechanisms Part II) (Eds J. D. Brain, D. F. Proctor and L. M. Reid) (Executive ed. Claude Lenfant), Marcel Dekker, New York and London.

5. Bateman, E., Emerson, R. and Cole, P. J. (1980). Mechanisms of fibrogenesis. In: *Lung Biology in Health and Disease*. Vol. II (*Occupational Lung Diseases*). (Eds. M. Turner-Warwick, and H. Weill) (Executive ed. Claude Lenfant), Marcel Dekker, New York and London pp. 237–90.

6. Cole, P. J. (1980), Immunological mechanisms in lung disease. In: *Recent Advances Respiratory Medicine*, **2**, (Ed. D. C. Flenley) Churchill Livingstone, Edinburgh pp. 1–8.

7. Cole, P. J. (1981), Immunity deficiency states. In: *Scientific Foundations of Respiratory Medicine*. (Eds J. G. Scadding, G. Cumming and W. M. Thurlbeck), William Heinemann Medical Books, London pp. 441–51.

8. Easmon, C. S. F., Cole, P. J., Williams, A. J. and Hastings, M. (1980), The measurement of opsonic and phagocytic function by Luminol-dependent chemiluminescence. *Immunol.*, **41**, 67–74.

9. Williams, A. J., Hastings, M. J. G., Easmon, C. S. F. and Cole, P. J. (1980), Factors affecting the *in vitro* assessment of opsonization using the technique of phagocytic chemiluminescence. *Immunol.*, **41**, 903–11.

10. Williams, A. J. and Cole, P. J. (1981), Investigation of alveolar macrophage function using Lucigenin-dependent chemiluminescence. *Thorax* (in press).

11. Pavia, D. *et al.* (1980), Techniques for measuring lung muco-ciliary clearance. *Europ. J. resp. Dis.* (in press).

12. Elliasson, R., Mossberg, B., Camner, P. and Afzelius, B. A. (1977), The

immotile-cilia syndrome. A congenital ciliary abnormality as an etiologic factor in chronic airway infections and male sterility. *New Engl. J. Med.*, **296**, 1–6.

13. Waite, D. *et al.* (1978), Cilia and sperm tail abnormalities in Polynesian bronchiectatics. *Lancet*, **ii**, 132–3.

14. Rutland, J. and Cole, P. J. (1980), Non-invasive sampling of nasal cilia for measurement of beat frequency and study of ultrastructure. *Lancet*, **ii**, 564–5.

15. Roberts, D. E. and Cole, P. J. (1980), The use of selective media in bacteriological investigation of patients with chronic suppurative respiratory infection. *Lancet*, **i**, 796–7.

CHAPTER THIRTEEN

Bronchoscopy and Cytology

D. C. Zavala

13.1 Types of bronchoscopes

13.1.1 The rigid bronchoscope

In 1897, an endoscope was used for the first time by Gustav Killian to remove a pork bone from the main right bronchus [1]. This was a remarkable feat considering the rather primitive methodology, the crude instruments employed, and the inadequate source of light. Modern bronchoscopy began with Chevalier Jackson in the early 20th century. This pioneer from Philadelphia, USA, was responsible for the development of the rigid, open-tube bronchoscope and for the establishment of bronchoscopy as a medical specialty [2]. The procedure was (and often still is) carried out in an operating room theatre under sterile conditions with the endoscopist and his team gowned and gloved.

At first, the rigid bronchoscope served a limited but vital role; that is, it was used primarily for the removal of inhaled foreign bodies, an art which was practised by some physicians, otolaryngologists, and surgeons. Gradually the application of rigid bronchoscopy widened to include its use in the diagnosis and treatment of many pulmonary diseases [3]. During the 1930s and 1940s, chest physicians, specializing in pulmonary tuberculosis, began to acquire the skill of rigid bronchoscopy. Soon they learned to appreciate the endoscopic view of the tracheobronchial tree and the unusual capabilities of the instrument, including the diagnosis of endobronchial tuberculosis.

Over the years, the basic design of the rigid bronchoscope has not changed; the instrument has remained a hollow, metal tube. But great advances have been made in the optical systems, forceps and accessory equipment (Fig. 13.1). Some of the more recent improvements include the following:

1. Fibreoptic telescopes with lenses at 0°, 30°, and 90° angles for superb vision of the large airways.

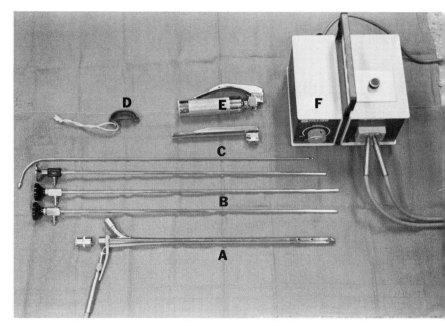

Fig. 13.1 The setup for rigid endoscopy: (A) rigid, open-tube bronchoscope; (B) bronchoscopic telescopes with angles at 180° (forward), 135° (oblique), and 90° (lateral); (C) metal aspiration tube, (D) rubber bite block, (E) laryngoscope with straight and curved blades, and (F) light source for the bronchoscope and telescopes [7].

2. Ventilation bronchoscopes and oxygen-venturi systems [4] for adequate gas exchange during anesthesia.
3. Optical (fibreoptic) forceps which enables the operator to see the jaws of the forceps and the biopsy site simultaneously.
4. A directable, optical forceps* which can be deflected at the distal end to biopsy previously inaccessible orifices of the upper lobes (Fig. 13.2).

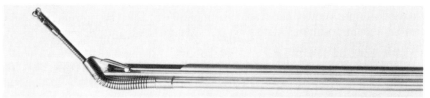

Fig. 13.2 The new, directable, optical (Karl Storz) forceps which can be passed through the rigid bronchoscope and deflected into the upper lobe for biopsy under visual control.

* Manufactured by Karl Storz KG, D-7200 Tuttlingen, W. Germany, Mittelstr. 8-P.O.B. 400.

5. Radio-opaque plastic tubing for aspiration biopsy.
6. Powerful cold light sources with excellent fibreoptic light transmission.
7. Fine paediatric ventilation bronchoscopes.
8. Effective suckers and on-line specimen collectors.
9. Aspiration biopsy needles to obtain cytological material from enlarged mediastinal lymph nodes compressing the carina or mainstem bronchi.
10. Teaching attachments and cameras.

13.1.2 The flexible fibreoptic bronchoscope

During the 1960s, a major event occurred in pulmonary medicine, namely, the introduction of the flexible fibreoptic bronchoscope by Dr Shigeto Ikeda, Tokyo, Japan [5]. This instrument, also called the bronchofibre-scope, proved to be an important advance in the diagnosis and management of pulmonary diseases (Fig. 13.3). Literally, the flexible fibreoptic bron-choscope has revolutionized pulmonary medicine! Open-tube broncho-scopy and surgical intervention are no longer the only options in diagnosing

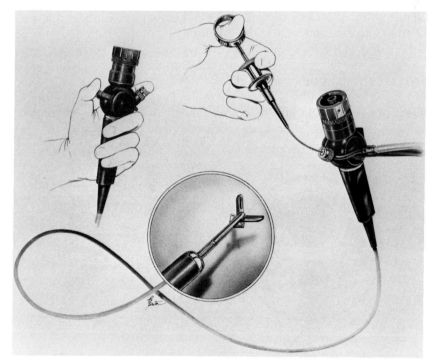

Fig. 13.3 An artist's drawing of the Olympus fibreoptic bronchoscope. The cup forceps, extending from the flexible distal tip of the bronchoscope, is ready for bronchial or transbronchial biopsies [7].

indeterminate chest disease. With few exceptions, the flexible instrument now plays a prime role in diagnosing a wide variety of lung densities and infiltrates [6, 7].

At the present time, the detection of lung cancer is one of the major diagnostic uses of the bronchofibrescope. Direct biopsy is performed on endoscopically visible lesions, i.e. vision through the fibreoptic bundles enables the operator accurately to position the inserted biopsy tool (brush or forceps) on target. Those lesions beyond the range of the fibreoptic instrument are biopsed indirectly under fluoroscopic control. In addition to cytopathological evaluation, culture specimens are obtained for the study of bacterial, mycobacterial, fungal and viral infections. Although the fibreoptic bronchoscope plays a vital role in diagnostic endoscopy, its therapeutic application in airway management has been equally important. It has been likened to a mobile 'seeing-eye' for the assessment of airway patency and the guided application of its suction tip to relieve atelectasis secondary to retained secretions and mucous plugs.

Currently there are five different makes of bronchofibrescopes: Olympus, Pentax, Machida, ACMI, and Fujinon. The operating head of each instrument has an adjustable eyepiece, plus a thumb/finger-controlled lever or knob to angulate and manoeuvre the distal end of the shaft. The insertion tube (shaft) of the standard fibrescope measures 5–6 mm in diameter, and contains a single operating channel (1.8–2.6 mm diameter) which serves both as a suction tube and a passageway for forceps, brushes, balloon catheters, or foreign body extraction tools. The distal end of the bronchofibrescope is shown in Fig. 13.4. Excellent sources of cold light (xenon or halogen) are available for illumination and photography.

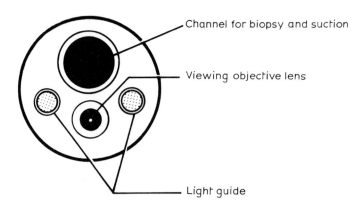

Fig. 13.4 The design of the bronchofibrescope as seen from the distal end (diameter approximately 5 to 6 mm). Note the close arrangement of the channel, viewing lens, and light guide [7].

13.1.3 Flexible versus rigid bronchoscopy

Since the advent of the flexible fibreoptic bronchoscope, the rigid (open-tube) bronchoscope is not being used as often as previously, but this does not mean that the technique of rigid endoscopy should be disgarded. This time-honoured instrument still plays an important diagnostic and therapeutic role. Thus, it is important for the physician to have a clear understanding of the indications, limitations, and contraindications of both the open-tube and flexible fibreoptic bronchoscopes. Selection of either bronchoscope is not simply a question of one technique against the other, but is a question of utilizing the advantages of each instrument. The proper usage of the two types of bronchoscopes is discussed in the following sections.

13.2 A comparison of the rigid (open-tube) and flexible fibreoptic bronchoscopes

13.2.1 Preferred uses of the rigid bronchoscope

(a) Paediatric cases

The open-tube, ventilating bronchoscope is the instrument of choice in paediatric bronchoscopy. In particular, foreign body removal in children remains the exclusive domain of the rigid, open-tube bronchoscope. The reason is rather evident, namely, the small size of the glottis and trachea preclude the passage of the adult bronchofibrescope with its solid, nonventilating shaft.

Miniaturized bronchofibrescopes have been tried in children as young as three to four years of age, but their use is limited. One technical drawback, almost impossible to correct, is that these tiny fibreoptic bronchoscopes either have no aspirating channel or have one which is too small for effective suction and the passage of instruments. On the other hand, they can be used to great advantage in infants and children for examination of the nose, nasopharynx, oropharynx and larynx; also, to verify the position of an endotracheal tube, to evaluate a cleft palate, and to appraise upper airway patency in an infant with the croup.

(b) Massive haemorrhage

The open-tube bronchoscope is mandatory for the control of life-threatening haemorrhage by suction, by application of adrenaline, by gauze tape packing, or by insertion of a Fogarty balloon catheter. Even the larger fibreoptic bronchoscopes with 2.6 mm diameter suction channels cannot effectively handle a major bleeding episode. In addition, when blood floods the airway, fibreoptic vision is completely lost.

(c) Profuse, thick secretions

At times, mucoid impactions and copious, sticky secretions cannot be handled by the small aspirating channel of the fibreoptic instrument. In such instances, open-tube bronchoscopy and utilization of a large sucker is the preferred method. Unfortunately, there are serious technical problems in attempting to use a rigid bronchoscope on a patient being mechanically ventilated. For such a situation, the flexible bronchofibrescope is ideally suited.

(d) Foreign body (centrally located)

For over half a century the open-tube bronchoscope has been eminently successful in the removal of endobronchial foreign bodies. This is especially true in the paediatric age group where most foreign body aspirations occur in toddlers and children up to four or five years of age. Today, rigid bronchoscopy remains exclusively the procedure of choice for the removal of foreign objects in the young. Also, in adults, the open-tube bronchoscope still is the standard approach [8]. There is, however, a small subgroup of adult patients in whom tiny aspirated objects become lodged in segmental bronchi, beyond the reach of the rigid bronchoscope, and are best retrieved with the flexible bronchofibrescope along with the aid of special extraction tools and fluoroscopy [7]. Otherwise, chest surgery must be carried out to prevent pneumonia, abscess formation, bronchopleural fistula or empyema. These complications are especially prone to occur if the object is organic rather than metallic.

(e) Bronchial adenoma

Although bronchial adenomas comprise only 1–5% of all primary lung neoplasms, special comment is warranted since these tumors (90% are carcinoids) may bleed briskly when disturbed. Some adenomas do not bleed when biopsied, but a conservative approach is best. If a bronchial adenoma is encountered during fibreoptic bronchoscopy, the endoscopist has two options: 1. call the surgeon for his visual confirmation and schedule the patient for thoracotomy without a forceps biopsy – a brush biopsy is non-productive, and 2. carry out forceps biopsy through the rigid, open-tube instrument. My preference is to obtain tissue via the rigid bronchoscope.

The diagnostic problem is to be aware that one may be dealing with a bronchial adenoma. A young adult with an abnormal chest radiograph and a history of recurrent pneumonia or haemoptysis certainly should arouse suspicion. Eighty per cent of these tumours are centrally located and frequently manifest their presence by atelectasis or an obstruction pneumonitis; 20% are present as peripheral coin lesions. The bronchoscopic appearance may be that of a pink, red, or greyish-yellow tumour whose overlying mucosa is intact. Sometimes the adenoma appears as a polyp, or as a submucous growth.

(f) Broncholith

Fortunately, broncholithiasis is rarely encountered. The stone (calcified lymph node) may be deeply incorporated into the wall of the bronchus, producing symptoms of obstruction. A rigid bronchoscope is absolutely necessary for insertion of a large forceps so that the intruding stone can be removed piecemeal.

(g) Narrowed trachea

If the diameter of the trachea is small (as normally occurs in a child, or abnormally occurs in an adult with tracheal or paratracheal pathology), then insertion of an open-tube, rigid instrument will ensure an adequate airway. On the other hand, passage of a flexible fibreoptic bronchoscope with its non-ventilating shaft will further occlude the airway. Examples of pathologic conditions which may result in significant tracheal occlusion are: tracheal tumours (rare), invading oesophageal carcinomas, enlarged paratracheal nodes secondary to metastatic carcinoma, benign or malignant thyroid disease, subglottic stenosis, and tracheal stenosis following tracheostomy.

(h) Photography

For photography of the tracheobronchial tree, nothing can compare with the superb pictures obtained through a rigid bronchoscope using a Hopkin's telescope (Karl Storz KG); the magnificent work of Stradling [3] is a fine example. The limitations of the flexible fibreoptic bronchoscope for photography are imposed chiefly by the image transmission characteristics of the fibre bundles [9, 10]. Any appreciable enlargement of the resulting tiny photomicrographs will produce a bothersome display of the fibre bundle network and indistinct pictures. Also, broken fibre bundles show up as black dots which further obscure the picture.

13.2.2 Optional uses of either bronchoscope

(a) Biopsy of central lesions

The biopsy of central lesions, under direct endoscopic vision, can be carried out by flexible or rigid bronchoscope with similar diagnostic yields of 94 to 98%. Using one or the other instrument, the recovery of tissue or cells may be accomplished by the forceps, brush, curette, needle (aspiration), or by lavage and suction. In this respect, the rigid bronchoscope has one advantage over the flexible instrument, namely, a large forceps can be utilized to obtain a generous piece of tissue for frozen section and prompt diagnosis.

Currently, however, most procedures are being performed with the flexible bronchofibrescope, primarily because of the comfort to the patient and the ease of the procedure. Flexible fibreoptic bronchoscopy can readily be performed under local anaesthesia using lignocaine and, unlike rigid bronchoscopy, rarely requires a general anaesthetic.

(b) Removal of secretions

Both rigid and flexible bronchoscopes are employed to assess airway patency and to clear troublesome secretions that fail to respond to conventional physiotherapy. Superior suction can be achieved with a wide-bore sucker via the rigid, open-tube bronchoscope, but the newer fibreoptic bronchoscopes with large-sized aspirating channels of 2.6 mm in diameter have greatly improved their suctioning capabilities. Currently, because of ease, convenience, and effectiveness, the flexible bronchoscope routinely is being used to achieve tracheobronchial toilet with clearing of atelectasis in 80 to 85% of the cases, and to obtain reversal of previously refractory hypoxemia [11, 12]. The controllable tip of the flexible instrument can be directed visually to the site of retained secretions, mucous plugs, exudate, or inspissated material. These problems commonly occur in patients following surgery or in those with chronic obstructive lung disease, asthma, cystic fibrosis [13, 14], allergic bronchopulmonary aspergillosis, or bronchocentric granulomatosis. Lavage with small boluses of sterile, normal saline facilitates the removal of putty-like material by suction. Occasionally, if the secretions are too abundant, too thick, or if the plugs are seemingly glued in place, then an open-tube bronchoscope with a large-bore aspirating tube is necessary.

(c) Transbronchial lung biopsy

As an initial diagnostic procedure in diffuse and localized lung disease, transbronchial biopsy (TBB) offers an attractive alternative to open lung biopsy (Fig. 13.5). In the past, TBB was carried out through a rigid bronchoscope with a diagnostic yield of 84%, bleeding in 1%, and a pneumothorax in 10 to 14% [15]. Insertion of a chest tube was necessary in approximately 50% of the patients with an air leak. At the present time, TBB is done almost entirely with the flexible fibreoptic bronchoscope. Properly done, the procedure has a good diagnostic yield, a low incidence of complications, and is well tolerated by the patient [7, 16]. In addition, flexible fibreoptic bronchoscopy not only has the advantage of being done under local anaesthesia, but also the mobile tip of the instrument can guide the forceps to *any* area of the lung. On the other hand, rigid bronchoscopy often requires general anaesthesia, and TBB is limited primarily to basal lung segments.

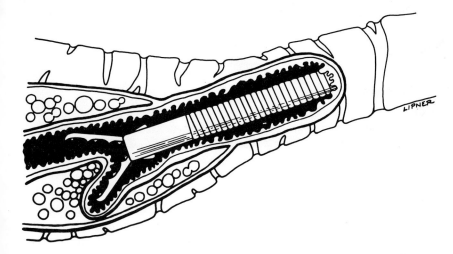

Fig. 13.5 An artist's impression of a transbronchial lung biopsy. Note the invagination of the bronchial wall (peripheral bronchus) into the jaws of the forceps [7].

TBB via the flexible bronchofibrescope is carried out by passing the closed forceps peripherally under fluoroscopic control to the area of involvement. In diffuse disease, a peripheral biopsy always is taken. Upon arrival at the periphery of the selected lung segment (usually anterior, lateral, or posterior basal segment of the lower lobe), the forceps are retracted 1–2 cm, opened on inhalation, gently advanced 1.0 cm as the patient lets out his air, closed at the end of exhalation, then slowly retracted. Routinely, several specimens are obtained from one lung only. The opposite lung is not biopsied because of the hazard of a bilateral pneumothorax. Fluffy, floating tissue in sterile saline solution is indicative of lung tissue, whereas bronchial tissue is dense and sinks (Fig. 13.6). *In localized disease*, the forceps are passed to the lung density or nodule with the aid of fluoroscopy, retracted 0.5 cm, opened, then advanced slowly until resistance is encountered or contract is verified fluoroscopically. Again, the forceps are closed and retracted. When dealing with localized lesions, 'blind' biopsies without fluoroscopic guidance result in an unacceptably low diagnostic yield and a greater potential for complications.

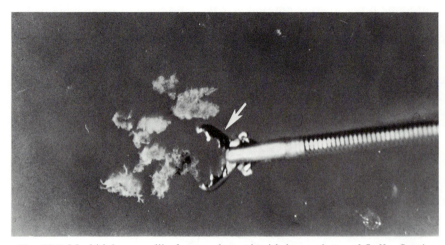

Fig. 13.6 Machida's crocodile forceps (arrow) with large pieces of fluffy, floating lung tissue obtained by transbronchial biopsy [7].

Immediately following biopsy, the forceps are withdrawn through the channel, but the tip of the fibreoptic bronchoscope is positioned firmly in the segmental bronchus to prevent blood from flooding the tracheobronchial tree. An important detail is that the bronchofibrescope be wedged *at the end*, and not the beginning, of exhalation since it is possible for air (under increasing pressure) to pass from the airway into a pulmonary vein [17]. If haemorrhage occurs, the bronchoscope is kept in the *wedge* position for four to five minutes to allow time for a clot to form [7]. Thus, haemorrhage as a result of TBB can be entirely confined to the segmental bronchus. In diffuse disease a peripheral biopsy always is taken since the arteries are smaller in this location and the danger of bleeding is less. One should not forget, however, that the risk of bleeding from pulmonary arterioles, capillaries, and bronchial vessels may be greatly increased by pulmonary hypertension.

(d) Lung abscess

Either the rigid or the flexible bronchoscope can be employed to drain a lung abscess, but one should not forget that the rigid instrument can allow greater suction. Thus, if the flexible bronchofibrescope is used, it is wise to have a rigid, open-tube bronchoscope handy in the event of a sudden outpouring of thick, purulent material which could drown the patient [18]. Flooding of the airway may occur during instrumentation, while inserting a biopsy tool into the abscess, or shortly following bronchoscopy. Any patient with a lung abscess should be kept under close observation after bronchoscopy, preferably in a recovery room.

13.2.3 Advantages of the flexible bronchoscope

The major advantages of the flexible over the rigid, open-tube broncho-scope are as follows [7]:

(a) Increased range of vision and biopsy

Upon comparison with the rigid bronchoscope, one important advantage of the flexible instrument is a considerable increase in the area of observation and biopsy as shown in Fig. 13.7. The white zone in the central airways represents the restricted area of biopsy possible with the straight tube bronchoscope. The stippled, gray zones (at the entrance to the upper lobes) represent the small added area of vision through a standard, rigid broncho-scope using forward-oblique and lateral viewing telescopes. The black, segmental bronchi in Fig. 13.7 represent the extended visual and biopsy

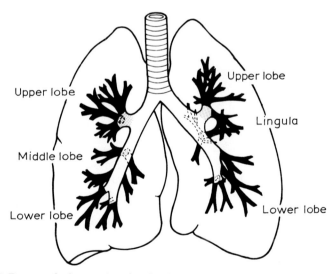

Fig. 13.7 Range of observation for flexible and rigid bronchoscopes. The black segmental bronchi illustrate the increased area of observation obtained by the flexible fibreoptic bronchoscope over the rigid bronchoscope [76].

range of the flexible fibreoptic bronchoscope. With the tip of a 5.5 mm bronchofibrescope, all third-order bronchi can be entered and all fourth-order bronchi can be inspected. In addition, 75% of the fourth-order bronchi can be entered, and as many as 68% of the fifth-order and 56% of the sixth-order bronchi can also be inspected [19].

(b) Manoeuverability

The difference in manoeuverability of each bronchoscope is emphasized in Figs 13.8 and 9. Fig. 13.8 illustrates the rigid, straight tube instrument overlaid on Ikeda's anatomical drawing of the tracheobronchial tree. The only movement possible is forward and backward, that is, in and out of the right and left mainstem bronchi. Fig. 13.9 shows the mobile shaft of the fibreoptic bronchoscope with the flexed distal tip directed into the right upper lobe.

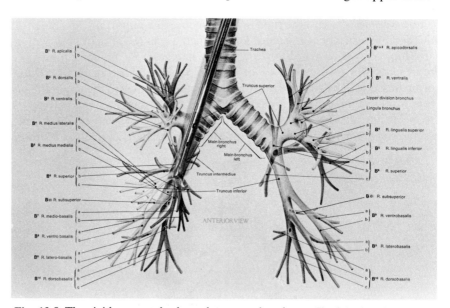

Fig. 13.8 The rigid, open-tube bronchoscope placed over Ikeda's drawing of the bronchial tree. Biopsy is chiefly restricted to central lesions. See Fig. 13.2 showing the new optical forceps which can be directed into the upper lobe [7].

(c) Patient comfort

The next major advantage of flexible over rigid endoscopy is the comfort of the patient. Fig. 13.10 illustrates the extended position of the patient's head necessary to introduce the straight bronchoscope. Under no circumstances should the upper teeth (or gums) be used as a fulcrum. Some operators

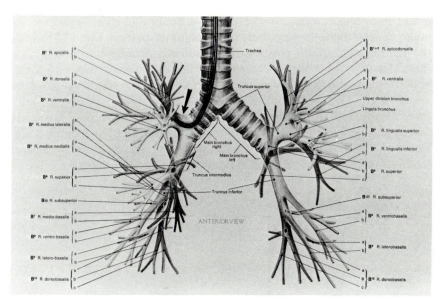

B¹ R. apicalis	a	
	b	
B² R. dorsalis	a	
	b	
B³ R. ventralis	a	
	b	
B⁴ R. medius lateralis	a	
	b	
B⁵ R. medius medialis	a	
	b	
B⁶ R. superior	a	
	b	
	c	
B⁺ʲ R. subsuperior		
B⁷ R. medio-basalis	a	
	b	
B⁸ R. ventro basalis	a	
	b	
B⁹ R. latero-basalis	a	
	b	
B¹⁰ R. dorsobasalis	a	
	b	
	c	

Trachea
Truncus superior
Main bronchus right
Main bronchus left
Truncus intermedius
Truncus inferior

ANTERIOR VIEW

a		B¹⁺² R. apicodorsalis
b		
c		
a		B³ R. ventralis
b		
c		
		Upper division bronchus
		Lingula bronchus
a		B⁴ R. lingualis superior
b		
a		B⁵ R. lingualis inferior
b		
a		B⁶ R. superior
b		
c		
		B⁺ʲ R. subsuperior
a		B⁸ R. ventrobasalis
b		
a		B⁹ R. laterobasalis
b		
a		B¹⁰ R. dorsobasalis
b		
c		

Fig. 13.9 The flexible tip of the fibreoptic bronchoscope (arrow) can be seen easily entering the right upper lobe. Thus, the range of biopsy is greatly extended [7].

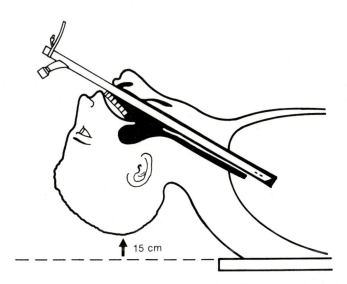

↑ 15 cm

Fig. 13.10 Rigid bronchoscopy. Note the uncomfortable, extended position of the head with the chin pointing vertically upward. This position would be difficult for a patient with cervical arthritis [76].

prefer local anaesthesia, but there is little doubt that rigid bronchoscopy under general anaesthesia is more pleasant for the patient. Fig. 13.11 shows the natural, comfortable position of the head in a recumbent patient for oral introduction of the bronchofibrescope through a previously inserted 8.5-mm endotracheal tube. The flexible shaft easily conforms to the curvature of the upper airway. The procedure is carried out under local anaesthesia. With practice, the operator of the flexible bronchoscope can become extremely fast in routine examination of the tracheobronchial tree, including all segments (B1 through B10) and subsegments. Biopsy of more peripheral lesions under fluoroscopic control does require additional time.

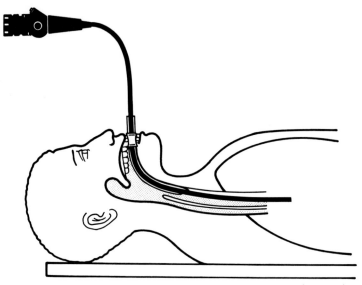

Fig. 13.11 Flexible fibreoptic bronchoscopy. The patient is shown resting comfortably on the table with the flexible fibreoptic bronchoscope inserted through an oral endotracheal tube [76].

(d) Detection of early lung cancer

Preliminary results from the Mayo Clinic Lung Project suggest that early bronchogenic carcinoma can be detected by a careful screening programme using the fibreoptic bronchoscope to identify radiologically occult tumours in male smokers with positive sputum cytology [20].

(e) Increased diagnostic accuracy

In comparison with the rigid bronchoscope, superior overall diagnostic results are obtained with the flexible fibreoptic bronchoscope. This is primarily because of the extended visual and biopsy range of the flexible instrument and the fact that fluoroscopy can be used to guide the biopsy tool to a peripheral lesion located beyond endoscopic vision. The combination of brush and forceps biopsy on all lesions produces the highest diagnostic yield. In fact, a variety of biopsy instruments should be available since no single instrument is adaptable to all situations (Fig. 13.12). In *central* fibreoptically visible bronchogenic carcinomas, the diagnostic yield is from 94 to 98% when using both the brush and the forceps on the same lesion [5, 21, 22]. In *peripheral* bronchogenic carcinomas, i.e. those beyond direct endoscopic vision, the overall yield drops to 60–70% [21–23]. In small, peripheral primary carcinomas the diagnostic accuracy of forceps biopsies (via the bronchofibrescope) drops to 50% if the lesion is less than 3 cm in diameter and to 30–40% if less than 2 cm [24].

In *metastatic* cancer to the lung the all-inclusive diagnostic success for the fibreoptic bronchoscope is only 30–40% [21]. The yield is much higher in malignant melanoma and genitourinary tract carcinomas, since these malignancies often metastasize to the lungs endobronchially where they are accessible to direct biopsy. In such circumstances, it is common for metastatic renal carcinoma to be mistaken for primary lung cancer because of its appearance when viewed during endoscopy.

In *diffuse lung disease* the diagnostic yield ranges from 60–80% with about 40% classified as aetiologic and 30% classified as non-specific [25]. Thus TBB via the flexible fibreoptic bronchoscope may be successful in providing the bronchoscopist with a specific diagnosis in a number of diffuse alveolar and parenchymal diseases, such as alveolar cell carcinoma, lymphangitic carcinoma, lymphoma (Hodgkin's and non-Hodgkin's), sarcoidosis [26, 27], fungal bacterial and mycobacterial infections, cytomegalic inclusion disease,

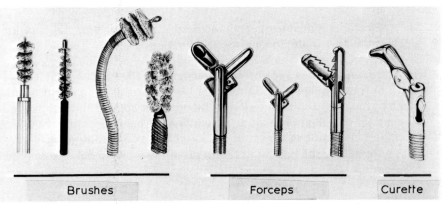

| Brushes | Forceps | Curette |

Fig. 13.12 Biopsy tools, including a variety of brushes, forceps, and a single-hinge curette. The curette is difficult to manipulate safely and is seldom used in the United States or England [21].

Pneumocystis carinii pneumonitis [28], pulmonary alveolar proteinosis, etc. In addition, biopsy tissue may show pathological changes consistent with the diagnosis of silicosis, asbestosis, collagen vascular disease, vasculitis (Wegener's granulomatosis), Goodpasture's syndrome, histiocytosis-X, eosinophilic pneumonia, drug-induced lung disease, etc. Unfortunately, finding non-specific inflammation, pneumonitis, or diffuse fibrosing alveolitis gives the physician no information regarding the cause of the disease process although it does provide a diagnosis.

13.2.4 Preferred uses of the flexible bronchoscope

Although the uses of the flexible fibreoptic bronchoscope are many and varied, as listed below, sound clinical judgement in the application of the instrument is essential.

(a) Diagnosis of lung disease (diffuse or localized)

The exceptions are mediastinal lesions which do not involve airway or lung parenchyma, and the peripheral nodule or subpleural density which is best approached by fine needle aspiration or thoracotomy.

(b) Assessment of airway patency

(c) Removal of retained secretions or plugs

(d) Special situations

The unique operational features of the flexible fibreoptic bronchoscope are ideally suited for the following special situations:

(i) *Haemoptysis with a negative chest radiograph.* The fibrescope, is a super sleuth in tracking down mild bronchial bleeding to its source. Bronchitis is one of the most common causes of blood in the sputum, but the reward of a careful examination may be an early laryngeal or bronchogenic carcinoma. If inspection of the upper and lower airway is non-productive, then it is important for the patient to return promptly for rebronchoscopy if the haemoptysis should recur.

(ii) *Positioning a Fogarty catheter (for control of haemorrhage).* In selected patients with intermittent, severe bleeding the fibreoptic bronchoscope can be inserted when bleeding temporarily ceases to position strategically a

Fogarty catheter and then occlude the orifice by inflating the balloon [29]. This technique can be especially helpful when the haemorrhage is from either upper lobe, an area extremely difficult to approach with the straight, open-tube bronchoscope.

(iii) *Positive sputum cytology for cancer with a negative chest radiograph.* Again, as above, it is important to pay close attention to the nasopharynx and larynx as well as the tracheobronchial tree. Any visible lesion, localized area of 'infection', oedematous spurs (subcarinae), and granular lack-lustre mucosa should be biopsied by brush and forceps. If visual examination is negative, then the operator has the option of performing meticulous, time-consuming, segmental bronchial brushing or else instructing the patient to return for periodic examination.

(iv) *Nasopharyngeal or laryngeal lesions.* No fibreoptic bronchoscopy is complete without a thorough examination of the airway above the trachea (Fig. 13.13). The normal anatomy of these sites, as seen by the bronchoscopist, is shown in Fig. 13.14. A history of hoarseness should lead one directly to

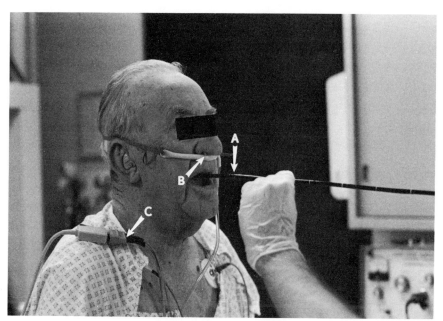

Fig. 13.13 Examination of the nasopharynx and larynx, just prior to bronchoscopy. The operator is positioned facing the patient. (A) Denotes the shaft of the broncho-fibrescope which is inserted intraorally. The patient is receiving prophylactic O_2 by nasal cannula (B) and is connected for cardiac monitoring (C) [7].

the larynx. Because of the high incidence of laryngeal carcinoma in smokers, sometimes occurring simultaneously with primary bronchogenic carcinoma, fibreoptic inspection of the larynx is essential in planning the overall management of the patient. A history of an adult suddenly developing a 'stuffy' or infected ear should alert the physician to possible involvement of the Eustachian tube and nasopharynx. One of several aetiologies to be considered is a nasopharyngeal tumour blocking the tube's orifice.

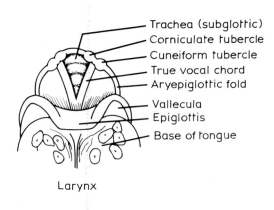

Larynx

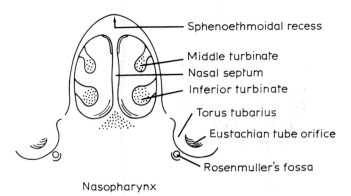

Nasopharynx

Fig. 13.14 The anatomy of the larynx and the posterior nasopharynx as visualized through the fibreoptic bronchoscope via oral insertion (see Fig. 13.13 showing the procedure) [7].

(v) *Small, peripheral foreign bodies.* In adults, the flexible fibreoptic bronchoscope is being recognized for its capability in removing small foreign objects located beyond the range of the rigid bronchoscope [21, 30, 31]. Recently developed techniques make use of new extraction tools (forceps, basket, claw, Fogarty balloon catheter) which are inserted through the biopsy channel. Metallic objects usually can be secured by the jawed forceps or wire basket (Fig. 13.15). Organic objects, however, may present technical problems in recovery because of an intense tissue reaction which results in impaction or entrapment of the object (e.g. peanut). In such a situation, the Fogarty catheter is directed beyond the foreign body, the balloon is expanded, and the catheter is pulled back to dislodge the object into a larger airway where it can be captured more easily with the appropriate extraction tool. Proper technique is essential to avoid trauma to the airway, fracture of the food material into small pieces, displacement of the foreign body to a more peripheral location, loss of the object in the subglottic area during extraction, and hypoxaemia.

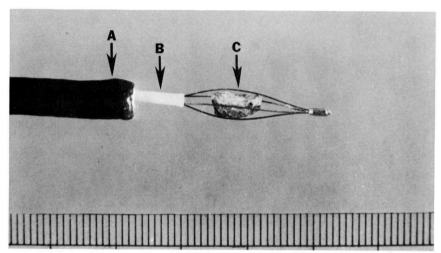

Fig. 13.15 Fibreoptic retrieval of a foreign body from the right middle lobe of a 69-year-old man: (A) the distal end of the bronchofibrescope; (B) the teflon tube which is passed through the channel of the bronchoscope and sheaths the closed basket, and (C) the dental filling captured by the basket. At bronchoscopy the foreign body was dislodged using a Fogarty balloon catheter, then secured with the wire basket [7].

(vi) *Certain predicaments.* Sometimes bronchoscopy is needed under difficult or unusual circumstances, such as when patients are on mechanical ventilators or when they have disease or trauma involving the skull, jaw, or cervical spine. The flexible shaft of the fibrescope is ideally suited to handle patients in any of these situations where use of a rigid, straight tube would be ill-advised. For intubated or tracheostomized patients on mechanical ventilators, a swivel tracheal tube adapter (Fig. 13.16) is utilized to facilitate passage of the bronchofibrescope for examination of the tracheobronchial tree and the removal of secretions.

Additional special applications of the fibreoptic bronchoscope not previously discussed include: performing therapeutic and diagnostic bronchoalveolar lavage; assessing resectability in lung cancer; obtaining selective cultures in pneumonia using special, double sheathed, sterile brushes (Meditech, Watertown, Mass., USA); determining the extent of respiratory tract injury in inhalation of noxious fumes, gastric aspiration, and thermal exposure; evaluating thoracic trauma; checking sutures on sleeve resections; determining the position of an endotracheal tube plus the condition of the adjacent mucosa; appraising a tracheoesophageal fistula; performing gastroscopy on a child; aspirating patients on frame beds or those wearing neck braces; and intubating patients with cervical spondylitis, dental problems, myasthenia gravis, acromegaly, achalasia, full stomach,

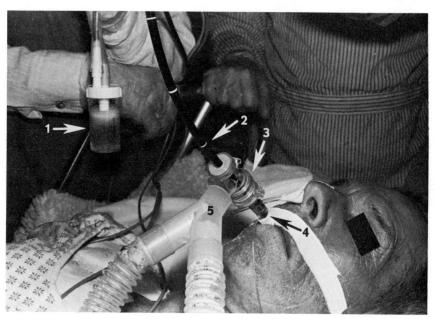

Fig. 13.16 Fibreoptic bronchoscopy on a patient who is being mechanically ventilated in the Intensive Care Unit: (1) suction trap; (2) shaft of the fibreoptic bronchoscope inserted through the tracheal tube adapter and the endotracheal tube; (3) T-tube adapter which is interposed between (4) oral ET tube and (5) connector leading to inspiratory and expiratory lines of the ventilator. A large plug of putty-like material was removed from the left mainstem bronchus, resulting in prompt clearing of massive atelectasis (left lung) and marked improvement in the blood gas values [7].

small bowel obstruction and pathology of the head, neck, oropharynx, larynx or trachea.

13.3 Indications

The indications for bronchoscopy are rather broad but reasonably clear [3, 7, 32]. Many of the indications are implied in the preceding discussion on the relative merits of the rigid and flexible bronchoscopes. Prolonged deliberations on whether or not to perform endoscopy, albeit flexible or rigid, represent wasted time and effort. With modern methods and in well-trained hands, the procedure is safe and rewarding, both from the standpoint of diagnosis and therapy. A single episode of haemoptysis in a smoker may be sufficient to warrant bronchoscopy, even if the chest radiograph is normal. A recent onset of unexplained cough, a change in the nature of a chronic cough, a unilateral wheeze, an expiratory stridor, a persistent or recurrent pneumonia, and an abnormal chest radiograph (atelectasis, infiltrate, density, localized hyperlucency, etc.) all raise strong suspicions of serious pulmonary disease and make such patients potential candidates for bronchoscopy.

13.4 Contraindications

There is no substitute for sound clinical judgement, but knowledge of high risk situations and contraindications can help the bronchoscopist to avoid doing great harm to the patient. Obviously, the hopeless, terminal cases and fragile patients of great age are unlikely candidates for endoscopy.

The *absolute* contraindications for rigid and flexible fibreoptic bronchoscopy are [7]: 1. lack of patient cooperation in diagnosis; 2. uncorrected bleeding diathesis; 3. nonreversible hypoxaemia with an arterial oxygen tension (P_aO_2) that cannot be corrected to at least 60 or 65 mmHg (about 8 kPa) with supplemental oxygen; 4. *acute* hypercapnia with a resting arterial carbon dioxide content (P_aCO_2) above 45 mm Hg (about 7 kPa); 5. serious cardiac arrhythmia, and 6. recent myocardial infarction (within six weeks).

For elective bronchoscopy, patients with untreated pulmonary tuberculosis can be started on specific drug therapy, then undergo a procedure two to three weeks later without danger of infecting the endoscopist or other members of the team. Patients with advanced obstruction of the superior vena cava are at risk because of laryngeal oedema. It is proving easier and safer to employ a flexible fibreoptic bronchoscope on these patients and to keep the subjects in a sitting position during and after the procedure. Closure of the glottis has been known to occur following rigid bronchoscopy. Another option is to first treat the patient with irradiation.

Other high-risk situations include: 1. asthma – danger of increased airways obstruction [33]; 2. uremia – major hazard of severe haemorrhage after biopsy [25]; 3. vascular tumour with haemoptysis – may be associated with significant postbiopsy bleeding; (4) lung abscess – danger of rupture with flooding of the airway; 5. immunosuppression – risk of postbronchoscopy infection.

13.5 Training

The flexible fibreoptic bronchoscope is responsible for a marked increase in the number of clinicians, medical and surgical, undertaking bronchoscopy. Medical pulmonologists, surgeons and otolaryngologists primarily are involved. Also, the specialized application of using a fibrescope for difficult intubations has caught the eye of anaesthetists. The paediatrician is showing some interest in miniaturized fibreoptic bronchoscopes, but the uses of these small instruments are definitely limited.

Thus, the modern chest physician needs to acquire the skill of flexible fibreoptic bronchoscopy in order to play an active and important role as a chest consultant. Fellowship programmes in the speciality of chest diseases should provide thorough instruction in the art of bronchofibrescopy; otherwise, the course of training will be incomplete. Not only may a poorly performed bronchoscopy without adequate safeguards do great physical harm to the patient, but lesions may be missed and the patient given false reassurance that 'everything is all right'. In 1921, Chevalier Jackson made a statement that is fully applicable today: 'Endoscopic ability cannot be bought with instruments'. Another way of expressing this thought is the statement of mine that 'the bronchoscope does not make the bronchoscopist'.

Some physicians have had extensive experience in rigid bronchoscopy, but this fact does not give them the privilege of carrying out flexible fibreoptic bronchoscopy without prior training, any more than a physician experienced in flexible fibreoptic endoscopy has the right to attempt rigid bronchoscopy *de novo* without supervision. *Ergo*, regardless of the instrument employed, bronchoscopy should be performed by experienced, qualified physicians in a hospital biopsy room or an intensive care unit where proper supportive equipment and trained personnel are readily available.

A difficult question to answer is: 'Should one learn fibreoptic bronchoscopy without being thoroughly trained in rigid, open-tube endoscopy?' Expertise in both techniques is theoretically sound and ideally desirable, but in practice may not be absolutely necessary. It is important, however, for the fibreoptic endoscopist to become familiar with rigid endoscopy, so that he or she may have a better appreciation of its uses and limitations. Also, while performing fibreoptic bronchoscopy, it is wise to have a rigid bronchoscope available to handle the unusual event of massive haemorrhage from a forceps biopsy or an outpouring of thick material from a ruptured abscess. In our experience of over 5000 fibreoptic bronchoscopies, it was necessary to terminate the procedure and insert a rigid, open-tube bronchoscopy on only four occasions. Specifically, these instances were as follows: two patients with excessive haemorrhage, one patient with copious, thick purulent material from a lung abscess, and one patient with a large oesophageal tumour invading the trachea. In the two instances of severe bleeding, one was the result of forceps biopsy of a highly vascular tumour near the carina, and the other was secondary to a transbronchial lung biopsy in an immunosuppressed, uraemic patient.

There are two aspects in the training of a competent endoscopist which are seldom mentioned. The first is education of the hands to manoeuvre the bronchoscope, and the second is education of the eyes to recognize the view. Manipulation of the instrument, rigid or flexible, should be natural and spontaneous. All of this takes *time, patience*, and *effort*. The trainee needs to become familiar with the anatomical variations of the tracheobronchial tree and the appearance of bronchial pathology. The abnormal must be distinguished from the normal. Particularly in flexible fibreoptic bronchoscopy, one needs to have a thorough knowledge of segmental lung anatomy (B1 through B10 plus subsegments) and to be able to correlate the location of the lesion on the chest roentgenogram with the bronchial route leading to the target area (Figs 13.17–13.20). Otherwise, it is like 'being on a fishing expedition while blindfolded'.

The use of lung models (Fig. 13.21), illustrations, coloured photography, and cinematography is helpful, but nothing can take the place of the real thing. The ratio of the skilled, dedicated teacher to the committed student must remain one to one. To become competent in bronchoscopy, the exact number of procedures which the trainee must perform over a finite period of time cannot arbitrarily be set. Each trainee differs in the acquisition of new skills; therefore, the operator's performance must be judged on an individual basis. In a fellowship training programme in chest diseases, most trainees develop an acceptable degree of competency after performing approximately a hundred bronchoscopies with the rigid or flexible instrument. Then, the endoscopist should continue to perform the art of bronchoscopy often enough to reinforce and further develop his talents [34].

13.6 Patient preparation

Following the history, physical examination and appropriate laboratory tests (our own check list is shown in Table 13.1), a complete explanation is made to the patient of the coming events and a written consent is obtained. The alleviation of the patient's anxiety and the proper use of premedications are essential. This statement applies to both types of endoscopy, rigid or flexible. For a morning procedure, the patient is kept without food or drink for eight hours overnight. A light liquid breakfast may be allowed if endoscopy is performed in the afternoon. The premedications are as follows:

The most important routine premedication is *atropine*, 0.6 to 1.0 mg, given by intramuscular injection 30 min prior to rigid or flexible bronchoscopy; a higher dose may be required by asthmatic patients. This rather substantial dose is required to achieve the following beneficial effects: block the vasovagal reflex, reduce bronchorrhoea, and neutralize the bronchospastic results of topical anaesthesia and bronchoscopy. The use of sedatives and hypnotics varies from centre to centre. *Morphine*, long known for its excellent hypnotic and antitussive effects, has a safety factor which is uni-

Table 13.1   Screening checklist for fibreoptic bronchoscopy

Patient's Name_____   Age_____   Hosp._____

1. ____   Operative Permit Signed_____

2. ____   Previous Bronchoscopy_____

3. ____   History of: Asthma_____   Drug Allergies_____

　　　　　 C-V Disease_____   Haemoptysis_____   Uremia_____

　　　　　 Immunoincompetence_____

4. ____   Time of Last Food or Drink_____

5. ____   Current Meds. (propranolol, Coumadin, nitroglycerin)

6. ____   Premedications: atropine_____   morphine_____

　　　　　　　　　　 other_____

7. ____   Chest radiographs_____

8. ____   PT, PTT, Platelets_____

9. ____   Arterial Blood Gases_____

10. ____   Spirometry_____

11. ____   EKG_____

12. ____   Blood Urea Nitrogen (optional)_____

13. ____   Sputum Smears: Cytology_____   AFB_____

---

que; namely, any respiratory depression from overdosage can rapidly be reversed by the intranvenous administration of naloxone. The morphine is given intramuscularly with atropine at the discretion of the physician. The dose may vary from 7.5 to 15 mg depending upon the age, size, and condition of the patient. Those with severely compromised pulmonary function should receive no morphine. If morphine is omitted, then sometimes

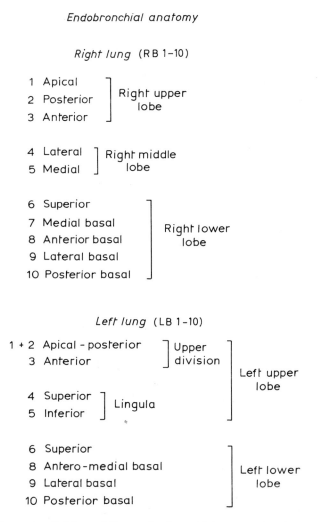

Endobronchial anatomy

Right lung (RB 1–10)

1 Apical ⎤
2 Posterior ⎬ Right upper lobe
3 Anterior ⎦

4 Lateral ⎤ Right middle lobe
5 Medial ⎦

6 Superior ⎤
7 Medial basal ⎥
8 Anterior basal ⎬ Right lower lobe
9 Lateral basal ⎥
10 Posterior basal ⎦

Left lung (LB 1–10)

1 + 2 Apical - posterior ⎤ Upper division ⎤
3 Anterior ⎦ ⎥
⎥ Left upper lobe
4 Superior ⎤ Lingula ⎥
5 Inferior ⎦ ⎦

6 Superior ⎤
8 Antero-medial basal ⎬ Left lower lobe
9 Lateral basal ⎥
10 Posterior basal ⎦

Fig. 13.17 The major divisions of the tracheobronchial tree are listed for both sides by name and corresponding number. It is convenient to refer to the segment by its number [7].

codeine 60 mg is given to suppress cough. *Barbiturates* are often used with atropine if the patient is being prepared for a general anaesthetic, but this type of sedation is seldom employed in flexible fibreoptic bronchoscopy. Instead, diazepam 10 mg orally or by injection is sometimes administered if the patient is unusually apprehensive.

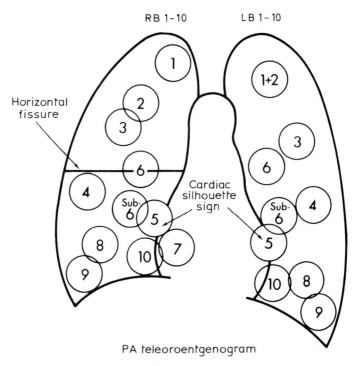

Fig. 13.18 The location of lung lesions on a PA chest film by segmental anatomy. This diagram and the one in the Fig. 13.19 will help the trainee to orient the chest lesion to the appropriate bronchial segment [7].

13.7 Anaesthesia

13.7.1 Rigid bronchoscope

Either a local or a general anaesthetic may be utilized for rigid broncho-scopy. Some operators prefer to insert the rigid bronchoscope using topical anaesthesia with moderate sedation. This is done in preference to employing a general anaesthetic which requires an operating room and the services of an anaesthetist and surgical nursing staff. But even in ex-

RB 1–10 and LB 1–10

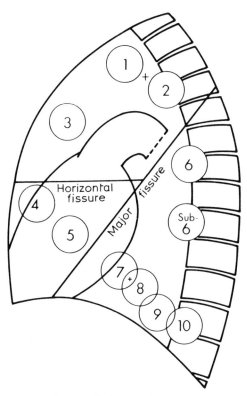

Lateral teleoroentgenogram

Fig. 13.19 The location of lung lesions on a lateral chest film by segmental anatomy [7].

perienced hands, rigid bronchoscopy under local analgesia may be a trying experience. Many patients who have had this procedure done while awake say, 'never again'. For this reason, general anaesthesia, often with an intravenous muscle relaxant, is commonly preferred in rigid bronchoscopy [35].

Briefly, the traditional method of local anaesthesia for rigid bronchoscopy is as follows. While the patient is in a sitting position, the pharynx is sprayed with 1.0 ml of 5% cocaine solution; pledgets of cotton (soaked in 5% cocaine) are applied to the pyriform fossae, and 1.0 ml of 5% cocaine solution is dropped on the vocal cords using a curved cannula and laryngeal mirror. At this point, many operators like to bend the patient to one side, then the other, while instilling additional cocaine (1.0 ml per side) through the glottis into the trachea. This last manoeuvre helps to achieve better anaesthesia in the areas of the right and left upper lobes.

13.7.2 Flexible bronchoscope

Unlike rigid bronchoscopy, general anaesthesia is rarely indicated in flexible fibreoptic bronchoscopy. The few occasions requiring a general anaesthetic for bronchofibrescopy are when the patient is sensitive to topical anaesthetics, and when a markedly prolonged fibreoptic bronchoscopy is required. One example would be for the identification of an occult lung tumour in a patient with positive sputum cytology and a negative chest radiograph. Such a procedure may last two or more hours and involves extensive segmental brushing and multiple spur (subcarinal) biopsies [20, 36].

Routinely, fibreoptic bronchoscopy is performed using local anaesthesia [7, 37, 38]. The methodology is similar to that employed for rigid bronchoscopy except that lidocaine is used in preference to cocaine. Although topical cocaine provides excellent anaesthesia and vasoconstriction, it does

Endobronchial anatomy

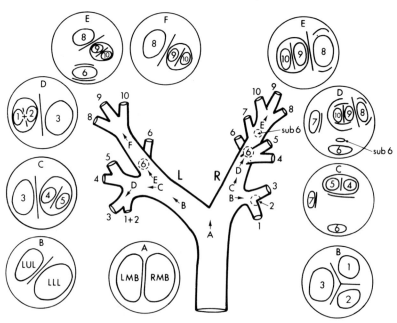

Fig. 13.20 The bronchial segments, B1 to B10 bilaterally, as they appear to the bronchoscopist standing at the head of the supine patient. The endoscopic picture changes 180° if the operator passes the bronchofibrescope transnasally while facing the patient [7].

have a reduced margin of safety and carries all of the security problems associated with any highly addictive narcotic. By contrast, lignocaine is a non-narcotic which, properly applied, is effective and safe. Normally, lignocaine is rapidly dissipated with 60% being metabolized in a single pass through the liver. Nevertheless, careless overdosage can result in central nervous symptoms and even cardiovascular collapse. Toxic levels start at venous blood levels of 5 to 6 $\mu m/ml$ [39]. Symptoms of muscle fasciculation, tremor, twitching, visual disturbances, and even convulsions occur more frequently at lignocaine concentrations greater than 9 $\mu g/ml$. To avoid

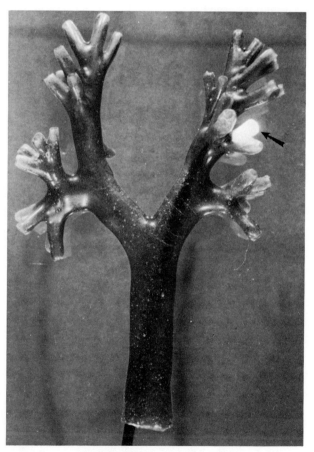

Fig. 13.21 A plastic model of the human tracheobronchia tree (Medi-Tech, Watertown, MA.). Arrow points to the RB4 segment, which is lighted by the distal end of the fibreoptic bronchoscope. Practice time spent on this reproduction will greatly facilitate the learning process [7].

adverse reactions, the total dosage of lignocaine employed during a procedure should not exceed 600 mg [7]. Even more conservative dosages should
be used in patients with congestive heart failure or serious liver disease.

The technique to achieve topical anaesthesia for flexible bronchoscopy
via an oral endotracheal tube is summarized from Zavala's training handbook [7]. First the patient gargles 30 ml of 0.5% dyclonine, followed by
spraying the oropharynx with approximately 5 ml of 4% lignocaine in an
atomizer. Cotton balls, soaked in 4% lignocaine are applied to each pyriform
sinus for one minute (Fig. 13.22). After blocking the internal division of the
superior laryngeal nerve (pyriform sinus), 5 ml of 1.0% lignocaine is delivered slowly through a curved cannula down the back of the tongue, over
the vocal cords and into the trachea (Fig. 13.23). The method of administering lignocaine by puncturing the thyrohyoid and cricothyroid membranes is
not recommended because of increased complications. Upon entering the
tracheobronchial tree, an additional 1.0% lignocaine (4–5 ml) is injected
through the channel of the bronchofibrescope into each upper lobe orifice.
Subsequently, small amounts of lignocaine are instilled in the airway.

If transnasal insertion of the bronchofibrescope is desired, a spray or a few
drops of a nasal decongestant are utilized to shrink the turbinates, thereby

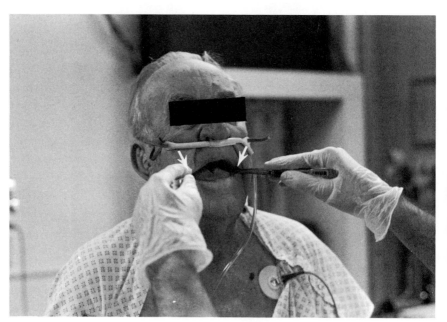

Fig. 13.22 Topical anaesthesia. The correct position of the Jackson forceps (arrows)
is shown at the corners of the mouth. The curved, distal ends of the forceps (not seen)
hold the medicated cotton balls in the pyriform sinuses [7].

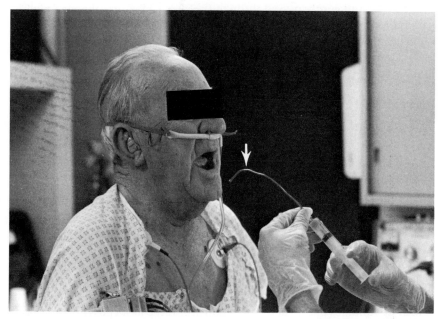

Fig. 13.23 Topical anaesthesia. The operator is ready to deliver 5 ml of 1% ligno-caine, contained in a syringe, through a curve cannula (arrow) [7].

facilitating passage of the instrument. This manoeuvre is followed by topical anaesthesia of the nares with 4% lignocaine. The remaining method is similar to local anaesthesia for oral insertion except that many bronchoscop-ists prefer to deliver the lignocaine on the vocal cords under direct fibreoptic vision.

13.8 Techniques of insertion

13.8.1 Rigid bronchoscope

An excellent detailed description of oral insertion of the rigid-tube bron-choscope is given by Stradling [3]. With the patient's head resting on a three to four inch thick pillow and the chin pointing vertically (as if shaving under the chin), the operator introduces the bronchoscope using the forefinger and thumb of the left hand to guide (and support) the tube. The position of the left hand is not unlike that of holding a cue stick in billiards. The broncho-scope is introduced almost vertically, then lowered towards the horizontal until the epiglottis is located. Care is taken to prevent injury to the mouth, especially the teeth and gums. The larynx is exposed by lifting the epiglottis forward. After inspection of the vocal cords, the tip of the rigid tube is rotated 90° and gently passed through the glottis by a twisting manoeuvre. Intubation is greatly facilitated by the routine use of a telescope which is inserted through the bronchoscope for improved vision.

13.8.2 Flexible bronchoscope

The routes of introducing the fibreoptic bronchoscope are many and varied (Fig. 13.24): 1. transnasal, usually without an endotracheal (ET) tube; 2. transoral, usually with an ET tube; 3. through a tracheostomy/tracheotomy tube or stoma; 4. through an open-tube bronchoscope (not shown in Fig. 13.22).

One needs to be thoroughly familiar with both the transnasal and transoral (via ET tube) methods of inserting the flexible bronchoscope, and should not use one technique to the total exclusion of the other. Each method has its advantages and limitations. Currently most of the bronchofibrescopic procedures in the United States, United Kingdom, and Europe are being performed transnasally without an endotracheal tube. Although the nasal route is convenient for examination of the tracheobronchial tree, this method of insertion fails to establish an airway. Other potential disadvantages of transnasal insertion are: 1. the nasal passages may be so restricted that insertion of the broncofibrescope is difficult, traumatic, or

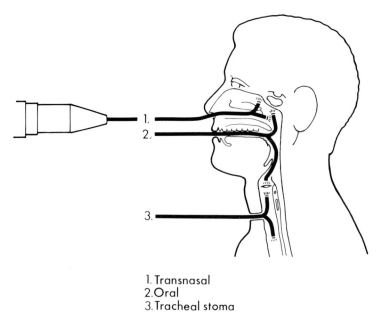

1. Transnasal
2. Oral
3. Tracheal stoma

Fig. 13.24 Insertion routes. Not shown in this illustration is passage of the fibreoptic bronchoscope through an ET tube, rigid bronchoscope, or tracheostomy tube [75].

impossible; 2. flooding of the airway with blood or purulent material cannot be handled effectively and safely; 3. considerable biopsy material can be lost by having to remove the brush through the channel of the bronchoscope; 4. the shaft of the instrument is subjected to greater angulation which may decrease survival of the fibrebundles; and 5. the vocal cords are rubbed almost continuously by the shaft of the bronchoscope, a factor which may contribute to the patient's cough and the need for increased amounts of lignocaine.

Situations do arise, however, in which transnasal passage of the fibreoptic bronchoscope (without an ET tube) is desirable: 1. in patients who bite during attempted oral insertion; 2. in patients who are extremely apprehensive, unco-operative, or refuse to accept oral passage; 3. in patients who need only an examination of the airway without any anticipation of biopsy.

The method of transnasal insertion is rather easy to learn [40, 41]. One simply passes the lubricated shaft of the bronchoscope through the floor of the nasal passageway. Care is taken not to make a forced entry. Once in the nasopharynx, the tip of the fibreoptic bronchoscope is flexed downwards and directed to the glottis.

The advantage of passing the fibrescope through a previously inserted endotracheal tube is that resuscitation can be given immediately if needed, a large bore sucker (catheter) can promptly be introduced to control haemorrhage or aspirate material from a ruptured lung abscess, and the bronchoscope may be rapidly withdrawn and reinserted with ease for multiple biopsies or clearing of the distal lens. This technique is indicated in transbronchial lung biopsy and in any high risk situation.

One of the most common methods employed to insert the ET tube is with the bronchofibrescope [36]. A number of plastic, flexible endotracheal tubes are available, but the important feature is to use one with an internal diameter of at least 8.5 mm to insure an adequate flow of air. The tube, with lubricant added, is passed into the trachea by gliding it over the shaft of the preinserted fibrescope, as shown in Fig. 13.25, and then secured externally with tape. Other methods of ET tube insertion are with a laryngeal mirror, with a laryngoscope, or blindly without any instrument.

13.9 Fluoroscopy

Fluoroscopy serves two valuable functions in *flexible fibreoptic bronchoscopy*: 1. to help perform transbronchial biopsies (TBBs), and 2. to help position the forceps when biopsying lung tumours which lie beyond endoscopic vision. When the biopsy tool is inserted through the long, restricted channel of the flexible instrument, tactile sensation is greatly reduced, especially when the distal tip of the bronchoscope is flexed. Thus, fluoroscopic control is necessary to make certain that the forceps do not penetrate the visceral pleura and that the jaws of the biopsy tool open properly. Unfortunately, physical limitations at many institutions make the routine use of fluoroscopic techniques difficult, so that TBB via the bronchofibrescope is performed without fluoroscopic guidance. Interestingly, fluoroscopy is not required when obtaining TBBs via a *rigid bronchoscope* [42]. The large 7–8 mm passageway of the open-tube instrument offers such little resistance to the inserted forceps that the operator can rely on tactile sensation to engage the biopsy tool gently in a small peripheral bronchus of the lower lobe.

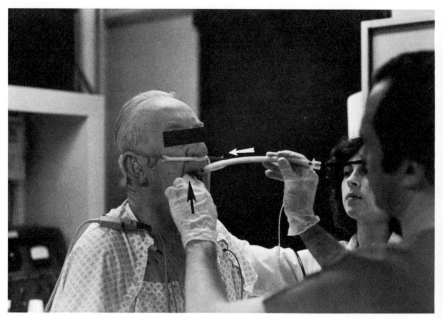

Fig. 13.25 Oral intubation. When the distal end of the bronchofibrescope is just above the carina, the operator hands the head of the bronchoscope to the technician and performs two manoeuvres: (1) the epiglottis is pulled forward with the index finger (black arrow) curved over the back of the tongue and (2) the ET tube is slid forward over the shaft of the preinserted bronchoscope (white arrow). [7].

Fig. 13.26 shows a Siemens C-arm fluoroscope, an image intensifier for TV fluoroscopy, and an image store unit. Although not essential there are three major advantages to having equipment of this type: 1. the C-arm can be rotated around the patient for oblique and lateral views so that the patient need not be turned; 2. a visual record of the position of the biopsy tool can be recorded and played back, and 3. the amount of radiation time can be reduced. Needless to say, it is vital for any physician operating a fluoroscope to be thoroughly trained in its proper usage. Fluoroscopy time must be kept to a minimum and protective lead aprons plus dosimeter badges worn by all personnel. Localization of the biopsy tool can be verified fluoroscopically by the following manoeuvres: 1. rotating the patient (or the C-arm) while checking for co-ordinated movement of the lesion and the forceps or brush, 2. having the patient perform respiratory manoeuvres and noting if the lesion and the biopsy tool move together, and 3. observing movement of the lesion while engaging it with the forceps or brush.

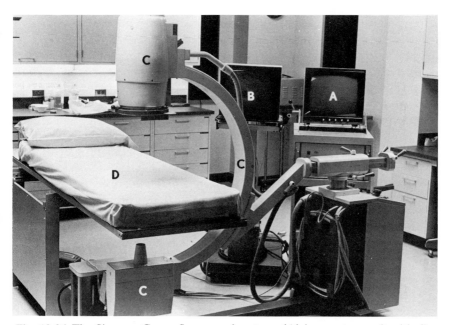

Fig. 13.26 The Siemens C-arm fluoroscopic set up: (A) image store unit with disc recorder; (B) fluoroscopic screen with image intensification; (C) C-arm fluoroscope, and (D) adjustable fluoroscopic table [7].

13.10 Endoscopic features

It is essential for the endoscopist to recognize mucosal abnormalities in the tracheobronchial tree and to appreciate even subtle changes. This visual knowledge comes only with adequate training and experience. The acutal view, as seen through the bronchoscope, is far superior to any written description, but a brief review of the salient endoscopic features of inflammatory and malignant disease is worthwhile.

The paramount features of acute bronchial inflammation are [43]: purulent exudates, mucosal erythema, mucosal oedema, and longitudinal ridges. *Purulent exudates* may appear as slightly cloudy mucus, mucopus, or frankly purulent material. Sometimes the exudate can be seen bubbling in bronchial orifices as the patient breathes. No movement of the mucus or pus signifies an occluded airway which is a signal for the bronchoscopist to remove the plug by suction and to look further for a possible obstructing carcinoma.

Erythema, a reddening of the bronchial mucosa, is one of the most frequent signs of inflammatory change. The reddening and increased vascularity should be differentiated from submucosal ecchymoses, secondary to suction or instrumentation, and from the prominent mucosal vessels seen in mitral stenosis.

Oedema of the mucosa is a common finding in inflammation. Moderate or marked mucosal swelling is readily recognized by blunting and thickening of the bronchial or segmental spurs (subcarinae) and a blurring of the longitudinal ridges.

Longitudinal ridges are a common sign of inflammatory change. They represent an infolding of the mucosa (hence the ridges) which is produced by the contraction of smooth muscle in the bronchial wall. Sometimes these ridges are seen only during expiration. As the inflammation progresses, the ridges become prominent and persist throughout the respiratory cycle.

The bronchoscopic features of chronic inflammation are characterized by *abundant mucus*, which must be removed by suction to provide a better view of the airway; *dilated ducts* of mucous glands, which appear as small pits or holes in the mucosa; *transverse ridges*, which are smooth muscle bands around the bronchial lumen, and *longitudinal light bands* which can be seen running in the longitudinal ridges down the mainstem bronchi out into the smaller divisions.

There is an important diagnostic point to be made between the significance of *generalized* and *localized* disease in the airways. In acute and chronic bronchitis the above signs of inflammation are generalized, but the confinement of these abnormal features to one area opens up many diagnostic possibilities. For example, a localized reaction may indicate infection (pneumonia, lung abscess, bronchiectasis, tuberculosis, fungal disease, etc.), carcinoma, or an aspirated foreign object.

The features of bronchogenic carcinoma can be subtle or gross [3, 44, 45]. At one end of the spectrum, it is possible for a carcinoma to produce only localized inflammatory changes without the tumour itself being visible. Other fine clues, suspicious for malignancy, are: a lack-lustre mucosa, i.e. loss of mucosal sheen; a finely granular mucosa, and a thickened spur. At the other end of the spectrum, the diagnosis of malignancy may be obvious. These gross changes include: a swollen, fixed carina, an externally compressed, distorted airway, thickened longitudinal ridges which converge into an eccentric, fixed bronchus, and an endobronchial tumour which presents as an ulcerating, fungating, fleshy, necrotic, or polypoid mass that may vary in colour from light to dark red or from dirty yellow, to cream, to white.

13.11 Lavage

Selected comments are indicated on the important subject of bronchoalveolar lavage:

1. The lavage is more readily carried out via the flexible fibreoptic bronchoscope, although at times the rigid bronchoscope may be necessary to remove large mucoid impactions or profuse, glue-like secretions.
2. The technique of lavage consists of injecting 30 ml boluses of normal saline solution, preceded by a single 5 ml bolus of adrenaline (1:20 000). Aspiration is then performed via a large-channel (2.6 mm) fibreoptic bronchoscope. It is important to keep the total amount of irrigating solution to a minimum, usually not over 200 to 300 ml. Otherwise, indiscriminate, extensive lavage may produce any of the following undesirable events: (a) temporary airway obstruction; (b) bronchospasm; (c) removal of surfactant; (d) postlavage fluid overload into the vascular bed, and (e) hypoxaemia.
3. Bronchoalveolar lavage via the bronchofibrescope could be overused in intensive care units and should not be employed as a substitute for day-to-day, conventional chest physical therapy.
4. It is advisable to give prophylactic oxygen to patients during and at least six hours following bronchial lavage.
5. The processing of lavage specimens is described in detail by Drew and associates [46].
6. The therapeutic results of lavage (with physiologic saline or 5% acetylcystein solution) are equivocal in the management of cystic fibrosis [13, 14, 47] but valuable for alveolar proteinosis.
7. In pulmonary research and the diagnosis of diffuse lung disease, segmental lung lavage is a useful technique to harvest alveolar macrophages for study and to analyse the effluents for cellular and protein components including immunoglobulins [48–51].

13.12 Staging lung cancer

Bronchoscopy plays a significant role in the staging of lung cancer. The extent of the tumour must be defined so that the surgeon can plan the appropriate operative procedure such as a lobectomy, pneumonectomy, sleeve resection, etc. Evidence of tumour within 2 cm of the main carina still is indicative of inoperability [52]. The value of biopsy from the main carina via the rigid and flexible bronchoscopes is well established, even when no visible abnormality of the carina is seen. The incidence of abnormal carinal biopsies via the flexible fibreoptic bronchoscope is 10% [53] as compared to a 11.5 to 13% positive yield using larger forceps via the rigid, open-tube bronchoscope. *The finding of malignant cells in the biopsy specimen of the carina dictates that the tumour is unresectable and that further staging procedures are unnecessary.*

The following guidelines are recommended to help the bronchoscopist determine the anatomic extent of a primary lung tumour:

1. Routinely carry out a biopsy of the main carina by forceps, especially if the tumour is located in either mainstem bronchus or in the right upper lobe.
2. If the tumour is located in a bronchus or a segmental bronchus, then perform a forceps biopsy of proximal spurs (subcarinae). The proximal spread of bronchogenic carcinoma can be more extensive than is visibly evident to the endoscopist.
3. In patients with enlarged mediastinal nodes causing external compression of the trachea or mainstem bronchi, carry out a transtracheal or transbronchial needle aspiration biopsy through the rigid or flexible bronchoscope.

13.13 Bronchoscopy in intensive care

Whereas rigid, open-tube bronchoscopy presents major problems in the management of poor risk patients on mechanical ventilators, flexible fibreoptic bronchoscopy can be readily performed through a swivel tracheal tube adapter (Fig. 13.16) without interruption of controlled ventilation. Nevertheless, critically ill patients are at increased risk [54] since even small changes in the ventilation pattern caused by bronchofibrescopy may cause serious cardiopulmonary distress. For example, insertion of the fibreoptic bronchoscope through a small diameter endotracheal tube can cause high airflow resistance with resulting barotrauma. Also with vigorous suctioning, arterial P_aO_2 may fall precipitously and the lung volume may decrease to below functional residual capacity.

In order to avoid the potential risks of fibreoptic bronchoscopy in patients being mechanically ventilated, the following recommendations are made [55]:

1. Use an ET tube which has an internal diameter (ID) of at least 8.5 mm, especially when employing a large-shafted bronchofibrescope such as the Olympus BF-1T or the Pentax FB-19A.
2. Increase the F_IO_2 to 1.0 (100%).
3. Discontinue PEEP.
4. Monitor the exhaled tidal volume.
5. Monitor the electrocardiographic pattern, heart rate, and rhythm.

6. Observe the patient's chest for adequate excursions.
7. Keep the procedure as short as possible.
8. Restrict suction to only brief periods.
9. When indicated, continually monitor the blood arterial oxygen by ear (Hewlett-Packard Ear Oximeter Model 4720A).
10. When indicated, obtain a follow-up chest radiograph to rule out pneumothorax and mediastinal emphysema.

13.14 Complications

Careful screening, proper preparation of the patient, and skilful biopsy techniques will prevent most complications. Even though bronchoscopy by rigid or flexible fibreoptic instruments is safe in experienced hands, problems occasionally arise [56–59]. The potentially serious complications are [7]: 1. reaction to the topical anaesthetic; 2. trauma secondary to insertion of a rigid-tube bronchoscope or an endotracheal tube; 3. laryngospasm; 4. bronchospasm; 5. hypoventilation; 6. pneumothorax; 7. haemorrhage; 8. cardiac arrhythmia; 9. myocardial infarction; 10. flooding of the airway with purulent material from a ruptured lung abscess; 11. postbronchoscopy fever/infection, and 12. hypoxaemia. From a physiological standpoint, many of these complications have a common end result namely a ventilation–perfusion ($\dot{V}/\dot{Q}$) mismatch which can result in a life-threatening hypoxaemia.

A *reaction to the local anaesthetic, trauma from faulty tube insertion, and laryngospasm* are virtually nonexistent when good procedural techniques are used. But *bronchospasm* is a real danger, especially when dealing with asthmatics. In such patients, rigid or flexible bronchoscopy may precipitate increased airways resistance with resulting hypoxaemia, hypercapnia, and even death. Trouble can be circumvented by the judicious use of bronchodilators. As a complication of the procedure *per se, hypoventilation* almost uniformly is caused by excessive premedication.

In transbronchial lung biopsy, *pneumothorax* occurs in 1 to 5% of the patients if the procedure is done via the fibreoptic bronchoscope and in 10 to 14% if the rigid bronchoscope is used. Usually this complication presents no serious threat if it is recognized early and is corrected (when indicated) by insertion of a chest tube with water-seal drainage. Generally a small air leak requires no therapy; nevertheless, the patient should be observed. If the patient develops symptoms or has serious underlying disease, then early recognition and removal of the air from the pleural space is imperative. One should be aware that a delayed pneumothorax can occur several hours after biopsy. Fortunately, tension pneumothorax is rare, but this complication can be fatal if not treated immediately.

Pulmonary haemorrhage is a matter of concern to all bronchoscopists. It is vital that the physician be aware of the extreme danger of life-threatening bleeding if bronchial or transbronchial biopsy is performed on patients with uraemia, abnormal clotting factors, thrombocytopaenia, or highly vascular tumours. For prophylaxis, an infusion of 6 to 12 platelet packs should be given, just prior to biopsy, to any patient who has a platelet count less than 50 000/mm^3 or has abnormally functioning platelets. Warning: although effective dialysis of uraemic patients may decrease the danger of haemorrhage, the risk is still substantial. To tamponade potential haemorrhage resulting from TBB via the fibreoptic bronchoscope, the 'wedge' technique (p. 346) has proven to be highly effective. As previously emphasized, major haemorrhage is more easily controlled with a rigid bronchoscope than a flexible fibreoptic bronchoscope.

The over-all prevalence of *cardiac arrhythmias* during bronchoscopy is not known. This is because many medical centres carry out cardiac monitoring only on high-risk patients or on those who have a history of cardiovascular disease. In our endoscopy suite, where *all* patients are monitored electrocardiographically, the occurrence of premature ventricular contractions (PVCs) is in the range of 0.5 to 1.0%. Such a low figure may be due to the fact that oxygen is given routinely to each of our patients, thus preventing oxygen desaturation and resultant rhythm disturbances. In over 5000 fibreoptic bronchoscopies we have not observed acute myocardial infarction, ST–T wave changes, or the onset of rhythm disturbances other than PVCs, but they are known to occur. Interestingly, the arrhythmias associated with bronchoscopy are generally well tolerated, self-limited, and rarely of haemodynamic significance [60, 61]. But regardless of statistics, it may be wise to use a cardiac monitor on all patients undergoing bronchoscopy to follow their electrocardiographic pattern, heart rate and rhythm.

Occasionally purulent material from a *ruptured abscess* can drown the patient [18]. The flooding may occur during instrumentation (e.g. inserting a biopsy tool into the abscess) or shortly following bronchoscopy. A rigid bronchoscope should be readily available to handle such a situation. Any patient with a lung abscess should be kept under close observation after bronchoscopy, preferably in a recovery room.

Bacteraemia had been known to occur following rigid bronchoscopy, but it is especially uncommon after fibreoptic bronchoscopy unless the patient is immunosuppressed. Our prevalence of postbronchofibrescopy pneumonia requiring antibiotic therapy has only been 1:500 cases. In each instance the patients were elderly and their airways narrowed or obstructed by tumour.

Hypoxaemia secondary to over-medication, to topical anaesthesia, to intubation, or to the bronchoscopic procedure itself, always is a potential danger [62–64]. A fall in the P_aO_2 of 10 to 20 mm Hg (2–3 kPa) commonly occurs during bronchoscopy. Normally this poses no problem, but such is not the case when dealing with patients who are elderly, immunosuppressed, being lavaged, undergoing transbronchial lung biopsy or are ill with pre-existing lung disease. In this high-risk group, prophylactic oxygen should be administered routinely to prevent the possible occurrence of hypoxaemia. Furthermore, oxygen by nasal cannula should be given after bronchoscopy (often for 6 to 12 h) to any patient with a borderline or reduced arterial oxygen tension prior to bronchoscopy. Those patients on mechanical ventilators who require fibreoptic bronchoscopy, should have their FIO_2 increased to 100% during the procedure. Since severe hypoxaemia may be induced by bronchial lavage with large volumes of saline, one should employ small aliquots (10 to 30 ml) and keep the total amount of irrigating fluid not over 200 to 300 ml. Finally, those patients with severe hypoxaemia (not corrected with supplemental oxygen) should be excluded from bronchoscopy.

13.15 Precautions

The prevention of trouble is the key message. In addition to using a preoperative check list (Table 13.2) and an operative report form, it is wise to take the following precautions on all patients [7]:

1. Carry out adequate patient screening;
2. perform the bronchoscopy in a well-equipped biopsy room;
3. have good technical assistance;
4. insert an 8.5-mm oral endotracheal tube for passage of the fibreoptic bronchoscope in all high-risk situations;
5. avoid excessive premedication, especially tranquillizers;
6. provide oxygen prophylactically as well as therapeutically;
7. continue nasal oxygen after bronchoscopy on any patient with a borderline or reduced P_aO_2 prior to bronchoscopy;
8. monitor the patients on a cardioscope;
9. apply adrenaline (3–5 ml, 1: 20 000) directly onto endoscopically visible tumours prior to biopsy;
10. utilize the 'wedge' technique when performing flexible fibreoptic TBBs;
11. give an infusion of platelet packs immediately before bronchoscopy in any patient who has a platelet count less than 50 000/mm³ or has abnormally functioning platelets;
12. avoid any biopsy procedure (brush or forceps) on a uraemic patient;
13. make certain that asthmatic patients are adequately protected with bronchodilators against increased airways obstruction, and
14. utilize a postbronchoscopy recovery room.

13.16 Care of the equipment

Cleansing the rigid or flexible bronchoscope is carried out in two stages: cleaning and sterilization or disinfection.

13.16.1 Cleaning

Although the cleaning techniques differ between the two instruments, one important, yet similar task is the meticulous removal of adherent material from the endoscope immediately after its use. This includes the passage of a brush, appropriately sized, through the channel of the rigid or flexible instrument to remove bits of tissue, blood, secretions, or inspissated material. One has the option of washing the open-tube bronchoscope entirely by hand, but it is more effective to clean the instrument thoroughly in activated detergent using ultrasound, followed by rinsing in water and drying. On the contrary, the flexible fibreoptic bronchoscope must be cleaned manually [7, 65]. The outer shaft of the instrument is gently washed with diluted soap, followed by 30% alcohol, then rinsed in distilled water. The cleaning process also consists of passing the soap solution, alcohol, then water through the channel of the flexible instrument by suction. Care is taken with the fibreoptic bronchoscope never to immerse the control head in any solution or damage may result.

13.16.2 Sterilization/disinfection

After cleaning, the next step is sterilization or disinfection. Whereas sterilization assures the total destruction of all micro-organisms, disinfection eliminates the risk of infection but does not necessarily sterilize the most resistant microbes such as bacterial spores. For this reason there was initial concern regarding the safety of disinfection for the bronchofibrescope and the possible need to sterilize the instrument between cases. Fortunately, disinfection procedures for the fibrescope have proven to be effective.

Routinely, the rigid, metal-tube bronchoscope is sterilized by *autoclave*, but the high temperatures and pressures which are generated by this method damage the fibreoptic bronchoscope. *Gas sterilization* with ethylene oxide (EtO) is safe and effective for the fibreoptic instrument, but unfortunately EtO avidly adsorbs to rubber and plastic and thus has the disadvantage of requiring a long aeration time.

The method of choice for the flexible fibreoptic bronchoscope is *cold disinfection* for 20–30 min [7, 65, 66]. This is accomplished by placing the shaft of the bronchoscope into a cylinder or tube filled with 2% alkalinized gluteraldehyde or a povidone-iodine germicide consisting of two parts surgical scrub solution (7.5%), one part alcohol (70%) and one part distilled water. The solution is drawn through the channel by a syringe connected to the biopsy port. After disinfection, the outer shaft and inner channel of the bronchofibrescope are thoroughly cleaned in a manner similar to the initial process, using alcohol, and then distilled water. Failure to remove the disinfectant may produce a chemical bronchitis. Finally, the bronchofibrescope is air-dried by connecting it to a sucker for several minutes, then hung vertically (head-up) in a dry storage cabinet. The biopsy tools (forceps and reusable brushes) are cleaned and autoclaved. The disposable brushes are replaced after each use.

The possible *transmission of hepatitis type B virus* by improperly cleansed endoscopes continues to cause some apprehension among those who use the instruments. What should one do when bronchoscopy is needed on patients who are carriers of hepatitis type B (HBsAg)? Until recently, use of the bronchofibrescope on such patients was thought to be an absolute contraindication since the flexible instrument, unlike the rigid bronchoscope, could not be sterilized by autoclave without ruining it. Unexpectedly, the Centre for Disease Control, Atlanta, Georgia [67], has indicated that disinfection of the flexible bronchoscope with an iodophore or 2% alkalinized gluteraldehyde is efficacious for patients with hepatitis B surface antigen. Nevertheless, direct evidence is still lacking since the virus cannot as yet be grown in tissue culture for inactivation studies. Presently, the only way to determine infectivity is by innoculations into chimpanzees but these animals not only are in short supply, but also they are an endangered species.

13.17 Handling the biopsy specimens

The manner in which biopsy specimens are handled is an important link in the diagnostic chain [7, 68]. The best approach is to utilize the skills of the pathologist, cytopathologist, and bacteriologist. The processing of the biopsy specimens is shown in Fig. 13.27.

Forceps biopsies via the rigid or flexible bronchoscope are submitted to the pathology laboratory in 10% formalin for processing, and, when indicated, one or two of the samples may be placed directly into a sterile tube containing a few millilitres of sterile saline (or Ringer's solution) and sent to the bacteriology laboratory for appropriate cultures. If the biopsy pieces are tiny, as often occurs in flexible fibreoptic bronchoscopy (because of the smaller forceps), they initially may be put in sterile saline, then transferred to a glass slide where a few drops of human plasma, rabbit brain thromboplastin, and 0.02 M calcium chloride are added to form a fibrin clot around the specimen. This technique consolidates the small pieces of tissue into a single specimen which is immersed in 10% formalin for subsequent processing.

The brush biopsy specimens, which routinely are obtained by bronchial brushing through the flexible bronchofibrescope, are handled in a different fashion. Upon completing each biopsy, the brush is drawn back to its exit porthole and the entire bronchoscope is withdrawn from the patient. The brush is then advanced from the bronchoscope to make smears directly on glass slides (promptly immersed in 95% alcohol), or the brush is placed in a tube of sterile saline and manually agitated to separate the cells and bits of tissue from the bristles of the biopsy tool. The tubes containing the brush biopsy material are promptly submitted to cytology for smears, millipore filter preparations, and cell buttons. Selective bronchial brush specimens may be helpful for fungal, mycobacterial and viral cultures. For this purpose the operator should employ sheathed sterile brushes. The most reliable collecting system, to obtain uncontaminated specimens, is a telescoping double catheter* with distal occlusion by a polyethylene glycol plug [69]. Upon arrival near the area to be sampled, the double catheter is inserted through the suction channel of the bronchofibrescope into the lumen of the airway. Then the inner catheter containing the sampling brush is advanced a few centimetres, displacing the protective polyethylene glycol plug. After advancing the brush and obtaining the specimen, the brush is withdrawn into the inner catheter and the entire double catheter removed from the bronchoscope. The prior application of lignocaine locally should be kept to

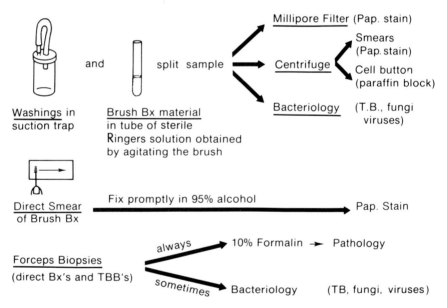

Fig. 13.27 Methods of handling and processing the specimens: washings, brush biopsy material, smears, and forceps biopsies [7].

* Meditech Division of Cooper Scientific Corp., Watertown, Mass., USA.

a minimum since this drug in concentrations higher than 0.5% to 1.0% has an inhibitory effect on the growth of organisms.

The smears and millipore filter specimens are stained using a modified Papanicolaou technique. The cell blocks and forceps biopsies undergo routine histopathologic preparation with haematoxylin and eosin. Grocott (silver methenamine) stains are done whenever *Pneumocystis carinii* pneumonia and fungal infections are suspected. Likewise, acid-fast stains are done when appropriate. A rapid, effective method of identifying *Pneumocystis carinii* organisms is to make touch preparations from one of the transbronchial biopsy specimens. The tissue is pressed on clean glass slides and stained by Giemsa, Gram-Weigert and Grocott techniques.

13.18 Cytology

Much emphasis has been placed on the experience of the operator and procedural techniques in achieving a high diagnostic yield. But cytologic and histologic evaluation are equally important factors. The skill of the cyto-pathologist and pathologist in examining cells and small fragments of tissue is paramount.

The first case report of a cytological diagnosis of lung cancer was made in 1945 by Papanicolaou [70]. Subsequently, with better methods of sputum collection, preservation, and processing, the diagnosis of lung cancer improved greatly. With the advent of modern cytological techniques, the identification of early stages of lung cancer (even carcinoma *in situ*) became entirely possible (see also Chapter 5). An extensive chapter on respiratory cytopathology is not germane to this discussion; however, appropriate comments are worthwhile regarding sputum sampling, cytologic criteria for malignancy, the classification of primary lung tumors, and the cellular changes associated with herpes and cytomegalovirus.

13.18.1 Sputum sampling

The patients should be carefully instructed on how to produce deep cough specimens [71]. After first rinsing the mouth with water, the sputum is collected upon arising for three to four consecutive mornings in wide-mouthed specimen jars which contain 50 ml of a mucoliquifying preservative. The sputum bottles are returned to the cytology laboratory where they are pooled into one specimen, processed and stained. As an alternative, fresh sputum samples may be collected in a clean container, smeared on slides without delay and immediately immersed in 95% ethyl alcohol. For the 10% of the patients who are unable to cough, the accepted practice is to obtain the specimens by continuous exposure to aerosolized tap water. Plain tap water seems to work as well as hypertonic saline or adding a mucolytic agent. After 20 min of aerosol by an ultrasonic nebulizer, the patient is directed to take several deep breaths, then to cough forcefully, and to expectorate into a specimen bottle before applying the lid tightly. When dealing with bronchogenic carcinoma, either the unaided deep cough or the aerosol technique of sputum collection should give a 75–85% positive yield. The yield is not improved by sampling further than three to four times.

The presence of 'dust' cells (alveolar macrophages) in the sputum is one indication that an adequate sample was obtained, otherwise the end product is spittle. Agreement between the types of malignant cells in the sputum and in necropsy specimens occurs in 80–84% of the cases. Sputum cytology screening is a helpful adjunct, especially when clinical or radiographic evidence suggests the possibility of a lung tumour. Screening for totally occult disease is not practical because of the time, effort, expense and poor yield (see Chapter 5).

In patients with undiagnosed chest disease, opinions vary as to the value of routine postbronchoscopy sputum sampling for malignancy. A reasonable approach is to forego collecting cough specimens following bronchoscopy in those patients with endoscopically visible tumours. In this situation, rarely, if ever, is the tissue biopsy (brush and forceps) negative and the sputum positive. Instead it makes good sense to obtain several samples during the immediate 24-h period after bronchoscopy in those patients who have mid-lung or peripheral tumours beyond the visual range of the bronchoscope. Even with fluoroscopy the diagnostic yield from a peripheral biopsy is reduced, so anything that improves the yield is helpful. In about 5% of these cases the postbronchoscopy sputum results are rewarding while the biopsy specimens are non-diagnostic.

13.18.2 Primary lung tumours

The classification of primary tumours of the lung by cell type is shown in Table 13.2. Of the group, the most common malignant tumour is squamous cell carcinoma. In the development of this tumour, significant cellular alterations occur which present a spectrum of progressive epithelial changes ranging from normal squamous metaplasia→atypical squamous metaplasia (mild→moderate→marked)→carcinoma *in situ*→invasive carcinoma. Unfortunately reactive hyperplasia and metaplasia can be confused with malignant changes. Some of the aetiological sources of error are pulmonary infarction, viral infections, acute smoke inhalation, artifacts, and degenerating columnar cells.

The *general criteria for malignancy* are as follows (Dept. Pathology, University of Iowa):

1. Increase in size and/or change in the shape of the cell and the nucleus.

Table 13.2 Classification of primary lung tumours

Cell type	% of total*
Bronchogenic Carcinoma	
Squamous (epidermoid)	30–50
Small cell undifferentiated†	20
Large cell undifferentiated	10–15
Adenocarcinoma‡	25–30
Mixed types	<5
Bronchiolo-Alveolar Cell	<5
Bronchial Adenoma	<5

* The percentages of the cell types depend on the cytological criteria and classification used.
† Oat cell and other variants (see WHO classification).
‡ Predominately in women; comprises only 5–9% of lung carcinomas in men.

2. Increase in the nuclear/cytoplasmic (N/C) ratio.
3. Changes in the internal structure of the nucleus.
   (a) Coarsening and clumping of chromatin, often with condensation at the nuclear membrane.
   (b) Folding or wrinkling of the nuclear membrane.
   (c) Increase in size and/or change in the shape of the nucleolus.
   (d) Frequent mitoses.
4. Changes in size, shape and staining characteristics of the cytoplasm.

13.18.3 Bronchogenic carcinoma

The basic cytologic features of bronchogenic carcinoma by cell type are as follows:

1. Squamous cell carcinoma (Figs. 13.28a, 28b), also called epidermoid carcinoma.
   (a) Nucleus is centrally located.
   (b) No nucleoli are in the keratinizing forms; large nucleoli are in the non-keratinizing forms.
   (c) Cytoplasm is often keratinized (orange) but may be non-keratinized (grey-green).
   (d) Cytoplasmic borders are distinct (keratinized forms) or hazy (non-keratinized forms).
   (e) Cells may occur singly or in sheets.
   (f) Miltinucleation, bizarre forms (tadpoles, spindles, pearls), or cannibalism may be present.

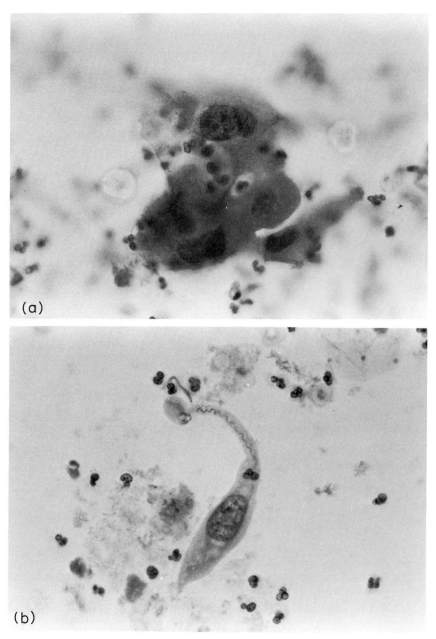

Fig. 13.28 (a) A sheet of malignant cells with abundant, keratinized cytoplasm and nuclear pleomorphism. Cytological diagnosis: squamous cell carcinoma. (b) A single, bizarre-shaped cell which often is referred to as a 'tadpole'. Note the large nucleus, abnormal chromatin, and a Herxheimer's spiral (in the tail). Cytological diagnosis: squamous cell carcinoma.

(g) Depth of focusing is flat.

(h) Intracellular bridging is present.

2. Adenocarcinoma (Figs. 13.29a, 29b).

    (a) Nucleus is eccentric.

    (b) Nucleolus is prominent.

    (c) Cytoplasm characteristically is foamy or finely vacuolated and does not take a strain.

    (d) Cytoplasmic borders are indistinct.

    (e) Cells may occur singly or in glandular, rounded or papillary groupings.

3. Small cell undifferentiated carcinoma (Fig. 13.30), which includes the 'oat cell' and other variants.

    (a) Nuclei are small, hyperchromatic, and sometimes have an 'india ink' appearance.

    (b) Nucleoli are virtually non-existent.

    (c) Cytoplasm is scanty and often scarcely visible.

    (d) Cytoplasmic borders are vague.

    (e) Cells may be strung out along mucous strands or occur in tightly packed clusters with nuclear 'moulding'.

    (f) A crush artifact appearance may be present.

4. Large cell undifferentiated carcinoma (Fig. 13.31).

    (a) Nuclei are large, rounded and hyperchromatic (coarse chromatin); multinucleation and nuclear moudling occur.

    (b) Nucleoli are prominent, often multiple.

    (c) Cytoplasm is variable in amount; its borders are well limited or indistinct.

5. Bronchiolo-alveolar cell carcinoma.

    (a) Nucleus is rounded, slightly enlarged and moderately hyperchromatic.

    (b) Single or multiple (small) nucleoli are present.

    (c) Cytoplasm is abundant and vacuolated; leukocytic ingestion may be present.

    (d) Cells form ascini or sheets and require a high depth of focusing.

    (e) Difficult to differentiate from benign reactive cells.

13.18.4 Viruses

The characteristic cytologic feature of *herpes* are demonstrated in Fig. 13.32. The nuclei are large and have intranuclear inclusions with a 'ground glass' appearance. Degenerative changes and giant, multinucleated cells with moulded, amorphous nuclei are common. The cytoplasm is scanty, often basophilic and has indistinct borders. In comparison, the cells affected by cytomegalovirus as shown in Fig. 13.33 are single, well preserved and

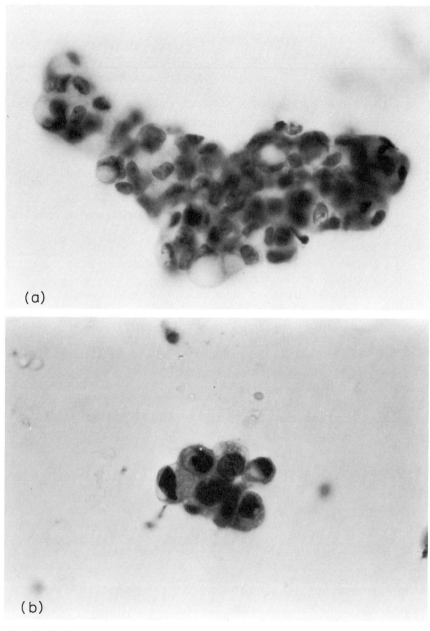

(a)

(b)

Fig. 13.29 (a) A papillary cluster of malignant cells showing prominent nucleoli, vacuolization, and nuclear moulding. Cytological diagnosis: adenocarcinoma. (b) A small cluster of malignant cells. Paramount features include eccentric location of the nuclei, prominent nucleoli, and diffuse vacuolization of the cytoplasm. Cytological diagnosis: adenocarcinoma.

have a basophilic intranuclear inclusion body surrounded by a clear halo, i.e. the 'owl's eye'. The cytoplasm is adequate, has distinct borders, and often contains inclusions.

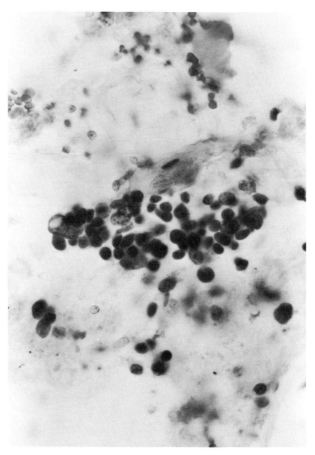

Fig. 13.30 A group of small, dark, malignant cells. Characteristic features are: 'india ink' nuclei, no nucleoli, and virtual absence of cytoplasm. Cytological diagnosis: small cell, undifferentiated carcinoma, 'oat cell' type.

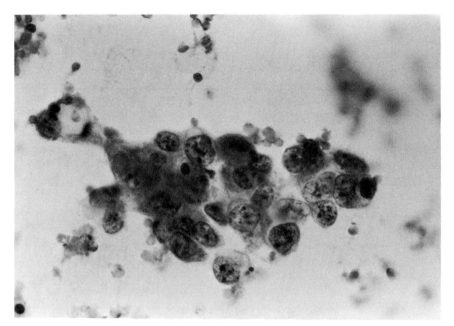

Fig. 13.31 A loose cluster of malignant cells showing large, rounded nuclei, abnormal chromatin pattern, prominent nucleoli, and indistinct cytoplasm. Cytological diagnosis: large cell, undifferentiated carcinoma.

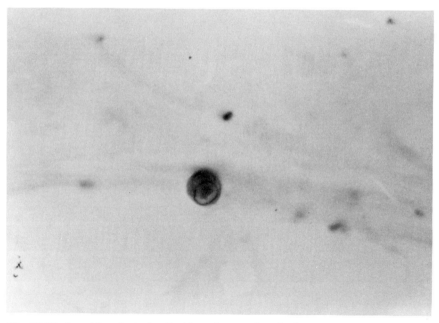

Fig. 13.32 A multinucleated cell with an intranuclear inclusion body which is much less dense than in cells infected by cytomegalovirus (see Fig. 13.33). Cytological diagnosis: herpes virus.

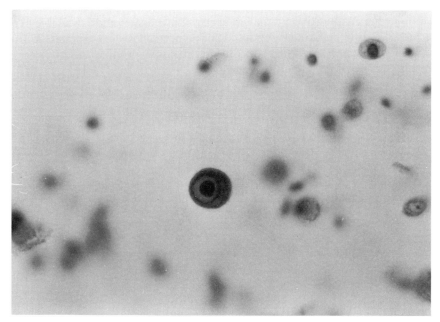

Fig. 13.33 A single cell with a large, dense intranuclear inclusion body (surrounded by a halo) which resembles an 'owl's eye'. Cytological diagnosis: cytomegalovirus.

13.19 Summary

Modern pulmonary medicine began with the introduction of the rigid, open-tube bronchoscope in 1897. Seventy years later the fibreoptic bronchoscope became commercially available. This flexible instrument has literally revolutionized pulmonary medicine. With few exceptions, the bronchofibrescope is now the instrument of choice in diagnosing a wide variety of lung densities and infiltrates. Whereas direct biopsy with brush and forceps is carried out on endoscopically visible lesions, lung densities or infiltrates beyond the range of the flexible fibrescope are biopsied indirectly under fluoroscopic control. Other diagnostic and therapeutic manoeuvres include: transbronchial lung biopsy, bronchoalveolar lavage, collection of material for microbiological study, assessment of airway patency, and removal of retained secretions, mucous plugs, or small foreign bodies.

Although the open-tube bronchoscope is not being used as often as previously, this time-honoured instrument still plays an important diagnostic and therapeutic role. Thus, it is essential for the physician to have a clear understanding of the indications, limitations, and contraindications of both the rigid and flexible bronchoscopes. The procedures always should be performed by experienced, qualified clinicians in an appropriate hospital setting where supportive equipment and trained personnel are available. To achieve skill in pulmonary endoscopy requires an ardent student and a dedicated teacher. Anything short of this goal may produce unsatisfactory results and even cause harm to the patient.

References

1. Zollner, F. (1965), *Archs Otolar.*, **82**, 656–9.
2. Jackson, C. and Jackson, C. L. (1950), *Bronchoesophagology*, W. B. Sanders Co., Philadelphia.
3. Stradling, P. (1976), *Diagnostic Bronchoscopy*, Churchill Livingstone, Edinburgh, London and New York.
4. Sanders, R. D. (1967), *Delaware med. J.*, **39**, 170–5.
5. Ikeda, S. (1974), *Atlas of Flexible Bronchofiberscopy*, University Park Press, London and Baltimore.
6. Sackner, M. A. (1975), *Am. Rev. resp. Dis.*, **111**, 62–88.
7. Zavala, D. C. (1978), *Flexible Fiberoptic Bronchoscopy: A Training Handbook*, University of Iowa Publication Department, Iowa City, Iowa.
8. Holinger, P. H. and Holinger, L. D. (1978), *Chest* (Supplement), **73**, 721–4.
9. Berci, G (1976), *Endoscopy*, Appleton-Century-Crofts, New York.
10. Berci, G. (1978), *Chest* (Supplement), **73**, 768–75.
11. Wanner, A. *et al.* (1973), *J. Am. med. Ass.*, **224**, 1281–3.
12. Weinstein, H. J., Bone, R. C. and Ruth W. E., (1977), *Chest*, **72**, 583–7.
13. Dahm, L. S. *et al.* (1977), *Chest*, **72**, 593–6.
14. Quick, C. A. and Warwick, W. (1978), *Chest* (Supplement), **73**, 755–8.
15. Andersen, H. A. (1978), *Chest* (Supplement), **73**, 734–6.
16. Ellis, J. H. Jr. (1975), *Chest*, **68**, 524–32.
17. Erickson, A. D. *et al.* (1979), *Ann. intern. Med.*, **90**, 937–8.
18. Hammer, D. L. *et al.* (1978), *Chest*, **74**, 306–7.
19. Kovnat, D. M. *et al.* (1974), *Am. Rev. resp. Dis.*, **110**, 88–90.
20. Fontana, R. S. *et al.* (1975), *Chest*, **67**, 511–22.
21. Zavala, D. C. (1975), *Chest*, **68**, 12–19.
22. Hanson, R. R. *et al.* (1976), *Am. Rev. resp. Dis.*, **114**, 67–72.
23. Richardson, R. H. *et al.* (1974), *Am. Rev. resp. Dis.*, **109**, 63–6.
24. Stringfield, J. T. *et al.* (1977), *Chest*, **72**, 474–6.
25. Cunningham, J. H. *et al.* (1977), *Am. Rev. resp. Dis.*, **115**, 213–20.
26. Whitcomb, M. E. *et al.* (1978), *Chest*, **74**, 205–8.
27. Koontz, C. H. (1978), *Chest*, **74**, 120–1.
28. Scheinhorn, D. J., Joyner, L. R. and Whitcomb, M. E. (1974), *Chest*, **66**, 294–5.
29. Saw, E. C. *et al.* (1976), *Chest*, **70**, 589–91.
30. Lillington, G. A. *et al.* (1976), *Am. Rev. resp. Dis.*, **113**, 387–91.
31. Fieselmann, J. F., Zavala, D. C. and Keim, L. W. (1977), *Chest*, **72**, 241–3.
32. Landa, J. F. (1978), *Chest* (Supplement), **73**, 686–90.
33. Sahn, S. A. and Scoggin, C. (1976), *Chest*, **69**, 39–42.

34. Faber, L. P. (1978), *Chest* (Supplement), **73**, 776–8.
35. Carden, E. (1978), *Chest* (Supplement), **73**, 697–700.
36. Sanderson, D. R. *et al.* (1974), *Chest*, **65**, 608–12.
37. Fry, W. A. (1978), *Chest* (Supplement), **73**, 694–6.
38. Perry, L. B. (1978), *Chest* (Supplement), **73**, 691–3.
39. Thompson, P. D. *et al.* (1973), *Ann. intern. Med.*, **78**, 499–508.
40. Smiddy, J. F. (1972), *Rhode Island med. J.*, **55**, 351–2.
41. Harrell, J. H. (1978), *Chest* (Supplement), **73**, 704–6.
42. Andersen, H. A. and Fontana, R. S. (1972), *Chest*, **62**, 125–8.
43. Rayl, J. E. (1979), *Bronchoscopic Features of Acute Inflammation* (Video-cassette), Veterans Administration Hospital, Lake City, Florida.
44. Marsh, B. R. *et al.* (1978), *Chest* (Supplement), **73**, 716–17.
45. Martini, N. and McCormick, P. M. (1978), *Chest*, (Supplement), **73**, 718–20.
46. Drew, W. L., Finley, T. N. and Golde, D. W. (1977), *Am Rev. resp. Dis.*, **116**, 215–21.
47. Ewing, C. W. (1978), *Chest* (Supplement) **73**, 755–8.
48. Mandel, M. A. *et al.* (1976), *New Engl. J. Med.*, **295**, 694–8.
49. Weinberger, S. E. *et al.* (1978), *Ann. intern. Med.*, **89**, 459–66.
50. Bell, D. Y. and Hook, G. E. R. (1979), *Am. Rev. resp. Dis.*, **119**, 979–90.
51. Hoidal, J. R. *et al.* (1979), *Am. Rev. resp. Dis.* (Program and Abstracts), **119**, 222.
52. American Joint Committee for Cancer Staging and End Results Reporting (1977), *Manual for Staging of Cancer*, Chicago, pp. 59–61.
53. Robbins, H. M. *et al.* (1979), *Chest*, **75**, 484–6.
54. Barrett, C. R. Jr. (1978), *Chest* (Supplement), **73**, 746–9.
55. Lindholm, C. E. *et al.* (1978), *Chest*, **74**, 362–8.
56. Credle, W. F. Jr., Smiddy, J. F. and Elliott, R. C. (1974), *Am. Rev. resp. Dis.*, **109**, 67–72.
57. Suratt, P. M., Smiddy, J. F. and Gruber, B. (1976), *Chest*, **69**, 747–51.
58. Zavala, D. C. (1976), *Chest*, **70**, 584–8.
59. Pereira, W. Jr., Covnat, D. M. and Snider, G. L. (1978), *Chest*, **73**, 813–6.
60. Shrader, D. L. and Lakshminarayan, S. (1978), *Chest*, **73**, 821–4.
61. Luck, J. C. *et al.* (1978), *Chest*, **74**, 139–43.
62. Albertini, R. E. *et al*, (1974), *J. Am. Med. Ass.*, **230**, 1666–7.
63. Karetzky, M. S., Garvey, J. W. and Brandstetter, R. D. (1974), *N.Y. St. J. Med.*, **74**, 62–3.
64. Dubrawsky, D., Awe, R. J. and Jenkins, D. E. (1975), *Chest*, **67**, 137–40.
65. Elford, B. (1978), *Chest* (Supplement), **73**, 761–3.
66. Spaulding, E. H. (March, 1978), In: *Endoscopes: Disinfection or Sterilization?*, Hospital Infection Control; Same-Day Surgery, Peachtree Park Dr., Atlanta, GA 30309.
67. Center for Disease Control (Sept. 1977), *Hepatitis Surveillance Report No. 41*, Atlanta, GA.
68. Kvale, P. A. (1978), *Chest* (Supplement), **73**, 707–12.
69. Wimberley, N., Faling, L. J. and Bartlett, J. G. (1979), *Am. Rev. resp. Dis.*, **119**, 337–43.

70. Papanicolaou, G. N. (1946), *J. Am. Med. Ass.,* **131**, 372–8.
71. Saccomanno, G. (1978), *Diagnostic Pulmonary Cytology*, American Society of Clinical Pathologists, Chicago.
72. Jackson, C. (1921), *J. Lar. Otol.,* **36**, 529.
73. Sanderson, D. R. and McDougall, J. C. (1978), *Chest* (Supplement), **73**, 701–3.
74. Zavala, D. C. and Rhodes, M. L. (1975), *Ann. Otol. Rhinol. Lar.,* **84**, 650–6.
75. Ollman, B., Lindholm, C. E. and Nordin, U. (1975), *Det Flexibla Bronkoskopet*, Medicinska Laromedia AB, Uppsala, Sweden.
76. Zavala, T. (1977), ACCP Audiographic Series, **14**

Acknowledgement

The author is grateful to Karen Rasmussen CT (ASCP), Department of Pathology, University of Iowa, for the Figs 13.28–33.

CHAPTER FOURTEEN

Biopsy Procedures

J. V. Collins

This chapter reviews the indications and methods for lung biopsy and compares open biopsy to transbronchial biopsy with the fibrescope and percutaneous needle biopsy using aspiration or cutting needle, punch biopsy or trephine methods. Thoracentesis is described including examination of the fluid for colour, protein content, other chemical constituents and cytology. The indications for pleural biopsy are described and the choice of punch or open biopsy is discussed. Finally lymph node biopsies are discussed including the indications for mediastinal, scalene and parasternal node biopsies.

14.1 Lung biopsy

Disorders requiring lung biopsy may be classified into two broad groups, circumscribed lesions and diffuse disorders. Universally recognized indications for lung biopsy are difficult to formulate and the threshold for acceptance of the need for lung biopsy for the same disorder varies widely between physicians. However, in general lung biopsy may be held to be necessary if the diagnosis cannot be made by non-invasive methods and knowledge of the true nature of the disorder is likely to alter management. The methods available for lung biopsy are open thoracotomy, percutaneous needle biopsy and transbronchial biopsy through a bronchoscope. The latter is dealt with in a separate chapter. There is a real need for studies in which several different methods of lung biopsy are compared, preferably by one operator. The method of biopsy chosen is in part influenced by the likely nature of the disorder under investigation. Thus for a solitary lesion, whether solid or cavitated, it is probably always worth attempting a percutenous needle biopsy before proceeding to thoracotomy, especially if when clear evidence of the diagnosis is obtained by this method, thoracotomy becomes unnecessary.

In general needle biopsy techniques probably give better results with discrete lesions than with diffuse disease, especially as in the latter type of disorder the histological features may vary in different parts of the lungs and the small samples obtained by needle biopsy may only be representative of part of the changes present. Lung biopsy in diffuse disease has also to be seen in relation to other investigations which usually are employed before a decision about biopsy can be made (Table 14.1).

Table 14.1   Investigation of diffuse pulmonary fibrosis

---

1. History to include occupation and pets
2. Clinical features: cough, dyspnoea, clubbing, crackles,
                      joints and other organs affected
3. Chest radiographs
4. Mantoux test
5. Sputum smear and culture for AFB's
6. Biochemistry: liver function, serum calcium
7. Immunology: immunoglobulins
              plasma proteins and electrophoresis
              rheumatoid factor
              antinuclear antibody
              immune complexes and complement
8. Biopsy of lymph nodes or liver
9. Lung biopsy: transbronchial by fibrescope, percutaneous needle or trephine
              open biopsy
10. Therapeutic trials of antituberculous drugs and corticosteroids

---

14.1.1 Needle biopsy of lung

Two types of needle biopsy of lung have been described, aspiration-needle and cutting needle.

(a) Aspiration-needle biopsy

This technique was first developed for diagnosis of acute pneumonias but was soon applied to cases of suspected malignant disease. At first long thick-walled needles were used but better results have since been obtained with thinner (18 gauge) angiographic or lumbar puncture needles [1]. Aspiration-needle biopsy is more useful for circumscribed solid or cavitated lesions especially at the periphery of the lung but is not much used for diffuse disorders except for acute pneumonias, the purpose for which it was originally described and is especially useful in the immunocompromised host [2].

Aspiration-needle biopsy should be done with the patient prone to minimize the risk of air embolism and fluoroscopic control of the positioning of the needle is advisable. With experience it is possible for the operator to be able to detect manually when the needle has penetrated a lesion. Because it is advisable for the patient to breath-hold for 15–30 s while the biopsy is taken it may be difficult to use the aspiration-biopsy technique in breathless patients. Once the needle has been seen to penetrate the lesion it is rotated while vigorous suction is applied with a syringe attached to it.

Very impressive success rates have been reported, diagnostic tissue being obtained in 80 to 90% of cases [3, 4]. The range of diagnostic accuracy in circumscribed malignant lesions has varied between 50 and 85% [5] but the incidence of false negative results has varied widely from 5 to 25%. It may be possible to reduce the number of false negative results by taking repeated biopsies. The success rate is very high with pancoast-type of tumours at the lung apex [6] and the method has been used with some success for cavitated lesions [7]. It can be used in conjunction with instillation of antifungal agents into mycetomas [8]. Major complications are uncommon with aspiration-needle biopsy; the most frequent complication, pneumothorax, occurs in about 20% of cases but most are small and only about one-third require an intercostal drain. Rarer complications include intrapulmonary and in-trapleural haemorrhage. Although it has been suggested that aspiration-needle biopsy may be used for pulmonary lesions which may be vascular most operators would probably avoid the technique in these circumstances. Implantation of tumour cells along the needle track has been reported [9].

(b) Lung biopsy with cutting needles

There are three different cutting needle techniques for biopsy of lung: punch biopsy, trephines and suction-excision needles.

(i) Punch biopsy

The first cutting needle used for lung biopsy was developed by Silverman [10]. Since then a number of modifications to this needle has been made and large series of percutaneous lung biopsies have been reported [11]. Two modifications of Silverman's needle the Vim-Silverman and the Vim-Tru-Cut disposable needles appear to give the best results. As with aspiration-needle biopsy the diagnostic yield is lowest in diffuse disease although lung tissue can be obtained in 80 to 90% of cases. Of these specimens about 50 to 65% were held to be representative of the histology of the underlying disorder [12].

As with aspiration biopsy the technique is unsuitable for breathless pa-tients who cannot manage to breath-hold for 15 to 30 s and it is difficult in those with troublesome cough. Other contraindications include pulmonary hypertension and cysts or bullae in the area to be biopsied. The procedure is safer and generally gives a higher diagnostic yield with solid lesions at the periphery of the lungs.

There have been wide variations in the incidence of reported complications. Wherever possible cutting-needle biopsy should be used for lesions within 3 cm of the lung surface as this will reduce the likelihood of serious complication. The commonest major complication is haemorrhage and this can be severe [12]. The incidence and severity of pneumothaces is similar to that with aspiration biopsy and implantation of tumour cells in the needle track is a rare occurrence.

(ii) *Trephine biopsy*

The applications of the trephine biopsy technique using a high-speed air drill for the diagnosis of lung disease was first reported by Steel and Winstanley [13]. The trephine provides larger and less distorted tissue specimens than those obtained with cutting needles and the tissue is adequate for histological study in 70 to 85% of cases. However, the success rate, judged by the number of specific tissue-diagnoses achieved is no greater than with other needle biopsy methods and is probably of the order of 50% [14]. Trephine biopsy appears to cause the patient less discomfort although the noise of the drill may be alarming. The complication rate is probably similar to that of other needle biopsy methods. Pneumothorax is quite common, reported rates varying from 25–65%, but although scanty haemoptysis is quite common, serious haemorrhage appears to be rare.

(iii) *Suction-excision needle biopsy*

Recently the Abrams pleural biopsy punch has been used to obtain lung tissue samples. Lung tissue can be obtained in about 90% of patients but specific histology was obtained in only about 60%. With this technique complications are rare, the incidence of pneumothorax is similar to that reported with other needle biopsy methods and severe haemorrhage appears to be uncommon. This technique is only applicable to diffuse lung disease in the immediately subpleural region. Because of the size of the cutting surface of the biopsy punch it is advisable to confine this method to lesions in the periphery of the lungs to avoid the risk of cutting through large pulmonary vessels.

14.1.2 Open lung biopsy

With open lung biopsy diagnostic tissue should be obtained in virtually all patients and in experienced hands the mortality rate should be no higher than with needle-biopsy techniques [15]. The morbidity is necessarily higher although control of postoperative pneumothorax and haemoptysis should be excellent. For diffuse disease a modified limited anterior thoracotomy through a small parasternal incision may be used to obtain small specimens of lung [16]. For circumscribed lesions a full thoracotomy is usually necessary for adequate access. Another modification of limited open lung biopsy has been described in which after dissection through the intercostal muscles under local anaesthetic a trochar and cannula is introduced through a small incision and a small section of lung is extracted with the cannula by asking the patient to blow up a balloon; the increase in intrathoracic pressure forces lung into the cannula and this is excised [17].

14.1.3 Thoracentesis (pleural tap)

A pleural effusion is usually diagnosed by the typical clinical signs and appearances on chest radiograph. Thoracentesis is indicated for relief of breathlessness, to prevent complications and for diagnostic studies (see Table 14.2). Unless the effusion is obviously caused by heart failure, pulmonary infarction or an acute pneumonia it is useful to combine pleural biopsy and thoracentesis with an Abrams punch biopsy. This can be done under local anaesthesia with the patient seated comfortably. The site chosen for biopsy and thoracentesis is usually the intercostal space corresponding to the area of maximum dullness to percussion over the posterior aspect of the chest or in the axilla. Fluid should be removed using a 3-way tap system and care should be taken to prevent air entering the pleural space through the chest wall or by accidental puncture of the lung. If no fluid is obtained at the first attempt the thoracentesis should be repeated above or below the original site. The quantity and rate of removal of the fluid should be controlled and certainly should not exceed 500 to 1000 ml at each thoracentesis as too rapid removal of large quantities may cause re-expansion pulmonary oedema [18]. The other dangers of pleural aspiration are air embolism where air enters a superficial pulmonary vessel through injury to the visceral pleura and pleural shock, circulatory collapse probably caused by vagal stimulation through pleural puncture.

Table 14.2   Investigation of pleural effusion

Clinical examination for: heart failure
                               liver disease
                               joint involvement
Chest radiographs
Aspiration and pleural biopsy for cytology and histology
Biochemistry: protein contents:>3 g/100 ml = exudate
                                    <3 g/100 ml = transudate
               glucose content: low in infections and rheumatoid
               lactic dehydrogenase: high in rheumatoid
               lipids: high cholesterol in rheumatoid
                    high in chylous effusions

14.2 Pleural fluid

14.2.1 Naked-eye appearance of pleural fluid

Blood-stained pleural effusion occurs with chest injuries, pulmonary infarction, tuberculosis and metastatic malignant disease. A turbulent fluid usually indicates an empyema or can occur with a high cholesterol content in tuberculosis or rheumatoid disease [19]. Both transudates and exudates usually produce a clear fluid, the depth of colour of which increases with the protein content. In rheumatoid disease, a pleural effusion may precede or follow the onset of other signs of the disease, is usually unilateral and is commoner in males. The fluid is an exudate, the colour varies considerably and it may be opalescent with a high cholesterol content. Both a low glucose content and high levels of lactic dehydrogenase are common. Rheumatoid factor may be present in the pleural fluid but this is not of diagnostic significance as it may be present in pleural effusions associated with several other conditions. At pleuroscopy there may be pleural nodules visible throughout the parietal pleura. Spontaneous resolution is usual but occasionally there may be gross pleural thickening with a persistent effusion.

14.2.2 Biochemical properties of pleural fluid

(a) Transudates

Pleural effusions with a low protein content (<3.0 g/100 ml) are termed transudates and occur with heart failure, renal failure with fluid overload or cirrhosis of the liver and other hypoproteinaemic states.

(b) Exudates

Fluid with a high protein content (>3.0 g/100 ml) is termed an exudate and is found with pulmonary infarction and other causes of pleural inflammation including pneumonias, tuberculosis and metastatic malignant disease.

(c) Glucose content of fluid

The glucose content of pleural fluid usually parallels that of the blood although it may be lower in tuberculosis, empyaema, malignant disease and rheumatoid disease.

(d) Fat content of fluid

A chylothorax is usually detected by the naked eye appearance of the fluid and the fat content is usually greater than 3.0 g/100 ml. The commonest cause of a chylothorax is malignant invasion or traumatic rupture of the intrathoracic lymphatic pathways but it can occur with lymphangiomyomatosis, filariasis and other rare disorders.

Occasionally there may be a high amylase content in pleural fluid especially in the pleural effusions accompanying acute pancreatitis and oesophageal perforation.

14.2.2 Biochemical properties of pleural fluid

The quantity of non-malignant cells in a pleural effusion may show considerable day-to-day variation [20]. The erythrocyte content of pleural fluid is no aid to diagnosis and high counts may occur with a variety of conditions. A high *neutrophil count* occurs with effusions secondary to bacterial infection, tuberculosis, malignant disease and pancreatitis. It has been suggested that when the neutrophil count is greater than 50% tuberculosis is unlikely. Conversely when the lymphocyte count is 50% or more the most likely causes are tuberculosis or malignant disease. Where the relative lymphocytosis is associated with a high red cell count the effusion is most likely to be neoplastic in origin [21]. A high eosinophil count in pleural fluid has been reported in a wide variety of diseases and is of little diagnostic significance although eosinophilic effusions are rare with tuberculosis or malignant disease [22]. Many pleural effusions associated with underlying malignant growths arise from secondary pneumonitis which develops distal to occlusion of a bronchus by tumour or from obstruction of lymphatics and the fluid may not contain recognizable tumour cells. Metastatic deposits form the commonest group of pleural malignancies but primary pleural mesotheliomas are increasingly recognized in patients exposed to asbestos. A variety of different cell types has been described and all carry a very poor prognosis. The diagnosis may be made by cytology of pleural fluid or biopsy of pleura, in most instances by thoracotomy. The prognosis is so universally bad and the risk of the tumour fungating through the scar so great that in most cases it is justifiable to leave the diagnosis unproven until autopsy.

14.3 Pleural biopsy

The methods available include needle biopsy, open excision biopsy and biopsy at pleuroscopy with a trochar and canula or fibreoptic bronchoscope.

14.3.1 Needle biopsy

There are at least three different types of needle which can be used for biopsy of pleura but in the United Kingdom the Abrams punch biopsy technique is probably almost universally favoured. As with other techniques the success rate of needle biopsy of pleura depends upon the operator's skill, the number of attempts at biopsy made and the type of problem under investigation. Thus at the time this method was first introduced tuberculosis was probably the commonest disorder for which pleural biopsy was undertaken and a high incidence of positive diagnostic histology was obtained. More recently with the decline in prevalence of tuberculosis the diagnostic yield from needle biopsy of pleura is often disappointingly low. The differing success rates were illustrated by the series reported by Cope and Bernhardt [23] where the diagnostic rate was 80% with tuberculous effusions but only 50% with neoplastic disease. The two other needles which have been used for pleural biopsy are the Vim-Silverman and Cope. Ideally needle biopsy of the pleura should be done whenever thoracocentesis is performed. Fluid is removed for cytology, culture and biochemical studies and this is followed by several biopsies of pleura. Complications such as mediastinal emphysema or pneumothorax should be uncommon; implantation of neoplastic cells along the needle track has been reported.

14.3.2 Open pleural biopsy

In general, because there is an added risk from a general anaesthetic, open biopsy of pleura should be reserved for those cases of pleural effusion where needle biopsy has failed to give a specific diagnosis and it is considered necessary to establish the nature of the underlying process. In the past when tuberculosis was more prevalent there was a strong case for treating all pleural effusions of unproven aetiology as tuberculous. With the decline in incidence of tuberculosis for most undiagnosed cases now, antituberculous therapy can reasonably be withheld for a further period of observation unless the tuberculin test is strongly positive.

14.3.3 Thoracoscopy

In the technique first described a rigid endoscope was inserted through an incision in an intercostal space and lung or pleural biopsy could be obtained. The introduction of the fibreoptic bronchoscope has led to renewed interest in the diagnosis of pleural disease. Provided that the instrument is carefully sterilized in ethylene oxide and is introduced using sterile conditions in an operating theatre the morbidity from the technique should not be increased. With the fibrescope the greater penetration possible and the increased mobility of the instrument allows inspection of the visceral and parietal pleura as well as the diaphragmatic and mediastinal surfaces. Biopsies can be taken from superficial pulmonary lesions as well as pleura [24].

14.4 Lymph node biopsy

14.4.1 Mediastinal nodes

Several different techniques have been developed for biopsy of mediastinal lymph nodes but generally the technique chosen will be dictated by the experience and practice of the individual surgeon.

(a) Thoracotomy

Using either a standard thoracotomy incision or a more limited parasternal incision [25] the mediastinal nodes can be viewed directly with the additional advantage that the extent of neoplastic invasion can be assessed more easily.

(b) Mediastinoscopy

This technique was originally described by Carlens. From a suprasternal incision the soft tissues around the trachea are dissected away and biopsy material removed under direct vision. The upper half of the mediastinum is accessible for exploration, including the tracheal bifurcation and the proximal part of the major bronchi. The incidence of complications should be of the order of 3 to 4%. Haemorrhage is the major danger but injury to the left recurrent laryngeal nerve and pneumothorax may occur [27].

(c) Bronchoscopic technique

At rigid bronchoscopy a needle is inserted into the mediastinal tissues through the bronchial wall and tissue can then be aspirated. The yield with this technique appears to be considerably lower than with others, positive histology being obtained in about 50% of cases [28].

(d) Free-catheter technique

A blunt cannula or catheter is inserted under fluoroscopic control in the region of the jugular vein or xiphisternum and guided to the mediastinum. Then with direct vision the biopsy instrument is passed through this introducer into the enlarged lymph glands [29]. Contrast mediastinography can be performed by insufflating carbon dioxide to separate the fascial plans and free cell material can be obtained for histology.

It is perhaps unfortunate that mediastinal lymph node biopsy has yet to become universally accepted as an essential part of the assessment of patients undergoing treatment for malignant disease, especially where they go on to thoracotomy or where the results of radiotherapy or chemotherapy are to be assessed. The other group in whom mediastinoscopy is of great benefit is patients with mediastinal lymph node enlargement from sarcoidosis where it has been shown that diagnostic histology can be obtained in over 80% of cases [30] but nowadays most clinicians prefer transbronchial biopsy of lung tissue through the fibrescope producing a similarly high diagnostic rate.

14.5 Scalene node biopsy

Removal of tissue overlying the scalene group of muscles including the fat pad and any lymph nodes therein was first introduced thirty years ago and although it has been widely used it is likely to yield inferior results to mediastinoscopy in cases where the mediastinal glands are involved. In general it should be reserved for those patients with palpable nodes and in experienced hands should have a low morbidity. It may occasionally be of value in patients with suspected sarcoidosis where there is no clinical or radiographic evidence of enlargement of the hilar lymph nodes and transbronchial biopsies are negative.

14.6 Parasternal lymph node biopsy

Biopsy of the parasternal or internal mammary lymph nodes may occasionally be helpful in determining the extent of spread of proven or suspected bronchogenic carcinoma [31] and has been advocated in cases of tuberculous pleural effusion where culture of the pleural fluid has proved sterile [32].

14.7 Conclusions

For a *solitary opacity*, the primary diagnostic procedure is now probably fibreoptic bronchoscopy with transbronchial biopsy; if this fails to provide adequate histology, it can be followed by a needle biopsy of the lesion. Where benign lesions seem improbable and the patient's age and condition justify open lung biopsy this remains the definitive investigation.

For *diffuse pulmonary disease* fibreoptic bronchoscopy is now probably the investigation of first choice for acquiring tissue for histology and it is especially likely to be diagnostic for sarcoidosis. Percutaneous trephine or cutting needle biopsies may also establish the diagnosis, but open biopsy may provide the only method to acquire sufficient and representative tissue for histology.

Thoracentesis: It is always worth attempting pleural punch biopsy at thoracentesis. It is not usually necessary to proceed to open biopsy for the diagnosis of pleural involvement.

Thoracoscopy: This is a much underused thoracic investigation, especially since the advent of the fibreoptic bronchoscope. It is particularly valuable for inspecting the lung in recurrent pnemothorax and for determining the spread of intrathoracic malignant disease.

Lymph node biopsy: Biopsy of lymph nodes both within and outside the chest is an important diagnostic method for the diagnosis of intrathoracic disease but blind biopsy of impalpable glands and scalene fat pads usually yield disappointing results.

References

1. Kling, T. S. and Neal, H. S. (1973), Needle biopsy. A pilot study. *J. Am. med. Soc.*, **224**, 1143.
2. Greenman, R. L., Goodall, P. T., and King, D. (1975), Lung biopsy in immuno-compromised hosts. *Am. J. med.*, **59**, 488.
3. Lalli, A. F., Naylor, B. and Whitehouse, W. M. (1967), Aspiration biopsy of thoracic lesions. *Thorax*, **22**, 404.
4. Rabinov, K., Goldman, H., Rosbash, H. and Simon, M. (1967), The role of aspiration biopsy of focal lesions in lung and bone by simple needle and fluoroscopy. *Am. J. Roentg.*, **101**, 932.
5. Zavala, D. C. (1973), The diagnosis of pulmonary disease by non-thoracotomy techniques. *Chest*, **64**, 100.
6. Walls, W. J., Thornbury, J. R. and Naylor, B. (1974), Pulmonary needle aspiration biopsy in the diagnosis of Pancoast tumours. *Radiology*, **111**, 99.
7. Millard, J. R. and Westcott, J. L. (1974), Percutaneous needle washings in the diagnosis of cavitary lesions of the lung. *Radiology*, **111**, 474.
8. Adelson, H. T. and Malcolm, J. A. (1968), Endocavitary treatment of pulmonary mycetomas. *Am. Rev. resp. Dis.*, **98**, 87.
9. Allbritten, F. F., Nealon, T., Gibbon, J. H. and Templeton, O. Y. (1952), III. The diagnosis of lung cancer. *Surg. clinics N. Am.* **32**, 1657.
10. Silverman, I. (1938), A new biopsy needle. *Am. J. Surg.*, **40**, 671.
11. Kremp, R. E., Klatte, E. C. and Collins, R. D. (1971), Technical considerations of percutaneous pulmonary biopsy. *Radiology*, **100**, 285.
12. Zavala, D. C. and Bedell, G. N. (1972), Percutaneous lung biopsy with a cutting needle. An analysis of 40 cases and comparison with other biopsy techniques. *Am. Rev. resp. Dis.*, **106**, 186.
13. Steel, S. J. and Winstanley, D. P. (1967), Trephine biopsy for diffuse lung lesions. *Br. med. J.*, **3**, 30.
14. Nicholson, D. P. and Mayfield, J. D. (1971), Trephine biopsy of lung. *Am. Rev. resp. Dis.*, **103**, 715
15. Gaensler, E. A., Moister, V. B. and Hamm, J. (1964), Open-lung biopsy in diffuse pulmonary disease. *New Engl. J. Med.*, **270**, 1319.
16. Andrews, N. C. and Klassen, K. P. (1957) *Eight years' experience with pulmonary biopsy*. **J.A.M.A.**, 1061.
17. Thompson, D. T. (1973), A new instrument and technique for lung biopsy using local anaesthesia. *Thorax*, **28**, 247.

18. Trapnell, D. H. and Thurston, J. G. B. (1970), Unilateral pulmonary oedema after pleural aspiration, *Lancet, 2*, 1367.
19. Roy, P. H., Carr, D. T. and Payne, W. S. (1967), The problems of chylothorax. *Mayo Clinic Proceed., 43*, 457.
20. Spriggs, A. I. and Boddington, M. M. (1968), *The Cytology of Effusions.* Grure and Stratton, New York, p. 1-39.
21. Light, R. W., Erozan, Y. S. and Ball, W. C. (1973), Cells in pleural fluid. Their value in differential diagnosis. *Archs intern. Med., 132*, 854.
22. Campbell, G. D., and Webb, W. R. (1964), Eosinophilic pleural effusion: A review with the presentation of seven new cases. *Am. Rev. resp. Dis., 90*, 194.
23. Cope, C. and Bernhardt, H. (1963), Hook-needle biopsy of pleura, pericardium peritoneum and synovium. *Am. J. Med., 35*, 189.
24. Senno, A. and Moallem, S. (1974), Thoracoscopy with the fibreoptic broncho-scope. *J. Thorac. Cardiovasc. Surg., 67*, 606.
25. Evans, D. S., Hall, J. H. and Harrison, G. K. (1973), Anterior mediastinoscopy. *Thorax, 28*, 444.
26. Carlens, E. (1959), Mediastinoscopy: a method for inspection and tissue biopsy in the superior mediastinum. *Dis. Chest, 36*, 343.
27. Editorial (1972), Mediastinoscopy, *Lancet*, i, 1219.
28. Schieppati, E. E. (1958), Mediastinal lymph node puncture through the tracheal carina. *Surgery, Gynec. Obstet., 107*, 243.
29. Nordenstrom, B. (1967), Transthoracic needle biopsy. *New Engl. J. Med., 276*, 1081.
30. Ross, J. K. *et al.* (1971), Mediastinoscopy. *Thorax, 25*, 312.
31. Villegas, A. H. and Naveiro, J. J. (1970), The diagnostic value of internal mammary lymph node biopsy in non-purulent pleural effusions: experience in 60 cases. *Chest, 58*, 345.
32. Burke, H. E., and Wilson, J. A. S. (1966), A new method for estimating the diagnosis of pleural disease – parasternal lymph node biopsy. *Am. Rev. resp. Dis., 93*, 210.

CHAPTER FIFTEEN

The Nose

N. Mygind, P. Borum and M. Pedersen

Many lung diseases also involve the nose and thus knowledge about investigation of nasal disorders can help clinicians when dealing with lung disease. For many years the larynx has posed an artificial barrier between the upper and lower airway leading to the development of separate specialities which often operate without sufficient knowledge of each other's potential contribution to patient care. This chapter sets out to provide insight into those nasal diseases which are of relevance to lung diseases and particularly concentrates on those nasal investigations which are of help to the chest physician.

15.1 Nasal protection of lower airways

The nose is the first line of defence against airborne threats: these include infective agents, allergenic particles, irritant gases, as well as unphysiological temperatures and humidity. It protects the delicate structures of the lower airways by acting as a filter, a humidifier, and a heating apparatus. In this respect, the narrow inlet to the nose, the bend of the airstream, and the slit-like passages are of importance (Fig. 15.1). In addition, the abundance of submucosal glands, arteriovenous anastomoses, and large venous sinusoids contributes to make the nose 'the air conditioner *par excellance*' [1]. After passage through the nose, virtually all particles larger than 10 μm are removed from the inhaled air as well as water-soluble gases; the air is warmed to 32°C and the relative humidity is raised to 98% [2]. When no environmental challenge exists, mouth breathing in normal subjects will only result in slight pharyngeal discomfort, but this substitute for normal breathing through the nose can be hazardous when inhaled air is heavily polluted, or the lower airways abnormal. An example of this is reflex bronchoconstriction in asthmatic subjects during exercise, induced by inhalation of unconditioned air through the widely opened mouth. This exercise-induced bronchoconstriction can largely be prevented, if patients can maintain nasal breathing during exercise [3].

The high prevalence rate of rhinitis diseases can be considered a consequence of the protection of the lower airways. Allergic rhinitis is related to the filter function of the nose, and rhinorrhoea and blockage in non-allergic rhinitis are consequences of malfunctioning of the 'nasal humidifier' and 'heating apparatus'.

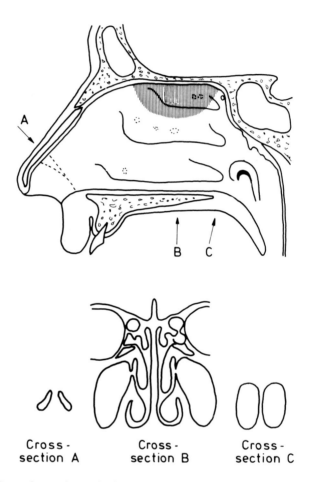

Cross-   Cross-   Cross-
section A   section B   section C

Fig. 15.1 Upper figure shows the lateral wall of the nasal cavity with the turbinates, the orifices to the Eustacian tube and the paranasal sinuses, and the olfactory region (hatched area). The cross-sections in the lower figure (A, B and C) show that the entrance to the nose is the most narrow part of the whole airway, and that the nasal cavity has a slit-like shape. Both qualities are important for the air conditioning function of the nose. The ethmoidal sinuses, from which nasal polyps originate, are seen above the nasal cavity, between the orbits [12]. (By courtesy of Blackwell Scientific Publications, Oxford.)

15.2 Allergic rhinitis and allied conditions

15.2.1 Seasonal allergic rhinitis

Seasonal allergic rhinitis or hay fever is rhinoconjunctivitis usually caused by pollen allergy. Subjects with hyperreactive bronchi may also develop asthma in the pollen season, but it is unclear how the allergens reach the bronchi as the large pollen grains are almost completely trapped in the nose.

15.2.2 Perennial rhinitis

This disease is characterized by watery/colourless discharge, sneezing attacks and/or blockage. It is generally accepted that an allergic and a non-allergic group exists, but it seems more appropriate to describe three groups. In the first, *perennial allergic rhinitis*, a relevant allergy can be demonstrated. In the second group, *perennial intrinsic rhinitis*, no allergy is found, but the disease is comparable with regard to symptoms, signs, and response to pharmacological therapy; the nasal mucosa is often pale bluish, the secretion contains eosinophils, steroids are effective, and many patients have or will develop nasal polyps and intrinsic asthma. In the third group, *perennial cholinergic rhinitis*, there is no asthma, polyps, or eosinophilia, and the response to steroid therapy is as a rule negative. This group is believed to be due merely to an imbalance in the autonomic nervous system, with a dominance of parasympathetic innervation, controlling the submucous glands. All three subgroups are characterized by increased mucosal reactivity in the nose; thus temperature changes, inhalation of dust, fumes, smell of cooking, washing powder, etc., will often provoke symptoms in perennial rhinitis.

15.2.3 Nasal polyposis

This disease is characterized by multiple polyps in both nasal cavities. Polyps are oedema-filled sacs, formed in the upper part of the nose, and especially in the ethmoidal sinuses. Contrary to widespread belief, positive allergy skin tests are not more prevalent in these patients than in the total population [4]. A non-allergic triad, consisting of polyposis, intrinsic asthma and aspirin intolerance is described by Samter and Beers [5]. Most patients with nasal polyposis probably belong to this entity, although only a minority of patients also suffer from asthma, and aspirin intolerance as a rule cannot be demonstrated [6]. Similar to perennial intrinsic asthma, the nasal secretion is characterized by eosinophilia, and the disease usually responds to steroid therapy.

While polyps are remarkably rare in children with allergic rhinitis, they are present in as many as 10–20% of patients with cystic fibrosis [7]. These polyps are characterized by neutrophil and not by eosinophil leucocytes, and steroid treatment is not useful. Polyps of a similar type also occur in some patients with Kartageners syndrome (see later).

15.3 Rhinitis symptoms

In the case record it is inadequate to state that 'the symptoms are typical for allergic rhinitis', or 'the patient suffers from severe symptoms of sinusitis'. A detailed description of distinct symptoms and of their severity is necessary. Rhinitis symptoms are composed of sneezing, rhinorrhoea and blockage, which causes snuffling, hyposmia, disturbed sleep, and dryness in the throat due to mouth breathing. Sinusitis symptoms include thick purulent secretions, postnasal secretions, a sensation of pressure over the cheeks and nasal bridge, and a nasal voice when the nose is patent [8, 9].

It is important to discover whether the secretion is predominantly watery/colourless as in perennial rhinitis, or purulent as in chronic purulent rhinosinusitis. Nasal obstruction caused by a swollen mucous membrane is bilateral, or alters from side to side, while a persistent unilateral obstruction is suggestive of a septal deviation. Unilateral symptoms, pain and haemorrhagic secretions should alert the physician to the risk of malignancy.

A considerable part of the total population suffers occasionally from slight nasal symptoms. Consequently, it is necessary to include quantitative criteria for making the distinction between a negligible disorder, and that requiring further investigation and therapy. The average number of hours with symptoms per day, multiplied by the average number of days with symptoms per week, is a clinically useful measurement of severity; patients can also count the number of sneezes and nose blowings per day.

15.4 Clinical investigation of rhinitis

15.4.1 Rhinoscopy

In rhinitis, inspection of the diseased mucous membrane takes a few seconds with a lamp, a mirror and a speculum being the only equipment required. Nasal patency, the septal position, appearance of the mucous membrane, and presence of secretion and of polyps can be assessed. Use of a vasoconstrictor before inspection is often necessary to improve the view, and when a more detailed examination of the posterior part of the nose is needed, a fibrerhinoscope can be used.

In clinical practice, rhinoscopy is useful for diagnosis and classification of the disease as well as for assessing the response to treatment. The importance of this simple examination has increased in the last years, as topical application of drugs has gained a more widespread use. Inspection of the nose, disclosing large polyps, pronounced septal deviation or enlarged turbinates, may explain an unexpected negative result with intranasal steroids.

15.4.2 Measurement of nasal airway patency

Nasal obstruction can be caused by dilatation of venous sinusoids, mucosal oedema, polyp formation, accumulation of secretion, septal deviation, or most frequently by a combination of these factors. Clinically, nasal patency can be estimated by rhinoscopy, and by getting the patient to breathe through each nostril separately. When a more exact measurement is needed, a rhinomanometer, a peak flow meter for nasal use or a body plethysmograph can be used [10]. Nasal patency can vary spontaneously within seconds and thus a single measurement is of limited value. While measurement of airway patency can provide useful information in asthma, it reflects only the contribution of one of three symptoms in rhinitis. In the context of precise measurement, it must be remembered that normal nasal patency is not synonymous with normal nasal airflow.

15.4.3 Radiography examination of paranasal sinuses

The main indications for this examination are suspicion of malignancy, and purulent rhinosinusitis. In the latter the following may be found: 1. a swollen mucous membrane, 2. an opaque cavity, or 3. a fluid level. Surgery can be helpful when a fluid level is present, the frontal sinuses are involved, and when, in addition, symptoms are severe, of long standing and resistant to conservative treatment.

Roentgenographic clouding of ethmoidal sinuses is usually found in nasal polyposis, as the polyps are formed in these sinuses. Although nasal polyps are not formed in the maxillary sinuses, these often look abnormal on radiograph. In patients with polyposis, puncture of the maxillary sinuses is only indicated when distinct sinusitis symptoms are present.

Perennial rhinitis produces minor radiograph abnormalities (marginal swelling) in about 20% of patients, but in another 20% significant changes with dense clouding are found [11]. These more pronounced changes are probably indicative of perennial intrinsic rhinitis, as paranasal sinuses are seldom involved in perennial cholinergic rhinitis.

15.4.4 Serum IgE

Most studies of perennial rhinitis are based on patients who suffer from both rhinitis and asthma. Such patients differ significantly from patients with perennial rhinitis without bronchial symptoms, with regard to serum IgE, blood eosinophils, and skin testing (Table 15.1). In the latter group, serum IgE will only be elevated in a small minority, while about half of the patients with rhinitis and asthma have an increased IgE level. When rhinitis is the only symptom, no reliable distinction can, therefore, be made between an allergic and a non-allergic group, based on a serum IgE determination.

Table 15.1   Results of investigations of patients with perennial rhinitis with and without concommitant asthma [11]

	Symptom-free subjects (N=75–141)	Perennial allergic rhinitis (N=58)	Perennial non-allergic rhinitis (N=87)	Perennial rhinitis and asthma (N=56)	All perennial rhinitis patients (N=201)
Positive allergen skin tests to 'perennial allergens' (in %)	6	100 (40 for these two groups together)	0	88	51
Serum IgE level determined by RIST (median, U/ml)	62	72	91	310	120
Eosinophils in blood (median, cells/mm³)	150	225	225	320	255
Eosinophilia in a nasal smear (≥10% of all leucocytes, % of subjects)	11	–	–	–	71

15.4.5 Eosinophilia in blood and smear

Eosinophilia is very characteristic in IgE-dependent diseases, but can occur in some airway diseases not associated with IgE antibody, e.g. nasal polyposis and intrinsic asthma. Eosinophil estimation will therefore not distinguish allergic from non-allergic disease; the distinction is made between allergic diseases and some allied conditions associated with eosinophilia, and infectious diseases and autonomic imbalance, not usually associated with eosinophilia.

In airway diseases eosinophil leucocytes are transported from the bone marrow to the mucous membrane by the blood, which merely acts as a transport medium for the white blood cell. In rhinitis and asthma eosinophils constitute seldom more than 10% of the total number of circulating leucocytes, and a normal differential count cannot provide an accurate measure; to achieve this a counting chamber is necessary. The blood eosinophil count depends on the amount of tissue involved in the disease; consequently, blood eosinophilia is only rarely found in rhinitis without concomitant asthma or dermatitis, and the test is of limited diagnostic value in patients with simple perennial rhinitis. An increased number of eosinophils is indicative of a subclinical affection of the bronchi and therefore provides a valuable clue to respiratory disease.

Following nasal allergen challenge, eosinophils migrate through blood vessels and lamina propria to the epithelial surface, where they can be demonstrated in a smear after 1–3 h, and persist for up to three days [12]. In contrast to the slight degree of eosinophilia, which occasionally is found in the blood, eosinophils will often constitute 50–100% of the leucocytes in a nasal smear. Nasal eosinophilia is therefore a constant finding in patients, recently exposed to allergens, but is also present in the majority of patients with perennial rhinitis and nasal polyposis without demonstrable allergy. Examination of a nasal smear is very simple; the result, available within minutes, is of importance for the correct classification of the disease, and also for treatment, as steroid-responsiveness by and large runs parallel with the presence of eosinophilia.

A nasal smear is collected by scraping the mucous membrane with a cotton applicator. Sufficient cellular material can be collected from adults by introducing the applicator two or three times on each side, but children prefer to blow the nose in a handkerchief. After drying the smear in air or on a hot plate (not in a flame) the slide is covered with 18 drops of May Grunwald stain, and after 30–45 s, 6 drops of Giemsa stain is added; 30–45 s later the stain is poured off by running water from the tap. Quick decolouration with alcohol, immediately followed by rinsing in water, will improve the quality of the staining. After drying, the specimen is ready for microscopy. An exact measurement of eosinophil percentage cannot be given, due to the uneven distribution of the cells; the test is therefore qualitative or semi-quantitative.

The following scale can be used:

> No eosinophilia: − (<5% eosinophils)
> Slight eosinophilia: +/− (<10% eosinophils)
> Moderate eosinophilia: + (<50% eosinophils)
> Marked eosinophilia: ++ (>50% eosinophils)

The values + and ++ are considered as pathological findings, present in patients with seasonal allergic rhinitis, and in most patients with perennial rhinitis and nasal polyposis; +/− has no significance, but indicates that a further examination may be required; − is found in the large majority of symptom-free subjects. A reliable characterization of the disease can be attained with 2–3 smears.

15.4.6 Metacholine/histamine tests

The typical rhinoscopy finding in perennial rhinitis is reduced nasal patency, accumulation of colourless secretion, and a pale bluish, swollen mucous membrane, but some patients can have a quite normal appearance of the mucous membrane in spite of marked symptoms. When, in addition, the microscopy of a nasal smear is normal and skin testing is negative, the diagnosis is merely based on the patient's statement. This is unsatisfactory because of the considerable individual variation in perception of symptoms, and there is a need for additional diagnostic tests.

In asthma, increased mucosal reactivity, which is a constant feature, can be demonstrated by metacholine and by histamine inhalation (see Chapter 11). This test can support the diagnosis of asthma in subjects with normal lung function. Clinical evidence suggests mucosal hyperreactivity as a consistent characteristic also of perennial rhinitis, and recent laboratory studies suggest that nasal metacholine challenge with subsequent measurement of the secretory response can serve as a simple test to support the diagnosis [13]. While metacholine is sprayed into the nose, histamine can also be given as a microdroplet; the number of sneezes is counted and the amount of secretion measured.

15.4.7 Allergen skin testing

As this topic is described in Chapter 10, only a few comments will be added. The allergen extracts, used for skin prick testing in asthma and in rhinitis are in principle identical. Positive reactions to fungi are rare in adult patients with rhinitis, and time-consuming examination for food-allergy is seldom indicated. Relevant extracts are usually confined to house dust mite, pollen, and animal danders. Compared with asthma, the allergen skin tests are less often positive, and skin reactions are usually smaller.

15.4.8 RAST and nasal allergen test

Positive skin test to pollen and to animal dander are as a rule confirmed by the case history, and no further examination is necessary. Although the case history regarding mite allergy is far less conclusive, an obviously positive skin test is in most cases of perennial rhinitis sufficient evidence for the diagnosis of mite allergy. However, when hyposensitization is considered for selected cases, it may be wise to confirm the skin test by RAST (radioallergosorbent test) or by allergen provocation test. The RAST test can also be useful, when high-quality extracts are not available for skin testing.

Nasal allergen provocation is a valuable test for research purposes, but in our opinion it is questionable whether it can be recommended for routine diagnosis. It is time-consuming, badly standardized, slightly unpleasant, and potentially hazardous. In addition, there is a risk of false positive results in patients with very hyperreactive mucous membranes. When a nasal allergen test is performed it is of importance to measure all three nasal symptoms, i.e. sneezing, discharge and blockage. It is easier to perform a nasal than a bronchial allergen provocation, but the nasal test is usually only marginally informative in patients without rhinitis and cannot serve as a substitute for the bronchial test in asthmatics [14].

15.5 Rhinitis and asthma

In extrinsic asthma, provoked by inhaled allergens, the nasal filter retains allergenic particles, which causes an allergic reaction and inflammation in the nasal mucosa. For unknown reasons, this will not always result in symptoms, but a high proportion of asthmatic subjects also have nasal symptoms. This is the rule in children, but they will often not complain, possibly because they are accustomed to having an itching, running and stuffy nose.

Perennial rhinitis occurs in extrinsic as well as in intrinsic asthma, while nasal polyposis is highly suggestive of the latter, and so is involvement of paranasal sinuses, especially of the ethmoidal sinuses.

In the sea-lion the effect of water on the nostrils causes apnoea and cardiovascular changes. Possibly, vestiges of this diving reflex exist in man which might explain why stimulation of the nasal mucosa can affect the bronchi [15]. It is a clinical experience that bronchial symptoms can deteriorate in parallel with nasal complaints, possibly due to a nasobronchial reflex; but it is also claimed that asthma appears when rhinitis disappears. For this reason it has been advocated that nasal polyps should not be removed, because 'the patient then gets asthma instead'. In our opinion, the nose should be treated for nasal symptoms, irrespective of bronchial symptoms, and *vice versa*.

In the past it has often been claimed that a quiescent allergic or infective focus in the paranasal sinuses can cause and perpetuate asthma. Although this statement has never been documented or disproved we have to accept that our knowledge is limited regarding the interplay between nose and bronchi, and between infection and allergy; for example a common cold, mainly affecting the nose, can cause an increase in bronchial reactivity, of importance in asthmatic subjects [16]. Thus a complex interaction exists between upper and lower airways making it important for chest physicians to develop an abiding interest in nasal diseases.

15.6 'The immotile cilia syndrome'

A few years ago it was shown that male infertility can be associated with immotile spermatozoa, lacking the ATP-ase containing dynein arms. As the first patient with this defect also had dextrocardia, this finding resulted in the demonstration of absence of dynein arms in airway cilia from patients with Kartagener's syndrome, a triad consisting of situs inversus viscerum, chronic rhinosinusitis, and chronic bronchitis with bronchiectases [18]. As these patients had no mucociliary transport in the nose or bronchi [19], it was logical to assume that their cilia were immotile, although this had not directly been observed. Eliasson *et al.* [20] proposed the name 'the immotile cilia syndrome' for male sterility and chronic infections of the upper and lower airways, irrespective of the presence of situs inversus, which these authors emphasized was present in only half of the patients. Consequently, a diagnosis cannot be based merely on case history and radiograph examination.

Based on experience with cystic fibrosis it can be assumed that early and active physiotherapy and antibiotic treatment can prevent the development of bronchiectases and lung damage also in 'the immotile cilia syndrome'. In the following we will shortly describe our attempts during the last few years to develop a test for making an early diagnosis of this disease. The results are described more in detail elsewhere [21]. Such is the pace of development that we expect further advances to have been made by the time this book is published as the subject is being intensively investigated with new techniques. In this review we can only provide a snapshot of what is happening at the time of writing.

It is highly characteristic that these patients have had daily nasal discharge and productive cough since infancy. They are 'born with a cold'. A constant finding by rhinoscopy is accumulation of mucopurulent secretions in the nose, especially under the inferior turbinate. Typically, these patients can provide a productive cough and nose blowing upon request. Clouding of the paranasal sinuses are often seen on radiography, and in some patients polyps are formed in the ethmoidal sinuses. This can result in broadening of the nasal bridge in children, and occasionally in nasal stenosis. Interestingly, the incidence of acute otitis media is not increased, but almost all patients have a history of chronic secretory otitis media. During infancy and childhood several visits have been paid to otologists and surgery has repeatedly been performed for 'sinusitis' and for 'adenoids'. Active surgeons have often placed tubes in the ear drums of these patients two to three times a year.

The mucociliary transport can be examined in the nose in children from the age of about 8 years by placing small saccharine-dye particles on the mucous membrane [22]. Typically, these patients will not get a sweet taste due to a severely impaired transport of saccharine to the pharynx, and after 30–60 min the blue-coloured secretion will run out from the anterior nostril. Repeated tests may be necessary, as infections probably in some cases can be a cause of impaired mucociliary function.

Epithelial cells can be obtained by gently scraping the nasal mucosa with a sharp spoon (diameter, 2 mm); this painless procedure can be performed without bleeding even in newborns. Specimens can be used for electron microscopy, which in typical cases will show lack of dynein arms and often an abnormal arrangement of microtubules (Fig. 15.2). However, this examination is too time-consuming for clinical routine.

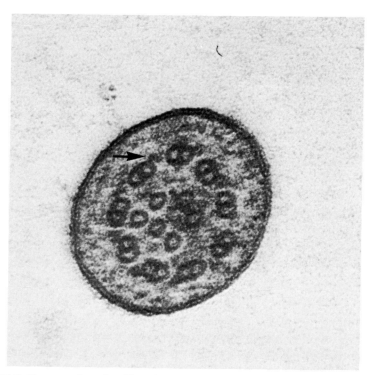

Fig. 15.2 Cross-section of a cilium from a patient with Kartagener's syndrome ('the immotile cilia syndrome'). There is an abnormal arrangement of central microtubules, but only a partial lack of dynein arms. An outer arm is shown by the arrow. Transmission electron micrograph ($\times$ 97 600).

Based on the first reports of absent mucociliary transport and ultra-structural defects of cilia in Kartagener's syndrome, it was believed that the normal effective-recovery stroke of cilia in the airways was replaced by a complete standstill. We decided therefore to study the living ciliated cells directly from a nasal scraping by a light microscope. Although the primary aim was to develop a simple diagnostic test, applicable to daily routine, the set-up described below is more complicated, as we also wanted to study the ciliary activity under standardized conditions.

With the sharp spoon, a sample of about 1000 cells is obtained and immediately placed in Ringer's solution in a perfusion chamber. In an anoptral contrast microscope the number of cells with motile cilia is counted, and the beating pattern is monitored in detail from 20 cells, using a microphoto-oscillograph. After focusing on the beating cilia of a single cell, a micro-aperture is introduced in the light beam. The changing intensity of the light signal, caused by ciliary activity is recorded by a photocell, connected to a writer. The frequency, amplitude, and degree of asynchrony can then be directly read on a curve, using a five-point scale for synchrony/asynchrony (Fig. 15.3).

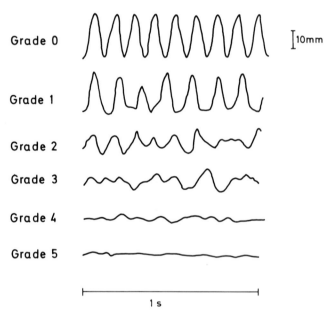

Fig. 15.3 Microphoto-oscillographic recording of cilia motility on single cells. Asynchrony is graded from 0 (= synchrony) to 5 (total asynchrony) [21].

The preliminary results are given in Fig. 15.4. It is remarkable that 10 of 11 patients, who clinically had 'the immotile cilia syndrome' had some motile cilia, and two of these patients had almost a normal number. On average a third of the ciliated cells was motile in patients, while normal controls had 90% cells with motile cilia (Fig. 15.4). In addition, the beating pattern was predominantly asynchronous, and more resembling the arm of a metronome than of a crawling swimmer, as in the normal effective-recovery stroke.

The results have shown that our present concept of 'the immotile cilia syndrome' is an oversimplification, and this term seems inappropriate when some of the patients can have a normal number of cells with motile cilia. It has been demonstrated that patients with Kartagener's syndrome lack the dynein arms in airway cilia, but the actual findings suggest that the lack of these ATP-ase containing structures is only partial. If this hypothesis, which is supported by some electron micrographs is correct (Fig. 15.2), it can explain why several of the cilia have a 'trembling motility'. We must assume that the normal effective-recovery stroke needs an equipment of energy-yielding dynein arms in the full length of the cilia; dynein arms in part of the cilia may only initiate incomplete ciliary motility.

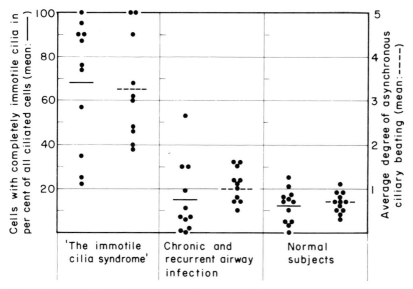

Fig. 15.4 Results of *in vitro* study of ciliated cells from nasal mucosa. Each point represents the mean value of recordings from 20 cells in one patient [21].

As this topic appeared to be more complicated than initially expected, it is unfortunately too early to describe precisely the recommended test for the diagnosis of this disease, or group of diseases; recent observations have suggested that some patients have other motility patterns with increased frequency of ciliary beating. At present it is also important to examine more in detail to what extent ciliary dysfunction is caused by a primary defect, and to what extent secondary factors, such as bacterial toxins and leucocyte enzymes contribute to the dysfunction observed. When these factors have been analysed we believe that the direct examination in a phase contrast microscope of nasal scrapings will be a diagnostic test, of similar usefulness as the sweat test for cystic fibrosis. In this way it will probably be possible to identify primary cilia dysfunction, based on inherited defects of the cilia, and secondary dysfunction, due to environmental factors and inflammatory reactions.

The nose is well suited for study and diagnosis of these diseases, as it has an impaired mucociliary transport in common with bronchial epithelium and is more accessible for diagnostic procedures.

15.7 Cystic fibrosis

Considering the abnormality of bronchial secretory function in this condition, it is remarkable that these children do not have an increased prevalence of secretory otitis media [23]. In contrast to the bronchial symptoms, however, complaints about nose and sinuses are not prominent. On the other hand a radiographic examination will often disclose sinus disease especially involving ethmoidal sinuses, which lead to the development of nasal polyps. These can be seen by rhinoscopy (after use of a vasoconstrictor) in as many as 10–20% of all patients [7]. They are not a sign of allergy, as microscopy shows infiltration with lymphocytes and not eosinophils [24]. The presence of nasal polyps in a child (a single choanal polyp excluded) strongly suggests a diagnosis of cystic fibrosis, and a sweat test, not allergy skin tests, is the relevant examination. A mucocele of paranasal sinuses in children is almost always connected with cystic fibrosis.

15.8 Sarcoidosis

In chronic sarcoidosis brown-yellow-bluish infiltrations are commonly seen in the skin of the outer nose. Similar infiltrations can in a few cases be seen in the nasal mucosa, but rhinoscopy is very seldom of value for the early diagnosis. Enlargement of the parotid glands with fever (uveoparotid fever) is occasionally an early sign of acute sarcoidosis, and about 5–10% of all patients with sarcoidosis have bilateral enlargement of parotid glands. Thus examination of nose and salivary glands may help in the diagnosis and management of pulmonary sarcoidosis [25].

15.9 Wegener's granulomatosis

This is a serious disease consisting of granulomata in the airways, which untreated, can lead to death within months or a few years (reviewed in [26], [27] and [28]) (also see Chapter 16). As treatment is occasionally effective, early diagnosis is important, and it is in most cases based on upper airway symptoms and signs. In the typical case, an adult patient will consult the physician complaining of prolonged and atypical nasal illness; the paranasal sinuses, middle ear and larynx can also be involved. Initially, the nasal discharge may be colourless, suggesting allergic rhinitis, but it is more often purulent, and the first diagnosis is then 'chronic rhinosinusitis'.

Rhinoscopy can at first show a swollen mucous membrane, but a later examination will disclose an inhomogenous mucosal picture with crusts, bleeding, anaemic areas, and a brittle mucous lining, which readily bleeds when attempts are made to remove the crusts. Repeated mucosal biopsies can be necessary, before the correct microscopic diagnosis is made by the pathologist, who often will describe 'non-specific inflammation', unless the clinician draws his attention to Wegener's granulomatosis. Symptoms and signs, the progressive course, and the microscopic picture are at this stage all necessary for a reliable diagnosis, and for commencement of therapy with a cytotoxic drug (cyclophosphamide) and prednisolone. Once treatment is started a microscopic diagnosis becomes more difficult. When the disease progresses, the destruction of mucous membranes and nasal skeleton becomes more prominent and saddle nose often develops; the nose and paranasal sinuses may be eventually transformed into one necrotic cavity. The destruction may extend to the orbits, and as mentioned earlier, the middle ear and larynx may be involved early in the disease; granulomas of the bronchial mucosa can be seen as infiltrates on radiography.

However, if only the nose is involved, problems may arise as to differentiating Wegener's granulomatosis from the 'non-healing granuloma of the nose' (malignant midline granuloma). Although the two entities may be variants of the same underlying disorder, their clinical course and response to treatment seems to differ. In contrast to Wegener's granulomatosis, the 'non-healing granuloma of the nose' usually remains localized and death is due to local invasion. Moreover, irradiation seems to be the treatment of choice in agreement with a histopathological picture dominated by an atypical histiocytic infiltrate with frequent mitoses, in contrast to the picture seen in Wegener's granulomatosis, where polymorphonuclear leukocytes are dominating. Unfortunately, however, many transitional cases are encountered, rendering the ultimate decision on diagnosis and therapy a matter for specialists.

15.10 Summary

A considerable number of patients with respiratory diseases will also suffer from symptoms from nose and paranasal sinuses. Some knowledge about diagnosis and management of rhinitis and sinusitis is therefore necessary for the chest physician. Examination of the nose and paranasal sinuses can also in some cases contribute to a correct diagnosis of bronchial diseases, and following that, to optimum therapy. Thus the demonstration of impaired ciliary function in the nose may be a simple way to diagnose 'the immotile cilia syndrome'. In children with obscure bronchial symptoms, the demonstration nasal polyps can alert the physician to the diagnosis of cystic fibrosis, and in asthmatic subjects the presence of polyps might suggest intrinsic rather than extrinsic asthma. Rhinoscopy followed by mucosal biopsies is a useful and common way to make a diagnosis of Wegener's granulomatosis, and an ENT examination may occasionally help in the diagnosis of sarcoidosis. The artificial separation of the airway by the vocal cords may have hindered the development of better methods in the management of diseases affecting both segments of the airway. A closer union between the specialities of thoracic medicine and otolaryngology should be to the benefit of both and to those frequent patients with diseases involving both lung and nose.

References

1. Proctor, D. F. (1977), The upper airways. I. Nasal physiology and defence of the lung. *Am. Rev. resp. Dis.,* **115**, 97–129.
2. Ingelstedt, S. (1956), Studies on the conditioning of air in the respiratory tract. *Acta Otolar.,* Suppl. 131, 1–80.
3. Shturman-Ellstein, R., Zeballos, R. J., Buckley, J. M. and Souhrada, J. F. (1978), The beneficial effect of nasal breathing on exercise-induced bronchoconstriction. *Am. Rev. resp. Dis.,* **118**, 65–73.
4. Caplin, I., Haynes, J. T. and Spahn, J. (1971), Are nasal polyps an allergic phenomenon? *Ann. Allergy,* **29**, 631–4.
5. Samter, M. and Beers, R. F. (1967), Concerning the nature of intolerance to aspirin. *J. Allergy clin. Immunol.,* **40**, 281–93.
6. Delaney, J. C. (1976), Aspirin idiosyncracy in patients admitted for nasal polypectomy. *Clin. Otolar.,* **1**, 27–30.
7. Mygind, N., Thomsen, J., Flensborg, E. W. and Weeke, B. (1977), Nasal immunoglobulins in cystic fibrosis. In: *Proc. First International Symposium on Infection and Allergy of the Nose and Paranasal Sinuses,* (ed. R. Takahashi), Scimed Publications, Tokyo, pp. 120–3.
8. Axelsson, A. and Runtze, U. (1976), Symptoms and signs of acute maxillary sinusitis. *ORL,* **38**, 298.
9. Evans, F. O. *et al.* (1975), Sinusitis of the maxillary antrum. *New Engl. J. Med.,* **293**, 735.
10. Cockcroft, D. W. *et al.* (1979), Nasal airway inspiratory resistance. *Am. Rev. resp. Dis.,* **119**, 921–6.
11. Mygind, N., Dirksen, A., Johnsen, N. J. and Weeke, B. (1978), Perennial rhinitis: an analysis of skin testing, serum IgE, and blood and smear eosinophilia in 201 patients. *Clin. Otolar.,* **3**, 189–96.
12. Mygind, N. (1979), *Nasal Allergy.* Blackwell Scientific Publications, Oxford.
13. Borum, P. (1979), Nasal methacholine challenge. A test for measurement of nasal reactivity. *J. Allergy clin. Immunol.,* **63**, 253–7.
14. Stenius-Arrniala, B. S. M., Malmberg, C. H. O. and Holopainen, E. E. A.

(1978), Relationship between the results of bronchial, nasal and conjunctival provocation tests in patients with asthma. *Clin. Allergy,* **8**, 403–9.

15. Drettner, B. (1970), Pathophysiological relationship between upper and lower airways. *Ann. Otol.,* **79**, 499–505.
16. Empey, D. W. *et al.* (1976), Mechanisms of bronchial hyperreactivity in normal subjects after upper respiratory tract infections. *Am. Rev. resp. Dis.,* **113**, 131.
17. Pedersen, H. and Rebbe, H. (1975), Absence of arms in the axoneme of immotile human spermatozoa. *Biol. Reprod.* **12**, 541–4.
18. Pedersen, H. and Mygind, N. (1976), Absence of axonemal arms in nasal mucosa cilia in Kartagener's syndrome. *Nature,* **262**, 494.
19. Camner, P., Mossberg, B. and Afzelius, B. A. (1975), Evidence for congenital nonfunctioning cilia in the tracheobronchial tract of two subjects. *Am. Rev. resp. Dis.,* **112**, 807–9.
20. Eliasson, R., Mossberg, B., Camner, P. and Afzelius, B. A. (1977), The immotile-cilia syndrome. *New Engl. J. Med.,* **297**, 1–6.
21. Pedersen, M. and Mygind, N. (1980), Ciliary motility in 'the immotile cilia syndrome'. First results of microphoto-oscillographic studies. *Br. J. Dis. Chest,* **74**, 239–44.
22. Andersen, I. *et al.* (1974), A comparison of nasal and tracheobronchial clearance. *Arch. environ. Hlth,* **29**, 290–3.
23. Bak-Pedersen, K. and Larsen, P. K. (1979), Inflammatory middle ear diseases in patients with cystic fibrosis. *Acta Otolar.,* suppl. 360, 138–40.
24. Sørensen, H., Mygind, N., Tygstrup, I. and Flensborg, E. W. (1977), Histology of nasal polyps of different etiology. *Rhinology,* **15**, 121–8.
25. Mayock, R. L., Bertrand, P. and Morrison, C. E. (1963), Manifestations of sarcoidosis. *Am. J. Med.,* **35**, 67–89.
26. Fauci, A. S. and Wolff, S. M. (1973), Wegener's granulomatosis: studies in eighteen patients and a review of the literature. *Medicine,* **52**, 535–61.
27. McDonald, T. J., DeRemee, R. A., Kern, E. B. and Harrison, E. G. (1974), Nasal manifestations of Wegener's granulomatosis. *Laryngoscope,* **84**, 2101–12.
28. Friedmann, I. (1964), Midline granuloma. *Proc. R. Soc. Med.,* **57**, 289–97.

CHAPTER SIXTEEN

Systemic Disease and Complications

P. D. B. Davies

A chest radiograph is a uniquely simple and informative investigation of a vital internal organ, the lung (together with the heart and in part the skeleton). While there can be no substitute for taking a full history and making a full examination of a patient, the chest radiograph rightly forms the starting point of virtually all investigation of pulmonary disease.

A clinician may approach the association of a respiratory disorder with a systemic disorder in one of three ways.

First, the clinician confronted with a particular systemic disorder may look to the respiratory system for the explanation; a very simple example might be clubbing of the fingers; more complex examples might be a neurologist's demonstration of polyneuropathy or an endocrinologist's recognition of inappropriate ADH secretion or the ectopic production of ACTH, in each case prompting the search for a lung tumour.

Second, the chest physician may invoke systemic disease as the basis of respiratory symptoms or signs; for example, the dyspnoea of anaemia or obesity and the cyanosis of cirrhosis of the liver; a history of severe recurrent chest infections might lead to investigation of the possibility of cystic fibrosis or hypogammaglobulinaemia. In general organic disease will be sought and found, but in some cases there may be a psychological explanation, for example in the hyperventilation syndrome or a persistent habit cough.

Third, the recognition of well established patterns of disease may prompt a dual search for respiratory and systemic lesions; this situation arises frequently in the connective tissue and other multisystem diseases. For example a chest radiograph is an essential part of the full investigation of a patient with polyarthritis or uveitis and the diagnosis of tuberculosis in any viscus should lead to a search for tuberculous disease in other viscera and most especially the lungs.

16.1 The systemic manifestations of respiratory disease

The discovery of metastases particularly those in the brain, bones, liver or skin will inevitably suggest the possibility of a primary site in the lung. Indeed a chest radiograph is a routine part of the investigation of all space-occupying lesions within the skull. In addition, carcinoma of the lung may be associated with a whole range of non-metastatic systemic syndromes which may on occasion present before the pulmonary lesions is detectable by chest radiograph, bronchoscopy or sputum cytology. In this situation the computerized tomographic (CT) scan and the fibreoptic bronchoscope have added new dimensions to the refinement of investigation.

In the same way the diagnosis of tuberculous disease of any viscus should always prompt the taking of a chest radiograph because of the likelihood of associated pulmonary lesions.

The systemic syndromes associated with carcinoma of the bronchus, tuberculosis and some other pulmonary diseases fall broadly into six groups.

16.1.1 Dermatological abnormalities

Acanthosis nigricans and dermatomyositis are the best known skin lesions which in adults suggest the need to search for an internal malignancy including lung cancer; much more rarely seen are pachydermoperiostitis and hypertrichosis lanugosa.

In addition to these non-metastatic dermatological manifestations of lung cancer, skin secondaries may be the presenting feature of the disease.

Pulmonary tuberculosis may be sought and found following the appearance of erythema nodosum or phlyctenular conjunctivitis at the time of development of tuberculin hypersensitivity four to six weeks after primary tuberculous infection. Tuberculous lesions of the skin such as ulceration at the mouth or anus, lupus vulgaris and papulo-necrotic tuberculides may all be associated with pulmonary disease.

16.1.2 Subcutaneous tissue and bony abnormalities

Clubbing is far and away the commonest non-metastatic disorder associated with carcinoma of the bronchus. It may be combined with hypertrophic osteoarthropathy, though curiously not in oat cell growths; this is manifested by soft tissue swelling, in some cases resembling acromegaly, pain and stiffness of joints even in severe cases affecting the spine and the deposition of subperiosteal new bone especially in the long bones, usually most marked close to the major joints. Benign lesions including fibroma of the pleura, suppurative lung disease and widespread pulmonary fibrosis may also be responsible for these disorders.

Tuberculous osteomyelitis may complicate pulmonary tuberculosis and, rarely, so may subcutaneous abscesses either appearing apparently spontaneously or at the site of injection of a drug. An ischiorectal abscess is always an indication for taking a chest radiograph.

16.1.3 Haematological abnormalities

Carcinoma of the lung like other malignant chronic and inflammatory diseases may be associated with a characteristic normocytic and normochromic anaemia in which both serum iron and iron-binding capacity are reduced; the bone marrow shows adequate iron stores, but reduced incorporation of iron into developing erythroblasts. Lung cancer, unlike carcinoma of the large bowel for instance, is not a common cause of the iron-deficiency anaemia of chronic blood loss. Bony metastases may be responsible for anaemia with or without a leucoerythroblastic picture. Some surveys have shown involvement of the marrow in up to 50% of cases of oat cell cancer at the time of presentation. Lung cancer may also be responsible for other abnormalities of circulating granulocytes. There may be an otherwise unexplained leucocytosis or even a leukaemoid reaction. On rare occasions carcinoma and leukaemia, particularly chronic lymphocytic leukaemia, coexist. Adenocarcinoma of the lung, like adenocarcinomas elsewhere, may be responsible for disseminated intravascular coagulation with or without the syndromes of thrombophlebitis migrans, microangiopathic haemolytic anaemia and non-bacterial endocarditis. Multiple venous thrombosis may lead to venous gangrene and endocarditis be the source of large systemic emboli.

Pulmonary tuberculosis may also be responsible for a variety of haematological disorders. Iron- or folate-deficiency anaemias as well as the anaemia of chronic disease are common at the time of diagnosis, the severity of the anaemia correlating roughly with the severity of the pulmonary disease; sideroblastic anaemia may develop during the course of treatment with isoniazid. Haematogenous spread of tuberculosis may cause pancytopenia, leucoerythroblastic anaemia, leukaemoid reactions or myelofibrosis. Search of a marrow aspirate for acid fast bacilli can be a critical investigation leading to the diagnosis of curable condition.

The intrapulmonary haemorrhages of idiopathic pulmonary haemosiderosis and Goodpasture's syndrome can be responsible for profound anaemia.

16.1.4 Neurological abnormalities

A whole range of non-metastatic neurological syndromes may precede or accompany the radiological appearance of carcinoma of the bronchus. The nervous system may be involved at any level from the cerebral cortex to limb muscles. Full neurological investigation may be required both to diffferentiate these conditions from other organic neurological disorders and from the effects of secondary spread. Investigation is important because treatment of the lung tumour may prevent deterioration or more rarely achieve actual improvement in the condition. There are five main types of syndrome.

1. Encephalomyelitis is characterized by inflammatory changes and neuronal destruction in the cerebral cortex especially the temporal lobes, brainstem, spinal cord and posterior root ganglia. These lesions may be responsible for a variety of syndromes including dementia and a disorder resembling motor neurone disease.

2. Cerebellar degeneration accompanies loss of Purkinje and ganglion cells in the cerebellar cortex; loss of function is usually bilateral and progressive.

3. Peripheral neuropathy is most often subacute in onset and sensorimotor in type, but either motor or sensory signs can predominate.

4. A myasthenic syndrome is most commonly diagnosed as the result of prolonged apnoea and paralysis following the use of a depolarizing muscle relaxant in general anaesthesia for rigid bronchoscopy.

5. Proximal muscle weakness and wasting is perhaps the commonest syndrome, the lesion is probably neural rather than truly myopathic. In these syndromes the cerebrospinal fluid may show an increased protein content and a raised lymphocyte count.

Metastases from lung cancer account for the majority of brain and spinal tumours; the lesions are frequently multiple. Secondaries in skull or vertebrae may involve the meninges and be responsible for cranial nerve lesions or spinal compression with a rapid clinical course consisting of back pain, progressive paralysis, sensory loss and sphincter disturbance.

Pulmonary tuberculosis may be the origin of tuberculous infection of the central nervous system. This may take the form of a tuberculoma having all the features of a tumour, meningitis or spinal compression due to tuberculous osteomyelitis in a vertebra.

Suppurative lung disease may be complicated by cerebral abscess, meningitis and osteomyelitis with spinal compression. Pneumonia can present as meningism in children and a toxic confusional state in old people.

16.1.5 Endocrine and metabolic abnormalities

Many of the non-metastatic consequences of lung cancer are the result of the tumour's elaboration of polypeptide hormones and other biologically active substances. These syndromes may be recognizable clinically, more often by the biochemical changes induced and most certainly by the identification and assay of the active compounds both in the blood and tumour substance. These measurements have proved of the greatest value in initial diagnosis, in tumour localization, in following the response to treatment and in the early detection of tumour recurrence.

(a) *Adrenocorticotrophic hormone (ACTH)*

This is generally associated with the presence of an oat cell lung carcinoma, much more rarely with a bronchial carcinoid or thymic tumour. The classical features of Cushing's syndrome are usually absent but may have time to develop if the tumour is exceptionally slow growing. The commonest finding is a profound hypokalaemic alkalosis. Plasma ACTH and cortisol levels are raised and circadian rhythm is lost.

(b) *Parathormone*

Surprisingly this hormone is synthesized by squamous carcinomas of the bronchus; in addition, they may manufacture prostaglandins which are also capable of producing the syndrome of non-metastatic hypercalcaemia. The symptoms are usually of acute onset and disturbances of cerebral function often predominate. The serum calcium is raised but can be lowered by corticosteroids (in contrast to primary hyperparathyroidism): 120 mg of hydrocortisone a day for 10 days should be given. Serum parathormone levels will be elevated in about 50% of cases.

(c) *Antidiuretic hormone (ADH)*

This syndrome of inappropriate antidiuresis is a common feature of oat cell carcinoma but may also be associated with non-malignant lung conditions particularly tuberculosis and suppurative infections. The diagnosis may be a biochemical one based on routine electrolyte determinations followed by measurements of osmolality in blood and urine together with urinary sodium. If serum sodium levels are exceptionally low there may be clinical features including profound disturbances of cerebral function.

(d) *Calcitonin, prolactin, gonadotropin*

High circulating levels of calcitonin are extremely common in both oat cell and squamous carcinoma of the bronchus but cause no obvious clinical or biochemical disturbance.

There are a few reports of galactorrhoea associated with the ectopic secretion of prolactin by lung tumours.

Gynaecomastia, sometimes associated with hypertrophic osteoarthropathy may be a consequence of elevated serum levels of gonadotrophin in patients with carcinoma of the bronchus. These effects can be reversed by the use of an oestrogen receptor blocker.

(e) The carcinoid syndrome

Most of the primary tumours responsible for this condition arise in the ileocaecal region but a small proportion arise in the lung (bronchial adenoma) and these may exhibit atypical clinical and biochemical features. These tumours release a variety of pharmacological active substances such as 5-hydroxytryptamine (5-HT), histamine, prostaglandins and kallikrein. The clinical diagnosis can be confirmed by the measurement of urinary excretion of 5-hydroxyindolacetic acid (5-HIAA) the major metabolite of 5-HT.

(f) Hypoglycaemia

Massive intrathoracic fibromatous and neurogenic tumours in children have presented with hypoglycaemia. There is, however, no evidence that they secrete insulin.

It is possible that lung tumours may secrete substances which may stimulate hormone release from normal endocrine tissues. There are reports of the association of lung cancer and thyrotoxicosis.

(g) Renal abnormalities

There are reports of glomerulonephritis and the nephrotic syndrome in the presence of lung cancer. The association is little understood but the assumption has been made that its basis is immunological perhaps involving the deposition of tumour antigen/antibody complexes. Sometimes it may present with Henoch-Schonlein disease.

Chronic suppurative or mycobacterial chest disease is now a comparative rarity in Britain, but may provide the explanation for the finding of proteinuria and renal failure due to amyloid disease.

The nephrotic syndrome has also been reported with pollen asthma and acute silicosis.

16.2 Functional disorders of ventilation with systemic features

Headache, somnolence, sleep disturbance, polycythaemia, venous thrombosis and embolism or cardiac failure may all occur in certain patients with alveolar hypoventilation without evidence of pulmonary disease. A proportion of the population have impaired central responses to hypercapnia and hypoxia; these people may develop sleep apnoea especially if they also have upper airway obstruction or they may develop respiratory and cardiac failure if they become obese (Pickwick syndrome).

Overventilation, which is usually psychologically determined, produces hypocapnia; this may lead not only to classical tetany but also to a whole range of systemic symptoms for which no organic cause can be found.

16.3 Respiratory disorders as a manifestation of systemic disease

Breathlessness is a symptom which may require the most detailed investigation to identify the responsible factors. As always in respiratory disorders, heart disease is an important differential diagnosis, but less obvious factors such as thyrotoxicosis or anaemia may have to be excluded. If the disturbance of ventilation is airways obstruction then it is likely that its basis is pulmonary though obstruction of the major upper airways can easily be confused; carcinoma of the trachea, vocal cord paralysis, massive enlargement of the tonsils in young children for example may all pose difficult problems of differential diagnosis.

Clinically, the detection of stridor can be vital and the characteristic changes seen in flow/volume curves can afford valuable confirmation.

A restrictive pattern of ventilatory impairment demands consideration of an extensive list of conditions. The basis of disturbance of function may be as remote as the central nervous system as in poliomyelitis, the peripheral nerves as in the Guillain-Barré syndrome, at the neuromuscular junction as in myasthenia gravis, the respiratory muscles as in polymyositis, or the chest wall in kyphoscoliosis or ankylosing spondylitis. The dyspnoea which may accompany scleroderma is seldom the result of involvement of the skin of the trunk; more usually it is a sign of pulmonary involvement by fibrosing alveolitis.

Pulmonary embolism is an important cause of dyspnoea. Major emboli may produce paroxsymal dyspnoea which may be accompanied by wheeze or complicated by pulmonary oedema (cardiac failure or myocardial infarction may be confusing features). Repeated minor emboli may be responsible for sustained dyspnoea when pulmonary hypertension develops. Ventilation/perfusion isotope lung scans and pulmonary angiography may be needed to establish the diagnosis especially in the absence of pulmonary infarction.

16.4 Drug-induced respiratory disease

Drugs may be responsible for disease throughout the respiratory tract. For example pituitary snuff may provoke rhinitis, asthma or alveolitis. The basis of their action may be toxic, idiosyncratic or allergic. The drugs may have been taken by ingestion, inhalation or injection.

16.4.1 Upper respiratory tract

Marihuana may cause sinusitis or a curious oedema of the uvula (interestingly there are also reports that it may relieve bronchospasm).

16.4.2 Bronchial tree

Asthma may be the result of direct irritation by inhaled drugs, this sometimes occurs with cromoglycate and is the reason for the formulation of Intal-Co which contains a small dose of isoprenaline to counteract the irritative effect suffered by a small number of asthmatics. Pharmacological activity of drugs may also be responsible for asthmatic reactions: the best example is perhaps the use of β-adrenergic blocking drugs such as propranolol. Drug induced asthma may have an allergic basis and be mediated by IgE, IgG or possibly IgD ('aspirin asthma' produced by prostaglandin antagonists); it may occur in isolation or as part of a generalized systemic reaction such as anaphylaxis or serum sickness.

16.4.3 Lungs

Drugs may cause pulmonary eosinophilia; nitrofurantoin is the commonest drug to do so (see Table 16.1). Another important adverse pulmonary reaction to drugs is fibrosis most often seen in cytotoxic therapy such as the use of busulphan (radiotherapy may do the same). There is a spectrum of

Table 16.1   Drugs reported to cause pulmonary eosinophilia

Aspirin
Furazolidone
Imipramine
Isoniazid
Mephenesin
Methotrexate†
Nitrofurantoin*†
Penicillin
Streptomycin
Sulphasalazine†
Sulphonamides

* Much the commonest.
† Also reported to cause pulmonary fibrosis.

histological change from fibrinous oedema leading to intra-alveolar fibrosis to an alveolitis leading to interstitial fibrosis (see Table 16.2). Perhaps the commonest and certainly the most serious drug-induced pulmonary disease is the progressive hyperplastic change produced by oxygen; this has always to be borne in mind when high concentrations of oxygen have to be administered for extended periods. Drugs may initiate systemic lupus erythematosus and polyarteritis and so set in train pulmonary disease (see Table 16.3). Oil-based compounds especially the contrast media used for bronchography may set up lipoid pneumonia. Pulmonary oedema may be a consequence of overdosage with heroin, methadone and other opiates, barbiturates and phenothiazines and curiously may lead to permanent bronchiectasis.

Table 16.2 Drugs reported to cause pulmonary fibrosis

Cytotoxic drugs
Nitrofurantoin
Sulphasalazine
Ganglion blockers
Beta blockers
Practolol
Pindolol
Methysergide

Table 16.3 Some groups of drugs reported to cause SLE

Antiarrhythmic drugs
Antibiotics
Anticonvulsants
Antihypertensives
Anti-inflammatory analgesics
Antituberculous drugs
β-adrenergic receptor blockers
Sulphonamides

16.4.4 Pleura

Pleural disease may also be attributable to drugs; effusions are a common manifestation of drug-induced lupus; more localized pleural reactions may result from the use of some β-blockers and methysergide which may also cause pulmonary or very rarely mediastinal fibrosis.

16.4.5 Mediastinum

Mediastinal lymph node enlargement may be part of generalized lymphadenopathy induced by phenylbutazone (a sarcoid-like reaction) or phenytoin (pseudolymphoma).

Chronic bronchitis, emphysema and carcinoma of the bronchus are of course related to abuse of the drug tobacco.

The identification of a drug as the cause of respiratory disease may demand careful history taking with a high index of suspicion and a general idea of the variety of drug-induced disease; sometimes the possibility is suggested by an associated finding either clinical such as a rash or from the laboratory perhaps the report of eosinophilia; often observation of the effect of withdrawal of drugs or provocation challenge may be needed. Rarely immunological investigation may prove the diagnosis; demonstration of antibody, histamine release from sensitized tissues, lymphocyte transformation or the inhibition of migration of white cells have all be used.

16.5 Pulmonary eosinophilia

Aspergillosis is the commonest cause of pulmonary eosinophilia in Britain, but systemic factors should be sought and may be identified. Loeffler's syndrome is a manifestation of larval migration, its diagnosis demands a search for parasites especially intestinal worms. Tropical eosinophilia can be confirmed by microfilarial complement fixation. Parasitization is accompanied by a high blood eosinophil count and high levels of IgE. Polyarteritis may present with asthma, transient lung shadows and moderate eosinophilia; there will be no rise of circulating IgE. Drugs have again to be considered as a possible cause.

16.6 Some systemic causes of pleural disease

Pleural transudates are a common manifestation of cardiac failure and hypoalbuminaemia due to liver and kidney disease. Occasionally other rare systemic factors may be responsible such as Meig's syndrome which consists of ovarian fibroma, ascites and pleural effusion, lymphatic deficiency with lymphoedema and yellow nails or acute inflammatory processes such as subphrenic abscess, amoebic liver abscess (diagnosed by identification of the organism and positive complement fixation test) and acute pancreatitis (the fluid will have a high amylase content).

16.7 Systemic disease associated with acute, recurrent or chronic chest infection

Severe or persistent chest infection will often suggest the need for detailed systemic investigation particularly in children. This may be reinforced by other findings either clinical, e.g. lymphadenopathy, or pathological, e.g. the report of anaemia or a markedly raised erythrocyte sedimentation rate. Increasingly frequently chest infections may develop in a host known to be compromised by a serious underlying disorder and its treatment such as haematological malignancy or transplantation. There may be dramatic deterioration in the clinical condition but with only vague respiratory symptoms and signs without a fever and only abnormal shadowing in the chest radiograph. Chest infection has then to be identified and treated as a matter of urgency and may be caused by a wide variety of opportunistic infecting agents; at the same time a number of important differential diagnoses have to be excluded such as spread of the original disease, haemorrhage, infarction and adverse reactions to drugs or radiation.

At times chronic or recurrent chest infection can be explained by some simple local lesion such as bronchiectasis or an inhaled foreign body (not always detectable radiologically) and both bronchoscopy and bronchography may be needed for diagnosis as well as a careful search for a source of infection in the upper respiratory tract. At other times the responsible factor may be found outside the respiratory tract, e.g. in the case of dysphagia pneumonitis due to repeated inhalation from a pharyngeal pouch or a dilated or immobile oesophagus. Here the pulmonary lesions will characteristically be found bilaterally in the axillary subsegments of the anterior and posterior segments of the upper lobes and in the apical segments of the lower lobes, that is to say predominantly in the mid-zones of the lung fields in straight radiographs. Examination of the sputum may demonstrate fat globules and even the saprophytic acid fast bacillus, *Mycobacterium butyricus*, the butter bacillus, which may abet the mistaken diagnosis of tuberculosis. Specialized contrast studies including ciné pictures may be needed to demonstrate the responsible alimentary lesions radiologically.

16.8 Chest infections and male infertility

Curiously, two important inherited conditions which present problems of chest infection are associated with infertility in the male. These are cystic fibrosis and the immotile cilia syndromes (see Chapter 15).

16.8.1 Cystic fibrosis

This condition, inherited as an autosomal recessive trait, occurs in about

1:2000 live births. Severity of chest infection more than any other factor determines the prognosis. A clue to the diagnosis may come from the family history or from the occurrence of meconium illeus, heat exhaustion, steatorrhoea or cirrhosis of the liver. Additional features may be nasal polyposis and allergic disorders. Increasingly good medical care leads to survival into adult life, or in mild cases the diagnosis may first be made in this age group. Infertility in the male is the result of hypoplasia or absence of the vas deferens. Sinus, bronchial and pulmonary infection leading to the development of bronchiectasis, fibrosis and spontaneous pneumothoraces are linked with failure of mucus clearance; the responsible organisms are usually *Staphylococcus aureus, Haemophilus influenzae* and *Pseudomonas aeruginosa*; aspergillosis may be superimposed. The vital investigation is the demonstration of raised levels of sweat sodium and chloride. Sweat is collected by iontophoresis of 0.2% pilocarpine; it is essential to collect an adequate weight of sweat. In children diagnostic levels are chloride 60 and sodium 80 mEq/l; in adults the figures are higher. Other tests may be needed to assess damage to the pancreas and liver.

16.8.2 Immotile cilia syndrome

Kartagener's syndrome consists of dextrocardia, bronchiectasis and sinusitis. Male sufferers from this condition are infertile: their spermatozoa are immobile because the flagella are immotile, resulting from lack of dynein arms in the microtubules of the flagella. The cilia of the respiratory tract are similarly immotile and the result is failure of mucus clearance in the bronchial tree and sinuses and in turn suppurative infection (Fig. 16.1). The beating of cilia determines the normal rotation of viscera in the embryo; its absence means that dextro- or laevocardia is a matter of chance; siblings of these patients may therefore have the same dysfunction but without situs inversus. Other syndromes link male infertility with respiratory infection; in some there are abnormalities in the ultrastructure of the flagella and cilia, in others there is disturbance of function without detectable anatomical abnormality; some have additional azoospermia due to functional obstruction in the vas deferens (there are cilia in the segment joining the epididymis to the vas).

16.9 Chest infection in the compromised host

Host defences may be impaired by quantitative and qualitative changes in the neutrophil leucocytes, immunoglobulins and cell mediated immune reactions (see Chapter 12). To these abnormalities may be added other less specific factors such as inadequacies in opsonins, interferon and complement, the debilitating effects of, for example, anaemia, uraemia, diabetes or

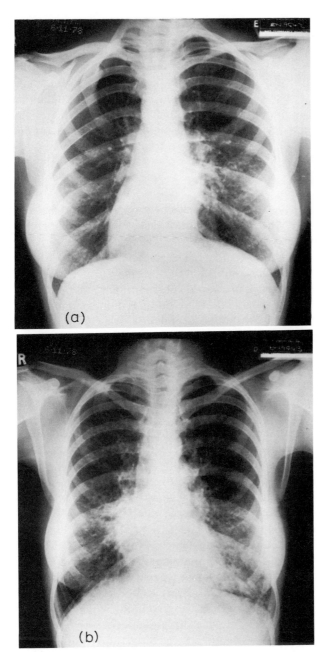

Fig. 16.1 Immotile cilia syndrome. Chest radiographs of two sisters age twenty-one and nineteen. Sister A (a) has severe upper respiratory symptoms with bilateral chronic otitis media and sinusitis. She has bronchiectasis in the left mid-zone and dextrocardia and situs inversus. This is the full Kartagener syndrome. Sister B (b) has relatively mild upper respiratory symptoms but severe bilateral bronchiectasis.

malnutrition and importantly the consequences of invasive procedures such as endoscopy, indwelling catheters, intravenous 'lines' and tracheostomy. In these respects the most important diseases are the leukaemias and lymphomas, the plasma cell dyscrasias and solid tumours; to their immunosuppressive effects may be added treatment with cytotoxic therapy, corticosteroids, antilymphocyte globulin and radiation. Immunosuppression is also employed for the purposes of organ transplantation.

16.9.1 Neutropenia and impairment of neutrophil function

If the absolute neutrophil count falls below $1 \times 10^9/l$ and especially if it falls below $0.1 \times 10^9/l$ the chances of infection become increasingly high. Most of the infections are caused by five organisms, *Pseudomonas, Klebsiella, E. coli, Staph. aureus* and *Candida*. The chief manifestations of such infections are stomatitis and septicaemia but the lung may be involved and indeed may be the origin of the generalized infection. The absence of granulocytes diminishes the clinical and radiological signs of inflammation, e.g. bacterial pneumonia may exist without consolidation. Diagnosis is difficult and treatment usually has to begin before the results of microbiological investigations are available. Any disease or drug which causes marrow suppression may be responsible but this devastating clinical problem is particularly a feature of the acute leukaemias.

The numbers of circulating granulocytes may be adequate and yet abnormalities of their function may contribute to susceptibility to infection. The functional disturbance may be impairment of neutrophil mobility; this is seen in some congenital conditions and in acquired disorders particularly metabolic failure and treatment with corticosteroids. Impaired ability to ingest organisms can have the same effect; an important example is patients with sickle cell disease rendered asplenic by infarction who are susceptible to pneumococcal and staphylococcal lung infections. A number of drugs may work in the same way.

Impaired intracellular killing of micro-organisms may also lead to susceptibility to infection. Chronic granulomatous disease is an X-linked disorder in boys (a less common autosomal recessive condition also exists in girls). The condition is due to the inability of the cells to generate hydrogen peroxide or superoxide which are responsible for the death of ingested bacteria; this is probably due to absence of the respiratory enzyme cytochrome b. The diagnostic test is the observation of the failure of the cells to decolonize the dye tetrasolium blue which is normally reduced during the respiratory activity which accompanies the killing of intracellular bacteria. The disease is characterized by recurrent infections especially by staphylococci and *E. coli*. Interestingly pneumococcal and streptococcal infections are seldom seen; these organisms produce hydrogen peroxide for themselves. The lungs become infiltrated with granulomas containing large histiocytes.

16.9.2 Defects in humoral immunity

Patients with deficiency of immunoglobulins may have recurrent bacterial infections especially pneumonia; usually common bacterial pathogens such as staphylococci and streptococci are responsible rather than opportunistic organisms. The deficiency of immunoglobulins may be primary or secondary. Primary hypogammaglobulinaemia is a sex-linked inherited condition; in these patients pneumonia is often caused by encapsulated organisms such as *H. influenzae* and *Ps. aeruginosa*; selective deficiency of IgA usually presents with recurrent respiratory infection. It is not uncommon for bronchiectasis to develop in these disorders. Measurement of immunoglobulins is an important routine investigation in chronic pyogenic respiratory disease. Secondary deficiency is common in the lymphomas especially in the lymphoproliferative disorders and the plasma cell dyscrasias such as myeloma. Many systemic disorders may lead to depression of immunoglobulins either by impairing synthesis as in renal failure, direct loss as in the nephrotic syndrome or by increasing catabolism as in thyrotoxicosis; immunosuppressive therapy has, of course, the same effect. In all there is an increased incidence of respiratory infection.

16.9.3 Impairment of cell mediated immunity

This abnormality may also be congenital or acquired. Congenital thymic hypoplasia (di George syndrome) is a pure form of the condition; the Wiskott-Aldrich syndrome, ataxia, telangiectasia and the chronic mucocutaneous syndromes combine this deficiency with that of immunoglobulins. Malignant disease may have this effect and it is particularly common in the malignant lymphomas, especially Hodgkin's disease. Acute viral infections such as measles may depress cell mediated immunity and so may cytotoxic drugs, corticosteroids, antilymphocyte globulin and radiation. The lungs may be invaded by a wide range of opportunistic organisms, often there are multiple infections with viruses, e.g. cytomegalovirus; fungi, e.g. *Nocardia* (strictly an actinomycete); nematodes, e.g. *Strongyloides* (hyperinfection syndrome); protozoa, e.g. *Pneumocystis carinii* (increasingly frequent and important because preventable and treatable) and mycobacteria (including atypical mycobacteria). This situation provides the chest physician with the most dramatic contemporary diagnostic dilemma. The physician is confronted with a very sick patient who has extensive shadowing in the chest radiograph; this may be due to the disease itself, to adverse reactions to drugs or to infection. In these circumstances lung biopsy becomes a matter of the greatest urgency for both histological and microbiological study.

16.10 Systemic and respiratory manifestations of multisystem disorders

16.10.1 Connective tissue disorders

The collagen/vascular diseases each present characteristic, though overlapping, patterns of both systemic and respiratory involvement. The respiratory component may involve specifically the airways, the alveoli, the vessels or the pleura. In addition there appears to be a non-specific susceptibility to respiratory infections.

In general the pattern of autoantibodies may usefully contribute to the precision of diagnosis in these overlapping syndromes; for instance, the exclusion from the diagnosis of systemic sclerosis of the relatively benign disorders mixed connective tissue disorder, eosinophilic fasciitis and CRST (calcinosis, Raynaud's, sclerodactyly and telangiectasia) which have superficial similarities to the much more serious disease (see Table 16.4). At the same time, though these disorders are categorized as idiopathic in many instances a careful search may reveal evidence of viral infection or drug taking as factors in the aetiology, e.g. influenza A infection or the use of penicillamine in Goodpasture's syndrome.

Table 16.4 The pattern of respiratory involvement in the collagen/vascular diseases

	Autoantibodies Clinical disorder	Lung pathology			
		Airways	Alveoli	Vessels	Pleura
Group I	Organ-specific autoantibodies				
	Goodpasture's syndrome	−	+	+	−
Group II	Organ-specific and non-organ-specific autoantibodies				
	(multiple) Sjögren's syndrome	+	+	−	−
Group III	Non-organ-specific autoantibodies				
	(multiple) SLE	−	+	+	+
	Rheumatoid arthritis	+	+	+	+
	Systemic sclerosis	−	+	+	−
	(fibrosing alveolitis)	−	+	−	−
Group IV	No autoantibodies				
	Polyarteritis	+	−	+	−
	Dermatomyositis, polymyositis	−	+	−	−

(a) Goodpasture's syndrome

The combination of a subacute glomerulonephritis with intrapulmonary haemorrhage causing haemoptysis and anaemia typically in a young adult male is virtually diagnostic. The chest radiograph may show abnormalities of three types; the first, at the time of bleeding into the lung, consists of transient opacities of any distribution according to the site and size of the bleed; the second, the result of many such haemorrhages, is a persistent fine dense stippling throughout the lung fields the result of the deposition of haemosiderin; and the third, comparatively rare, is seen in patients who undergo a prolonged phase of idiopathic pulmonary haemosiderosis before renal disease makes itself evident; these patients may show the appearances of widespread pulmonary fibrosis. The most sensitive index of intrapulmonary haemorrhage is the measurement of transfer coefficient which may be raised at a time when the chest radiograph shows no abnormality. The continued finding of iron-laden macrophages in the sputum is suggestive of the diagnosis which may be confirmed by the demonstration of circulating antiglomerular basement membrane autoantibody and its deposition in a diffuse linear fashion in that site in renal biopsy specimens.

(b) Sjögren's syndrome

About half the cases give a history of enlarged salivary and lacrimal glands; in about a third the glands are enlarged at the time of presentation. At this stage biopsy shows infiltration with plasma cells and lymphocytes not only of the glands but also along the length of the lamina propria of the respiratory tract. Later the picture is simply that of atrophy and this is associated with the finding of autoantibodies directed against salivary and bronchial mucous duct cells and the histological appearances of widespread pulmonary fibrosis. In many such cases other disorders are found which have organ-specific autoantibodies and the same histology; these include autoimmune thyroiditis, idiopathic hypothyroidism, pernicious anaemia, diabetes, Addison's disease and premature ovarian failure. Two-thirds of the patients also have a systemic connective tissue disorder mediated by non-organ specific autoantibodies; rheumatoid factor and antinuclear factor are found in the majority of cases. Just as these patients have dry eyes and a dry mouth – the sicca syndrome – so they may have a dry respiratory tract and with it a high incidence of non-specific disorders such as infection and atelectasis. Interestingly two-thirds of the patients are allergic to penicillin.

(c) Systemic lupus erythematosus

In this disease there is a whole range of autoantibodies directed against various nuclear, cytoplasmic and membrane antigens, blood cells and clotting factors; most specific are antibodies to double strand native DNA which may be assayed by antigen binding. Some of these antibodies are undoubtedly tissue damaging and can be demonstrated as immune complexes with complement in the kidney and dermoepidermal junction (reduction of complement levels is a valuable guide to the activity of the disease). Lung involvement is common and often recurrent, especially pleurisy with bilateral small effusions often accompanied by pericarditis but also pulmonary vasculitis presenting a picture of infarction, pneumonia or oedema (Fig. 16.2). A 'shrinking lung' syndrome can also occur with progressive elevation of the diaphragm and reduction of lung volume; surprisingly this syndrome is not usually the result of widespread pulmonary fibrosis, though rarely that may be found, but of extensive multifocal atelectasis which may result from

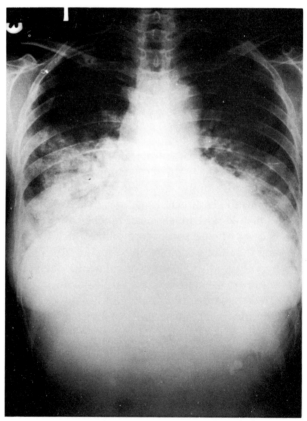

Fig. 16.2 Systemic lupus erythematosis. Woman aged 45 who presented with a clinical and radiological picture resembling pulmonary oedema.

diaphragmatic dysfunction. Drug-induced SLE is frequently seen; it represents at least 20% and perhaps up to 40% of all cases and has a particular predilection for the lung.

(d) Rheumatoid arthritis

The standard tests for rheumatoid factor detect an IgM immunoglobulin; in seronegative cases it may be possible to demonstrate an IgG antibody also reacting with the Fc portion of the IgG molecule. On the whole the titre of rheumatoid factor correlates well with the presence of pulmonary disease; routine lung function studies in patients with rheumatoid arthritis show a correlation between reduction of transfer factor and rise of titre of rheumatoid factor. There are exceptions: rheumatoid pulmonary or pleural lesions may precede the appearance of rheumatoid factor; in some cases rheumatoid factor is only demonstrable in the pleural fluid.

Effusions are the commonest manifestation of rheumatoid lung; usually there is pale green fluid with a characteristically low glucose content but sterile empyemata also occur containing much debris, pus cells and epithelioid cells. Fibrosing alveolitis is also seen and necrobiotic nodules with the typical palisading of histiocytes with (Caplan's syndrome) or without coexisting pneumoconiosis; the nodules are frequently multiple, appear in crops and often cavitate (Fig. 16.3). The airways may be involved in a progressive bronchiolitis with a poor prognosis. (It has been suggested but not confirmed that penicillamine and gold may play a part in the aetiology.)

Non-specific bronchial and pulmonary infections are unduly common in rheumatoid arthritis and may be a most serious complication of Felty's syndrome, that is to say, rheumatoid arthritis, splenomegaly and neutropenia.

(e) Systemic sclerosis

When a patient presents with Raynaud's phenomenon, scleroderma, radiological abnormalities of the oesophagus and perhaps evidence of disease elsewhere in the alimentary tract, kidneys and heart, it is reasonable to attribute concomitant fibrosing alveolitis or progressive pleural thickening to the same disease. More difficult to recognize are the comparatively rare cases presenting as pulmonary hypertension without lung fibrosis which suggest that the primary lesion of the disorder may be vascular.

In systemic sclerosis as with other connective tissue disorders, for example Sjögren's syndrome, there is an increased incidence of malignant disease including alveolar cell carcinoma which may also complicate other widespread pulmonary fibroses.

Dysphagia pneumonitis in patients with oesophageal involvement may be a troublesome feature.

(f) Fibrosing alveolitis

Fibrosing alveolitis is not itself, of course, a multisystem disorder but it is closely associated with connective tissue multisystem disorders, Sjögren's syndrome, rheumatoid arthritis, systemic sclerosis and more rarely systemic lupus erythematosus, polyarteritis and dermatomyositis and polymyositis. In addition there is an associated with coeliac disease, ulcerative colitis, renal tubular acidosis and chronic active hepatitis.

There is evidence that it is an immune complex disease; there is a high yield of autoantibodies even in the cases without a related multisystem disease; ANF is found in about a third of cases, and in about a tenth rheumatoid factor is found and in a similar proportion smooth muscle and mitochondrial antibodies are present.

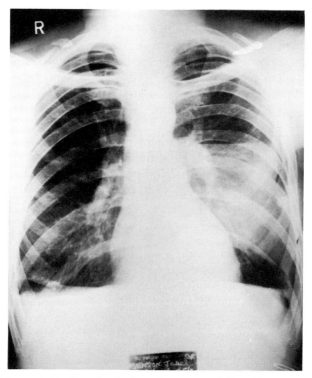

Fig. 16.3 Rheumatoid pleural effusion. A man aged 57 with severe rheumatoid arthritis who presented with a spontaneous pyopneumothorax. The original film shows a nodule in the left mid-zone the lung biopsy revealed fibrosing alveolitis.

In general the diagnosis can be made on simple clinical, radiological and physiological grounds based on a history of progressive breathlessness, the finding of clubbing and gravity-dependent crepitations, the appearance in the chest radiograph of widespread nodular shadowing with small ring shadows in the chronic cases, usually but not invariably appearing first and most predominantly in the lower zones, and the demonstration of a restrictive impairment of ventilation with reduction of transfer factor. If lung biopsy is thought to be necessary, e.g. in the exclusion of an industrial lung disease such as asbestosis, probably open lung biopsy is desirable for adequate pathological assessment. Drug-induced alveolitis, e.g. related to cytotoxic therapy, is an important differential diagnosis.

(g) *Polyarteritis*

Polyarteritis nodosa is the exemplar of a group of conditions to which the general term polyarteritis may be applied; they are characterized by necrotizing vasculitis. Polyarteritis nodosa itself comparatively rarely affects the lung; when it does it involves medium-sized arteries and produces pulmonary infarction. Some variants of polyarteritis more often affect the lung and may involve the respiratory system for weeks, months or even years before there appears evidence of systemic disease. Two examples of polyarteritis which may exhibit such a 'presystemic' phase are Wegener's granulomatosis and the Rose and Spencer type of polyarteritis.

Wegener's granulomatosis involves smaller vessels than classical polyarteritis nodosa involving both arteries and veins, and forms destructive granulomatous lesions. The disease usually begins in the upper respiratory tract with ulcerative lesions of the nasal septum, sinuses or middle ear; the major airways may be involved and the chest radiograph may show intrapulmonary masses, frequently multiple, often cavitated (Fig. 16.4). The combination of upper and lower respiratory lesions may suggest the disease but biopsy is required for definitive diagnosis (see Chapter 15).

The Rose and Spencer variant of polyarteritis sometimes called allergic granulomatous angiitis is also a disorder of small vessels and is characterized histologically by granulomas containing numerous eosinophils. Clinically the typical features are asthma, transient lung shadows and a raised blood eosinophil count. A useful investigation which may help to differentiate this condition from other causes of pulmonary eosinophila is the measurement of blood IgE levels which are high in disorders in which there is hypersensitivity to an extrinsic agent such as *Aspergillus fumigatus* or tropical worms. However some cases of allergic or hypersensitivity angiitis are induced by drugs. There is an association between polyarteritis nodosa and the presence of Australia antigen (hepatitis B surface antigen, HBsAG) in about a third of cases; complexes of the antigen, immunoglobulin and complement have been demonstrated in polyarteritic lesions.

(h) Dermatomyositis and polymyositis

The main features of these conditions are in the muscles and the skin. Proximal muscle weakness is the commonest presenting symptom; pharyngeal, laryngeal and respiratory muscles may be involved and cause dysphagia, dysphonia and respiratory difficulty. About half the cases show skin lesions typically consisting of a curious heliotrope rash associated with oedema most easily seen on the face and hands. The diagnosis is confirmed by muscle biopsy, electromyography and estimation of muscle enzymes in the blood, creatine phosphokinase (CPK), transaminases (SGOT, SGPT)

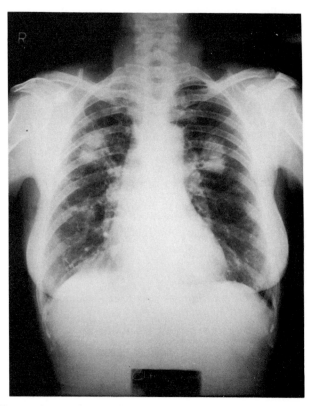

Fig. 16.4 Wegener's granulomatosis. A woman of 67 who presented with haemoptysis and unilateral middle ear deafness of sudden onset. The chest radiograph shows bilateral macronodular opacities. She later developed episcleritis, mononeuritis and finally kidney disease.

and aldolase.

Apart from respiratory difficulty due to muscle weakness there may be aspiration pneumonias due to pseudobulbar palsy. More specifically a small proportion of cases develop fibrosing alveolitis or a condition resembling it clinically, radiologically and physiologically, but with the histological appearances of an organising pneumonia (Fig. 16.5). In adults dermatomyositis and polymyositis may herald the discovery of visceral malignant disease including lung cancer.

(i) Seronegative arthritides

These forms of arthritis are certainly multisystem disorders; they include

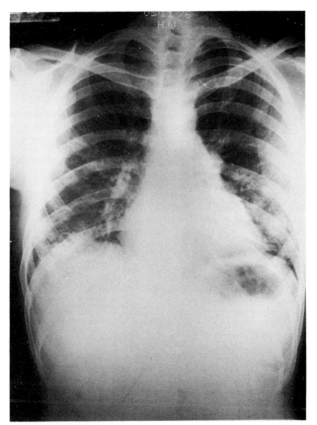

Fig. 16.5 Polymyositis and fibrosing alveolitis. A man aged 24, while on large doses of prednisolone as treatment for severe polymyositis with cutaneous vasculitis, developed the clinical, radiological and physiological picture of fibrosing alveolitis (confirmed by biopsy). This responded to treatment with cyclophosphamide.

ankylosing spondylitis, Reiter's syndrome, psoriatic arthritis, Behçet's syndrome and Still's disease; they are frequently associated with non-specific bronchial and pulmonary infections. Ankylosing spondylitis may be responsible for a progressive reduction in vital capacity due to increasing immobility of costovertebral and transverse joints but it is remarkable how little most patients are disabled in this respect and how rare is respiratory failure; the diaphragm can compensate considerably for the absence of chest expansion. Another pulmonary feature of the disease is progressive upper zone fibrosis with ring shadows easily mistaken for tuberculosis and frequently complicated by the development of aspergilloma. Ankylosing spondylitis both in its idiopathic form and when associated with either the other seronegative arthritides or inflammatory bowel disease is highly significantly correlated with the finding of HLA antigen B27.

(j) Inherited disorders of connective tissue

These include disorders of fibrous elements both primary and secondary to metabolic defects and the mucopolysaccharidoses. Most of them are rare, some extremely so, but Marfan's syndrome among them is not uncommon. The pulmonary manifestations include bullous emphysema, with recurrent spontaneous pneumothorax, anatomical abnormalities of the major airways or pulmonary arteries and effects resulting from deformities of the skeleton, e.g. kyphoscoliosis; and diaphragm, e.g. hernia or eventration. From the respiratory point of view there is much interest in the relationship between Marfan's syndrome and the extremely common syndrome of spontaneous pneumothorax in tall, thin, otherwise fit, young men who may certainly share the Marfan habitus.

(k) The phakomatoses

This group of conditions is characterized by the development of multiple hamartomas involving the nervous system, the skin and other viscera. Neurofibromatosis and tuberous sclerosis are the most common. In all of them widespread pulmonary fibrosis leading to a picture of honeycomb lung may be seen. A variant of tuberous sclerosis occurring in women may first appear in adult life, be confined to the lung and be rapidly progressive.

In neurofibromatosis intrathoracic neurogenic tumours may develop. Typically they arise on the intercostal nerves posteriorly but may involve the vagus nerves; more rarely they occur within the mediastinum or the lung itself. These tumours may be multiple, become malignant, grow through the intervertebral foramen producing 'dumbell' tumours compressing the spinal cord; those growing more laterally may be responsible for rib notching.

(*l*) Lipid storage diseases

The lungs may be involved in both Gaucher's disease and Neimann-Pick disease. Recurrent pulmonary infections may be a feature but most often the pulmonary lesions are asymptomatic, widespread mottling being discovered by routine radiograph.

(*m*) Whipple's disease; Crohn's disease

Both these diseases which are characterized by involvement of the alimentary tract may present respiratory features. Whipple's disease may include pneumonia and pleurisy. The diagnosis is made by the finding of PAS-positive granulomas in macrophages. Crohn's disease has been known to involve the larynx and upper airways. The histological picture is one of non-caseating epithelioid granulomata with giant cells. Inflammatory bowel disease (Crohn's) and ulcerative colitis may be associated with the development of fibrosing alveolitis and widespread bronchiectasis.

(*n*) Hereditary haemorrhagic telangectasia

The presence of the characteristic superficial lesions and a family history make easy the diagnosis of the associated pulmonary arteriovenous fistulae which are often multiple (Fig. 16.6). They may cause recurrent haemoptyses, which may be severe, or high output cardiac failure.

(*o*) Histiocytosis X

Arbitrarily on the basis of a common feature, the presence of numerous histiocytes, three disorders are grouped together under this title. They are Letterer-Siwe disease, Hand-Schuller-Christian disease and eosinophilic granuloma. Most often the lungs are involved as a solitary manifestation of the disease in adults, particularly men (Fig. 16.7), but rarely the pulmonary disorder may be accompanied by granulomatous lesions as with Hand-Schuller-Christian disease, e.g. when posterior pituitary lesions may produce diabetes insipidus. Another example is the osteolytic lesions of classical eosinophilic granuloma of bone usually seen in children.

The acute diffuse pulmonary lesions are often accompanied by relatively minor systemic symptoms, fever, malaise and loss of weight rather than specific respiratory symptoms but in the chronic stage respiratory insufficiency and recurrent spontaneous pneumothorax may predominate. At the time of presentation the chest radiograph shows indistinct nodular shadowing involving particularly the middle of the lung fields in the mid and upper zones being bilateral and roughly symmetrical and then followed by indistinct irregular small ring shadows. About a third of cases clear spontaneously within a few months, about a third slowly develop widespread pulmonary fibrosis with dilated bronchioles forming the non-specific feature of honeycomb lung with recurrent spontaneous pneumothorax and respiratory failure, and in a third the acute disease leads on to progressive bullous emphysema usually most marked in the upper zones. Biopsy is the only available diagnostic investigation, there being no specific biochemical or immunological features.

(p) Sarcoidosis

Sarcoidosis is by definition a multisystem disorder. The diagnosis depends upon the finding of compatible features together with the demonstration of

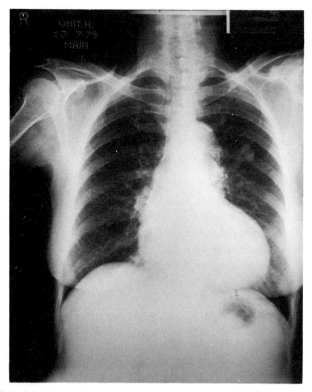

Fig. 16.6 Pulmonary arteriovenous fistula. A woman of 71 with hereditary haemorrhagic telangectasia (lesions on lips, tongue and nasal mucous membrane). She had a long history of epistaxes and a strong family history of the disease.

non-caseating epithelioid cell granulomata by biopsy of either a spontaneous lesion or a Kveim reaction.

It is comparatively rare for a patient to present with respiratory symptoms such as breathlessness or wheeze; most frequently the pulmonary disease is asymptomatic at the time of diagnosis being discovered either by a truly routine radiograph or one taken specifically in a patient with for example erythema nodosum. The radiological features comprise either enlargement of hilar and mediastinal lymph node, usually but not invariably bilateral, or pulmonary abnormalities again most commonly bilateral and roughly symmetrical, or a combination of the two.

Histological confirmation of the nature of the pulmonary lesions may demand bronchoscopy, percutaneous or open lung biopsy, mediastinoscopy or mediastinotomy as well as less direct methods such as liver or scalene node biopsy and histological examination of specimens obtained from

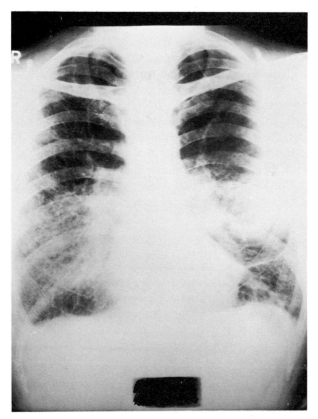

Fig. 16.7 Histiocytosis X. A man of 43 with histologically proved eosinophilia granuloma of the lung. He developed progressive bullous emphysema.

obvious systemic lesions or reactions at the site of the Kveim test; confirmation can be obtained in about three-quarters of the cases. Useful supportive tests include tuberculin testing which is found to be negative in about two-thirds of patients, reflecting depression of delayed-type hypersensitivity; measurement of serum angiotensin-converting enzyme which is raised in active sarcoidosis; demonstration of hypercalcaemia or hypercalciuria and measurement of serum immunoglobulin levels which are found to be raised in the majority of patients. Detailed lung function testing including measurement of transfer factor may help to decide the need for treatment and assess the response.

(q) Amyloid disease

The lungs are seldom involved in secondary amyloid disease though pleural effusions may accompany the hypoalbuminaemia of renal or more rarely hepatic or alimentary failure. The lungs may be involved in primary amyloid disease and indeed the disease may be confined to the respiratory tract; there may be solitary or multiple masses in either the larynx, trachea or major bronchi or the lung parenchyma. A diffuse type of pulmonary disease does occur with involvement of intra-alveolar septa giving widespread nodular opacities. Pleural disease is an extreme rarity. Primary amyloid disease may also involve the heart and present all the pulmonary features of cardiac failure. Pleurisy may be the dominant complaint in Familial Mediterranean Fever in which the development of amyloid is a notable feature. Of course chronic suppurative or mycobacterial disease of the lung may be responsible for amyloidosis. In general rectal biopsy confirms the presence of amyloid in about 75% of cases but in disease localized to the respiratory tract bronchoscopy or lung biopsy may be necessary.

(r) Malignant disease

A chest radiograph is an essential part of the staging of systemic malignancy; involvement of the lungs is of course a very common complication and may be the presenting feature, the primary lesion being quite occult. Tomograms including conventional whole lung tomography and more especially computerized axial tomography may be extremely revealing not only of the condition of the lung itself but also of the pleura and mediastinum (see Chapter 6).

(s) The leukaemias

Histological evidence of leukaemic infiltration of the lungs is common particularly in the lymphocytic and chronic varieties, in which it is found in over 80% at postmortem, but radiological evidence of this is less common. Enlarged hilar and mediastinal lymph node enlargement may be seen, perhaps in 50% of cases of chronic lymphocytic leukaemia; less frequent are intrapulmonary abnormalities and pleural effusions. Opportunistic infection, intrapulmonary haemorrhage and drug-induced lung disease are difficult differential diagnosis and may make lung biopsy essential; this is most safely performed by fibreoptic bronchoscopy. Rarely there may be extensive lung involvement without radiograph change presenting as dyspnoea and confirmed by reduction of transfer factor (after due correction for anaemia).

(t) The lymphomas

The thorax is often involved at the time of presentation of lymphoma; rarely the disease may be confined to the lung at this stage and may be treated successfully by resection; more commonly pulmonary involvement is associated with hilar and mediastinal lymph node enlargement, the lesions being usually bilateral. During the course of the disease spread to the lung, pleura or mediastinum is almost inevitable. A whole variety of radiological appearances may be seen. They include solitary masses which may be cavitated, lobar consolidation and miliary mottling. After radiotherapy the lesions may calcify; a characteristic appearance is narrowing over a considerable length of a bronchus due to external compression; rarely the involvement of the bronchus is intraluminal. As with the leukaemias the differential diagnosis of lymphomatous pulmonary infiltration is formidable; it includes haemorrhage, infarction, infection, radiation damage and drug-induced reactions. Bronchial, mediastinal (mediastinoscopy, mediastinotomy), lung or pleural biopsy may all be required.

(u) Solid tumours

The precise diagnosis of secondary involvement of the lungs by malignant growth may be of the utmost importance (Fig. 16.8). The primary site of the tumour may not be readily apparent but both primary and secondary lesions may prove to be amenable to treatment; the growth may be hormone-dependent or sensitive, susceptible to chemotherapy or on rare occasions both the primary and secondary lesions may be resectable. Usually the nature of the disease is determined histologically or cytologically but may depend on the identification of tumour markers such as acid phosphatase, α-foetoprotein, carcinoembryonic antigen or chorionic gondatrophin. Carcinoma of the thyroid is unique in that its secondaries may be identified by their uptake of radioactive iodine.

Malignant pleural effusions may present most difficult diagnostic problems; in addition to repeated examination of the cytology of the fluid more than one needle biopsy of the pleura may be needed and even sometimes thoracotomy and open biopsy. In the lung the appearance of a rounded opacity is an indication for tomography both conventional and axial to decide whether the lesion is truly solitary and not one of a number not readily seen by simple radiography; sputum cytology will be done and biopsy either by fibreoptic bronchoscopy, needle aspiration or at open thoracotomy. Lymphangitis carcinomatosa or the comparatively rare miliary carcinomatosis again may be investigated by sputum cytology or the selected technique of biopsy. The uncommon pattern of pulmonary hypertension without radiologically visible metastases sometimes seen in chorioncarcinoma will be diagnosed by the finding of tumour markers and elevated hormone levels; in this way it may be distinguished from idiopathic pulmonary hypertension, thromboembolic disease, or a drug-induced disorder. Hilar and mediastinal lymphadenopathy may require mediastinoscopy or mediastinotomy to make a tissue diagnosis.

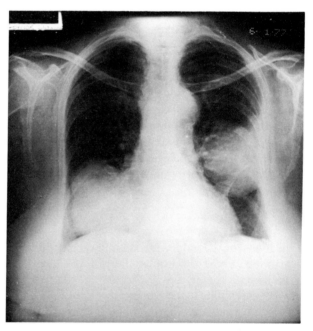

Fig. 16.8 'Cannon-ball' secondaries. A woman of 51 treated for carcinoma of the cervix by radiotherapy 12 years before.

16.11 Summary

In no other speciality do so many disciplines impinge as in the speciality of thoracic medicine. The lungs are peculiarly exposed to the environment; the surface area of the lungs in contact with the atmosphere is enormous (the surface area of the lungs is said to be roughly the size of a tennis court); the lungs are exposed to the environment more directly than the alimentary tract and even in a sense more intimately than the skin whose outer layers consist of dead cells which act as a protective cover absent from the respiratory epithelium.

In addition the lungs are unique in that they receive the entire cardiac output; what is more the first organ reached by material returned to the great veins in the neck by the lymphatics following ejection from the right heart is again the lung. It follows that the study of respiratory disease and the investigation of respiratory disorders may involve the whole of medicine. A textbook of thoracic medicine has in effect to be almost a textbook of medicine.

Further reading

Bayless, T. M., Knox, D. L. (1979), Editorial. Whipple's disease. A multisystem infection. *New Engl. J. Med.*, **300**, 920.

Davies, P. D. B. (1975), Drug-induced respiratory disease. *Medicine*, 2nd series, (22), 67.

Davies, P. D. B. (1971), The clinical presentation of tuberculosis. *Br. J. hosp. Med.*, 749.

Eliasson, R. *et al.* (1977), The immotile-cilia syndrome. A congenital ciliary abnormality as an etiologic factor in chronic airway infections and male sterility. *New Engl. J. Med.*, **297**, 1.

Hardwicke, J., Soothill, J. F., Squire J. R. and Holti, G. (1959), Nephrotic syndrome with pollen hypersensitivity. *Lancet*, **i**, 500.

Henson, R. A. (1972–74), Malignant disease and the nervous system. *Medicine*, 1st series, (32) 1890.

Hunninghake, G. W. and Fauci, A. (1979), Pulmonary involvement in the collagen vascular disease. *Am. Rev. resp. Dis.*, **119** (3), 471.

Jeffreys, D. B. Painful gynaecomastia treated with tamoxefen. *Br. med. J.* **1**, 1119.

Leading article (1978), Inhaled silica, the lung, and the kidney. *Lancet*, **ii**, 22.

Loughridge, L. and Lewis, M. G. (1971), Nephrotic syndrome in malignant disease of non-renal origin. *Lancet*, **i**, 256.

Lum, L. C. (1975), Hyperventilation. *J. psychosom. Res.*, **19**, 375.

Mitchell, D. M. and Hoffbrand, B. I. (1978), Relapse of Henoch-Schonlein disease associated with lung carcinoma. *J. R. Soc. Med.*

Rees, Lesley H. (1978), Endocrine manifestations of cancer. *Medicine*, 3rd series, (10), 485.

di Sant Agnese, P. A. and Davis, P. B. (1979), Cystic fibrosis in adults. *Am. J. Med.*, **66**, 121.

Turina, G. M. and Golding, R. M. (1978), Editorial. Sleeping and breathing. *New Engl. J. Med.*, **299**, 1009.

Turner-Warwick, M. (1974), Immunological aspects of systemic diseases of the lungs. *Proc. R. Soc. Med.*, **67**, 541.

Ward, P. H. and Goodman, M. L. (1978), Case records of the Massachusett's General Hospital. Hoarseness, dyspnoea and dysphagia in a young woman with Crohn's disease. *New Engl. J. Med.*, **299**, 538.

CHAPTER SEVENTEEN

Occupational Lung Disease

A. J. Newman Taylor and P. Sherwood Burge

The investigation of occupational lung disease is directed particularly towards the identification of a causal relationship between disease and occupational exposure. The confidence with which a disease in an individual can be attributed to a particular occupational exposure depends upon whether or not the relationship can be validated in the individual, the presence or absence of any features of the disease specific to the occupational cause, and the relative frequency of the disease in those with and those without the exposure. In diseases such as occupational asthma and extrinsic allergic alveolitis, the relationship between disease and exposure in the individual patient is potentially capable of validation by inhalation testing with the specific causal agent. Causal relationships between disease and occupational exposures are not generally susceptible to such direct testing. Disease can, however, be confidently attributed to an occupational exposure where the disease has some features of the occupational cause specific to it. The clinical features, functional abnormalities and appearances on the chest radiograph of asbestosis and cryptogenic fibrosing alveolitis are often indistinguishable. However, where pleural plaques can be seen on the chest radiograph in addition to the changes in the lung, asbestosis becomes the more probable diagnosis.

Often the relationship between exposure and disease cannot be validated in the individual, and the disease has no features specific to an occupational cause. The association between exposure and disease is based upon evidence from epidemiological investigations. Identification of the relationship between disease and exposure in an individual, has to be based on obtaining a history of sufficient exposure to a specific occupational agent known to be associated with an increased risk of the particular disease. Confidence in the association as cause and effect in the individual is related to the relative frequency with which the disease is found in those occupationally exposed and in those without the occupational exposure. Those occupationally exposed to asbestos have an increased risk of developing both lung cancer and pleural and peritoneal mesothelioma. Whereas lung cancer occurs frequently in the general population, mesotheliomas do not.

In the absence of other asbestos related diseases, such as asbestosis, a mesothelioma can be attributed to an exposure to asbestos with more confidence than can a lung cancer.

An accurate history of occupational exposure to a specific agent known to be associated with a particular disease is the basis upon which many occupational diseases are diagnosed. Not only the job name, but its description as well as the nature of the materials worked with and the circumstances in which exposure occurred should be obtained. The diagnosis of occupational lung disease often can only be based on a history of appropriate exposure to an occupational agent, where other possible causes of the disease have been excluded. For these reasons great emphasis in this chapter has been placed on the clinical (particularly radiographic features) of the different occupational lung diseases, the other important illnesses from which they have to be differentiated, and the nature of exposures which cause these diseases.

17.1 Pneumoconioses

Pneumoconiosis literally translated means 'dusty lungs'. It is defined for legal purposes in the National Insurance (Industrial Injuries) Act as 'fibrosis of the lungs due to silica dust, asbestos, or other dust, and includes the condition known as dust reticulation'. For medical purposes the pneumoconioses have been better described by Parkes [1] as 'the presence of inhaled dust in the lungs, and their non-neoplastic reaction to it'. It is usual to consider beryllium disease as a pneumoconiosis although it can follow exposure to beryllium fume as well as dust, and may cause systemic in addition to pulmonary disease.

17.1.1 Classification of the pneumoconioses

The pneumoconioses can be classified by cause into those due to inhalation of inorganic dusts and those due to organic dusts (Table 17.1). It is important to differentiate those dusts (such as asbestos and silica) which provoke a fibrotic reaction in the lung, from those (such as tin or iron) which are retained without provoking such a reaction. Those which do provoke an inflammatory or fibrotic reaction in the lung can conveniently be divided according to the pattern of the reaction.

17.1.2 Diagnosis of the pneumoconioses

The diagnosis of a pneumoconiosis often rests on the appearances of the chest radiograph in conjunction with an appropriate occupational history, although additional clinical features (such as finger clubbing and basal end inspiratory crackles in the lungs in asbestosis) and investigation findings (such as abnormalities of lung function in asbestosis, and serum precipitins to *M. faeni* in farmer's lung) can also be very valuable in making the diagnosis. It is very important to appreciate that there are no radiographic abnormalities specific for a pneumoconiosis, and that even if a suggestive occupational history is obtained, other non-occupational causes of the abnormalities observed must be considered before making the diagnosis of a pneumoconiosis.

Table 17.1 Classification of pneumoconiosis

	Effect on lungs	*Dusts*
Inorganic dusts	1. Retention	Iron (siderosis) Tin (stannosis) Barium (baritosis) Coal (simple coal worker's pneumoconiosis)
	2. Granulomatous reaction	Beryllium
	3. Fibrosis: nodular diffuse	Talc* Silica† Asbestos
	massive	Beryllium Coal
	Caplan nodules	Silica Coal Silica
Organic dusts	Extrinsic allergic alveolitis → Acute granulomatous ↓ Chronic fibrosis	*M. faeni* (farmer's lung) *T. sacchari* (bagassosis) *A. clavatus* (malt worker's lung)

* Industrial talc may contain silica and asbestos, and 'talc pneumoconiosis' can be due to the effects of these dusts as well as to talc.
† Inhalation of non fibrogenic dusts (most commonly iron oxide) with silica can modify the effects of silica producing a 'mixed dust fibrosis'.

The ILO/UC 1971 classification of radiographic abnormalities is now widely used to classify the appearances of the chest radiograph in the pneumoconioses. It can be used to classify the radiographic appearances of all pneumoconioses, including asbestosis. The full classification is based on a twelve point continuous scale of profusion; only the short classification will be discussed here. Opacities are divided into small (up to 10 mm) and large (greater than 1 cm). Small opacities are further divided into rounded and irregular opacities, and are categorized according to their profusion into categories 0, 1, 2 and 3 as below:

Small opacities

Category	Rounded	Irregular
0	Absent or less profuse than category 1	Absent or less profuse than category 1
1	Definitely present but few in number	Definitely present but few in number. Normal lung markings still visible
2	Numerous. Normal lung markings still visible	Numerous. Normal lung markings partly obscured
3	Very numerous. Normal lung markings partly or totally obscured	Very numerous. Normal lung markings totally obscured

Small rounded opacities are also classified according to their approximate diameter into 'p' opacities (less than 1.5 mm), 'q' opacities (between 1.5 mm and 3 mm) and 'r' opacities (between 3 mm and 10 mm). Small irregular opacities are divided according to their thickness into 's' opacities (fine irregular), 't' opacities (medium irregular) and 'u' opacities (coarse irregular).

Large opacities are divided into categories A, B and C according to their size:

Category A   An opacity whose greatest diameter is between 1 cm and 5 cm, or several such opacities the sum of whose greatest diameter does not exceed 5 cm.

Category B   One or more opacities whose combined diameter is greater than 5 cm but whose combined area is less than one-third of one lung.

Category C   One or more opacities whose area exceeds one-third of one lung.

A set of standard chest radiographs is available from the ILO which shows the different types of opacity and the grades of profusion.

The diagnosis and differential diagnosis of the pneumoconioses are usefully approached in relation to these different patterns of abnormality produced on the chest radiograph. Some of the important occupational causes of these patterns of radiographic abnormality, and the more important non-occupational causes from which they must be distinguished are given in Table 17.2. It is useful to consider the causes of the pneumoconioses

Table 17.2 Patterns of abnormality seen on chest radiograph in pneumoconioses

Opacities	Occupational causes	Non-occupational causes

1. Small rounded	Siderosis
	Stannosis
	Baritosis
	Coal worker's pneumo-
	  coniosis
	Silicosis
	Talc pneumoconiosis
	Acute beryllium disease
	Acute extrinsic allergic
	  alveolitis (e.g. farmer's
	  lung)
		Sarcoidosis
		Tuberculosis
		Acute extrinsic alveolitis
		  (e.g. bird fancier's lung)
		Pulmonary metastases (e.g.
		  from breast and thyroid
		  cancers)
		Healed chicken pox pneumonia
		Haemosiderosis
		Histoplasmosis

2. Small irregular	Asbestosis
	Talc pneumoconiosis
		Left heart failure
		Cryptogenic fibrosing
		  alveolitis
		Fibrosing alveolitis associated
		  with:
		    Rheumatoid disease
		    Scleroderma
		    SLE
		    Sjogren's syndrome

3. Small rounded with large opacities	Coal worker's pneumo-
	  coniosis complicated by:
	    Progressive massive
	      fibrosis
	    Caplan's syndrome
	Silicosis complicated by:
	    Conglomerate silicosis
	    Pulmonary tuberculosis
	    Caplan's syndrome
		Any of 1. with:
		  Lung cancer
		  Tuberculosis

4. Small rounded which may progress to upper lobe fibrosis	Extrinsic allergic
	  alveolitis (due to
	  occupational causes)
	Beryllium disease
	Silicosis complicated by
	  tuberculosis
	Mixed dust fibrosis
	  (which may or may not
	  be complicated by
	  tuberculosis)
		Sarcoidosis
		Extrinsic allergic
		  alveolitis (due to non-
		  occupational causes)

in relation to the appearances of the chest radiograph in the following groups:

1. Dusts which cause small rounded opacities alone.
2. Dusts which cause small rounded opacities which may be complicated by massive lesions.
3. Dusts which cause small irregular opacities.
4. Dusts which cause small rounded opacities which may progress to upper lobe fibrosis.

17.1.3 Dusts which cause small rounded opacities alone – siderosis, stannosis and baritosis

Retention in the lungs of sufficient quantity of inert but radio-opaque mineral dusts such as iron, tin and barium, produces widespread small rounded opacities on the chest radiograph which are particularly dense in baritosis and stannosis (Fig. 17.1). Accumulation of these dusts provokes a local proliferation of reticulin, but not of collagen fibres. Lung function is not impaired and life is not shortened. The diagnosis of siderosis, stannosis

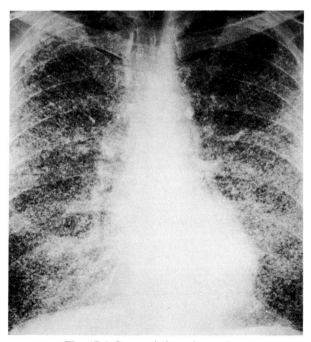

Fig. 17.1 Stannosis in a tin smelter.

and baritosis is made by recognition of the radiographic changes in a patient with an appropriate occupational history.

Some of the circumstances in which occupational exposure to iron, tin and barium may occur is given in Table 17.3.

Table 17.3 Dust retention without fibrosis

Dust	*Circumstances of exposure*
Metallic iron or iron oxide dust or fume (siderosis)	1. Mining of iron ore (haematite, magnetite and limonite) 2. Fettling (i.e. removal of burnt-on moulding sand with pneumatic hammers from iron castings) in iron foundries 3. Electric arc and oxyacetylene welding (welding temperatures liberate iron oxide fume – heavy exposure occurs particularly in enclosed and poorly ventilated spaces) 4. Boiler scaling (cleaning of coal-fired boilers which contain a high concentration of iron and carbon as well as quartz) 5. Silver polishing with iron oxide powder (jeweller's rouge)
Metallic tin or tin oxide fume or dust (stannosis)	Bagging of tin ore Tin smelting
Barium sulphate (barytes) – baritosis	Mining barytes Bagging dry barytes

It is important to appreciate that miners of these materials may also be exposed to a significant silica hazard, which can produce similar changes on the chest radiograph. Furthermore, haematite miners, fettlers, welders and boiler scalers may also be exposed to silica, which can cause a 'mixed dust fibrosis' (see p. 468).

17.1.4 Dusts which cause small rounded opacities which may be complicated by large opacities – coal workers' pneumoconiosis silicosis (and mixed dust fibrosis)

Coal workers' pneumoconiosis (CWP) and silicosis both produce small rounded opacities on the chest radiograph (simple CWP and simple silicosis). Both may also be complicated by the development of large opacities, in coal workers due either to progressive massive fibrosis or Caplan's syndrome, and in silicosis to conglomerate silicosis, pulmonary TB or Caplan's

syndrome. Commercial talc containing a high silica content may also produce small rounded opacities on the chest radiograph which may be complicated by the development of large opacities.

(a) *Coal workers' pneumoconiosis (CWP)*

Coal workers' pneumoconiosis is caused by the inhalation of coal dust.
Those exposed to the highest concentrations have been men working underground, particularly at the coal face. However, men in other underground
jobs, such as those transporting coal from the face to the pit shaft, and those
making and repairing underground roadways are also exposed to coal dust.
Surface workers such as those sorting and grading the coal on the 'screens'
are less exposed. Coal trimmers who loaded and distributed coal in the holds
of collier ships were exposed to high dust concentrations, but this work is
now done mechanically.

With improved measures of dust control the numbers affected by CWP
has fallen considerably in recent years. The prevalence of all categories of
CWP in 53 UK collieries was 15.7% in 1959 and 9.7% in 1970.

Pulmonary disease attributable to coal dust exposure is detected and
followed by the changes produced on the chest radiograph. The different
diseases due to coal dust exposure – simple CWP, progressive massive
fibrosis and Caplan's syndrome – are distinguished and classified according
to their radiographic appearances.

(i) *Simple CWP*

Simple CWP is characterized by the presence of widespread small rounded
opacities on the chest radiograph due to retention of coal dust in the lungs.
The profusion of these opacities correlates well with both coal dust exposure
and the coal dust content of the lungs. The dust is retained in the alveoli in
the walls of the first and second order respiratory bronchioles, and provokes
a local proliferation of reticulin fibres and to a lesser extent of collagen
fibres, which may be associated with some dilatation of these respiratory
bronchioles ('focal emphysema').

Simple CWP is probably not a cause of respiratory symptoms or disability
and does not produce physical signs in the chest. Small changes in lung
function test measurements have been identified in studies of groups of
miners with simple CWP when compared with groups of non-miners, but it
is unlikely that changes of this magnitude alone are responsible for respiratory symptoms. Simple CWP does not shorten life, and unlike PMF does not
progress if further exposure to coal dust is avoided, although rarely where
past coal dust exposure has been heavy simple CWP may progress to PMF

without further exposure. Its importance is as a precursor of PMF which may impair lung function, cause severe disability and shorten life.

The diagnosis of simple CWP is made on the finding of small rounded opacities on the chest radiograph in a coal worker who has had an adequate history of coal dust exposure. It is now unusual in men with less than 15 years' exposure underground. The presence of respiratory symptoms, physical signs in the chest and significant abnormalities of lung function in a man with simple CWP require an alternative explanation, and the other causes of similar radiographic abnormalities (Table 17.2) should be excluded. Respiratory symptoms in those with simple CWP are most commonly due to airway diseases such as chronic obstructive bronchitis or asthma, which should be identified so that appropriate treatment may be given.

(ii) *Progressive massive fibrosis (PMF)*

PMF produces large (greater than 1 cm in diameter) opacities which initially develop in the upper lobes (Fig. 17.2). They are ill defined and in the early stages, are irregular in outline. PMF usually develops on a background of category 2 or category 3 simple CWP. The opacities increase in size slowly over years, and become better defined. They can come to occupy a whole lobe and may cavitate. Histologically they are found to contain coarse bundles of collagen fibres separated by considerable quantities of coal dust.

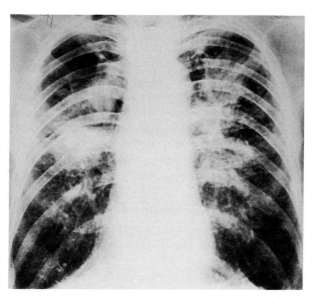

Fig. 17.2 Progressive massive fibrosis in a coal worker.

Why PMF develops in some coal workers and not others remains unclear. It seems in part to be a dose-dependant effect with an attack rate in one study of 0.7% per annum in those with category 1 CWP, 2.6% per annum in category 2 and 4.2% per annum in category 3 [2]. The attack rate is also related to age – the younger a man develops category 2 simple CWP the more likely he is to develop PMF – and shows a widespread geographical difference in prevalence, being high in South Wales, but low in Scotland and in the Midlands of England.

Early (category A) PMF causes no symptoms and little abnormality of lung function. More advanced PMF (categories B and C) not only occupy space in the lung, but also distort pulmonary architecture causing narrowing of adjacent airways. Those affected become increasingly disabled by shortness of breath, and may develop cough and sputum with intermittent episodes of infective bronchitis. FEV_1 and FVC which are usually normal in category A PMF, are reduced in categories B and C PMF with evidence of airway narrowing (i.e. a low FEV_1/FVC ratio). The carbon monoxide gas transfer test is also reduced in PMF in proportion to the size of the lesions. Rupture of the liquified contents of a massive lesion into a bronchus is coughed up as a jet black fluid, 'melanoptysis', which is associated with radiographic evidence of cavitation.

Unlike simple CWP, PMF may progress after removal from exposure to coal dust; the younger a man develops PMF the more likely it is to progress. Categories B and C, but probably not category A PMF, in addition to impairing lung function and causing respiratory disability, may shorten life.

PMF is diagnosed by the finding of the characteristic large opacities initially in the upper lobes of a coal worker with simple CWP, usually category 2 or 3. Such opacities should be distinguished from Caplan's syndrome (*vide infra*) and from other unassociated conditions, particularly pulmonary TB and lung cancer. Melanoptysis is diagnostic of PMF. Pulmonary TB like early PMF predominantly involves the upper zones and should always be looked for by examination of the sputum. An opacity increasing rapidly in size is more likely to be due to lung cancer than to PMF, although Caplan lesions may also progress rapidly. Where doubt exists a histological diagnosis should always be made.

(iii) *Caplan's syndrome*

Large opacities developing on the chest radiographs of coal miners with rheumatoid arthritis were first distinguished from PMF by Caplan in 1953 [3]. Since his original description similar opacities have been described on the chest radiographs of those with rheumatoid arthritis who have not been coal workers, and in some, such lesions can be the sole manifestation of the disease.

They are usually rounded well defined opacities of between 0.5 and 5 cm in diameter. They frequently develop on a background of category 1 simple CWP or less, and are typically distributed peripherally throughout both lung fields at the junction of the middle and outer thirds. They can appear in crops, progress in size over months and then remain stationary. They may cavitate.

Histologically the nodules consist of a central area of necrosis containing a variable amount of coal dust surrounded by a concentric ring of lymphocytes or plasma cells. Peripheral to this are fibroblasts and concentrically arranged collagen fibres. An associated obliterative endarteritis may occur.

A positive rheumatoid factor is found in the majority of coal workers with Caplan's syndrome. The disease causes only a small impairment in ventilatory function, even when widespread opacities are present on the chest radiograph.

The characteristic radiographic features, particularly in the presence of a positive rheumatoid factor, should allow differentiation of Caplan's syndrome from PMF. However, an opacity or opacities rapidly increasing in size may need to be distinguished from a primary or secondary lung cancer, for which a histological diagnosis is required.

(b) *Silicosis*

Silicosis is caused by the inhalation of respirable dust which contains more than about 10% free silica (silicon dioxide). Silica occurs in nature in three forms: quartz, cristabolite and tridymite. Quartz is the commonest mineral, and is a constituent of many rocks, including granite, sandstone and slate, but not of chalk or limestone.

Silica is extremely toxic to alveolar macrophages destroying those which phagocytose it, initiating a fibrotic reaction. Unlike asbestos which causes a diffuse fibrosis in alveolar walls, silica provokes a discrete nodular fibrosis. The collagen fibres in a silicotic nodule are arranged in a characteristic concentric pattern ('whorled' or 'onion skin' fibrosis), which allows them to be identified in histological sections of the lung.

Silicosis can occur in those employed in many different occupations [1]:

1. Mining, quarrying and tunnelling. Gold, tin, copper and mica are mined from rock with a high quartz content. Sandstone, granite and slate quarrying exposes those working the quarries to silica dust. Tunnelling through quartz containing stone produces a dust with a high silica content. The introduction of mechanized equipment into these processes has increased exposure to silica dust particles of a respirable size.
2. Stone cutting, dressing, polishing and cleaning monumental masonry where the stone used is sandstone or granite.

3. Sandblasting. Sand propelled by compressed air is used as an abrasive for scaling metal surface. When uncontrolled it is a major silica hazard. Sandblasting is outlawed in the United Kingdom.
4. Foundry work. Knocking out, shotblasting and fettling of casts moulded in quartzose sand.
5. Pottery workers. Powdered flint is used in the manufacture of earthenware. Grinding the flint and fettling the pot before it is fired produces silica dust. Grinding flint used to support chinaware during firing, and its removal from the chinaware after firing, was a major cause of silicosis in UK until the 1940s, when silica was replaced in this process by alumina.
6. Boiler scaling. Cleaning coal-fired boilers which contain a high silica content in the ash.

Three different types of silicosis are recognized, which are related primarily to the dose of silica inhaled:

Chronic silicosis follows exposure to moderate amounts of free silica, such as may occur in foundrymen and in potters. Changes on the chest radiograph seldom appear until after twenty years of exposure, and the average duration of life from first exposure is about forty years.

Accelerated silicosis follows heavy exposure to free silica such as may occur in sandblasting and tunnelling. The changes on the chest radiograph appears within four to eight years of exposure, and death occurs on average within about ten years.

Acute silicoproteinosis which follows very heavy exposure to free silica such as may occur in sandblasters. Symptoms develop within months of first exposure. The disease progresses rapidly, with death occurring from intractable respiratory failure within a short period.

Pulmonary tuberculosis may complicate each of these types of silicosis, and conglomerate silicosis and Caplan's syndrome can complicate simple and accelerated silicosis.

The number of persons compensated for silicosis in the United Kingdom has fallen in recent years: 721 cases were compensated in 1957, 162 cases in 1969 and 113 cases in 1975.

As with CWP, silicosis and its complications are detected and followed by the abnormalities it produces on the chest radiograph, with the exception that complicating tuberculosis should be diagnosed where possible bacteriologically.

(i) *Simple silicosis*

Simple silicosis is diagnosed by the presence of small rounded opacities on the chest radiograph. Initially these develop in the upper lobes but may progress, even in the absence of further exposure, to involve the whole lung. The opacities are classified in the same way as in simple CWP according to their profusion and size. The extent of the radiographic abnormalities in simple silicosis is related to total dust exposure. Calcification of the opacities can occur as can calcification of hilar glands, which gives them an 'egg-shell' appearance on the chest radiograph. The speed of appearance and progression of these small rounded opacities depends primarily upon the amount of respirable silica inhaled.

Unlike simple CWP, in which the appearances on the chest radiograph are due to the focal accumulation of coal dust in the lungs, the radiographic abnormalities in simple silicosis are due to fibrotic nodules in the lung and in draining lymph nodes. Studies of those with simple silicosis have shown that a small decrease in lung volumes (total lung capacity (TLC) and forced vital capacity (FVC)) occurs in categories 2 and 3, but not in category 1 silicosis.

Simple silicosis is diagnosed on the appearances of the chest radiographic in conjunction with an appropriate occupational history. The radiographic appearances are not specific for silicosis, and silicosis must be distinguished from other diseases producing similar radiographic abnormalities (Table 17.2). Of these, sarcoidosis can on occasions be particularly difficult to differentiate. Profuse small rounded opacities on the chest radiograph with bilateral hilar gland enlargement (which may on occasions develop 'egg-shell' calcification) can occur in both silicosis and sarcoidosis. In both diseases those affected may have no symptoms or abnormal physical signs and measurements of lung function can be either normal or only minimally abnormal. The distinction is important as sarcoidosis, unlike silicosis, may benefit from treatment with corticosteroids. Where a diagnosis of sarcoidosis cannot be made either from the presence of one or more of the extrathoracic manifestations of sarcoidosis or from a positive Kveim test, lung biopsy is justifiable.

(ii) *Complicated silicosis – conglomerate silicosis, silicotuberculosis and Caplan's syndrome.*
Simple silicosis may be complicated by massive fibrotic lesions (conglomerate silicosis), tuberculosis (silicotuberculosis) and by Caplan's syndrome.

Massive fibrotic lesions (conglomerate silicosis), which usually develop initially in the upper lobes, arise by the conglomeration of silicotic nodules. The nodules, which may retain their whorled appearance, are matted together by collagen fibres. They contain obliterated blood vessels and airways.

Conglomerate silicosis is diagnosed by finding large opacities on the chest radiograph, which usually, but not invariably, develop initially in the upper zones. These may increase slowly in size until they come to occupy a large part of both lung fields. Cavitation is rare in the absence of complicating tuberculosis. An opacity which increases rapidly in size is usually due to complicating tuberculosis, but may be due to a lung cancer or Caplan's syndrome.

Increasing limitation of activities by breathlessness is the principal symptom of silicosis. In the absence of coexisting airways obstruction due to other causes, breathlessness due to silicosis seldom occurs in the absence of conglomerate silicosis. Progression of conglomerate silicosis produces increasing distortion of lung architecture, and can lead to the development of hypoxic respiratory failure.

Conglomerate silicosis causes a marked reduction in lung volumes and a decrease in the carbon monoxide gas transfer test ($DLCO$) which is due to loss of alveolar volume.

Complicating tuberculosis can develop insidiously and may be difficult to recognize. It should be thought of particularly when fever, weight loss or haemoptysis occur, or when rapidly progressing or cavitating lesions are seen on the chest radiograph.

Caplan's syndrome in silicosis is no different from that seen in CWP (*vide supra*).

Massive lesions on the chest radiograph due to conglomerate silicosis need to be distinguished not only from complicating tuberculosis but also from lung cancer and Caplan's syndrome. Tuberculosis should always be suspected and the sputum examined for tubercle bacilli. In some cases of silicotuberculosis the infecting organisms have been found to be atypical mycobacteria, such as *M. kansasii*. Lung cancer generally produces an opacity on the chest radiograph which is better defined and which increases in size more rapidly than conglomerate silicosis. Where doubt exists lung tissue should be obtained either bronchoscopically or if necessary by open lung biopsy.

(iii) *Acute silicoproteinosis.*

Acute silicoproteinosis is an unusual reaction to silica exposure. It follows very heavy exposure to respirable silica as may occur in sandblasting or in tunnelling. Symptoms, which may develop within six months of first exposure, are of fever, weight loss, cough and increasingly severe breathlessness. The appearances of the chest radiograph are very similar to those of acute pulmonary oedema and alveolar proteinosis, with perihilar confluent 'bat's wing' shadowing, often showing air bronchograms. The disease progresses rapidly, with those affected dying from intractable respiratory failure.

(c) *Mixed dust fibrosis*

The term 'mixed dust fibrosis' is given to the pulmonary disease caused by the inhalation of silica dust simultaneously with another non-fibrogenic dust. Non-fibrogenic dust inhaled with silica appears to modify the fibrogenic effect of the inhaled silica. When the proportion of free silica to the non fibrogenic dust is low, the characteristic nodular fibrosis of silicosis does not occur; instead, irregular stellate fibrous lesions are produced. Complicating massive fibrosis can also occur, and tuberculosis occurs as frequently as in silicosis.

Mixed dust fibrosis has occurred most commonly in occupations where there is a mixed exposure to silica and iron, such as in haematite miners, iron foundry workers, electric arc and oxyacetylene welders in iron foundries, and in fettlers and boiler scalers.   Increasingly severe breathlessness on exertion, together with a cough productive of reddish-brown sputum develops particularly in those with massive lesions. Respiratory failure with pulmonary hypertension can develop in those with massive fibrosis.

Widespread small rounded opacities similar to those in silicosis, which predominantly affect the upper lobes, may be seen on the chest radiograph. Irregular opacities in the middle and upper zones, similar to the changes seen in postprimary tuberculosis, however, are more usual. Massive fibrotic lesions similar to those found in coal workers' pneumococniosis, usually in the upper lobes, may develop.

Radiographically the appearances of mixed dust fibrosis can be difficult to distinguish from tuberculosis, which may in any case complicate it (Fig. 17.3). It is therefore important even in the presence of an appropriate

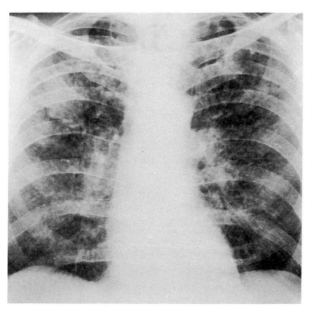

Fig. 17.3 Mixed dust fibrosis in an iron foundry worker.

occupational history to look for evidence of tuberculosis. The diagnosis of mixed dust fibrosis, however, should be made, even if evidence of tuberculosis is obtained, in a person with a history of appropriate occupational exposure.

17.1.5 Dusts which cause small irregular opacities – asbestosis and talc pneumoconiosis

(*a*) *Asbestosis*

Exposure to asbestos dust can cause one or more of several separate diseases of the lungs or pleura:

1. Benign pleural diseases
      diffuse pleural thickening
      pleural plaques
      pleural effusion
2. Malignant mesothelioma of pleura (and of peritoneum)
3. Diffuse pulmonary fibrosis – asbestosis
4. Lung cancer

It is important to appreciate that the term *asbestosis* refers to diffuse pulmonary fibrosis due to the inhalation of asbestos dust, and not to any of the other asbestos-related diseases (which can, however, occur in association with asbestosis). Also, of these different diseases only asbestosis is a pneumoconiosis. Malignant mesothelioma and lung cancer attributable to asbestos exposure are considered later in this chapter.

The term *asbestos* describes a number of naturally occurring fibrous silicates. They are found in nature in two main forms: as a *serpentine*, crysotile (white asbestos), and as *amphiboles*, which include crocidolite (blue asbestos), amosite, anthopyllite and tremolite. Ninety per cent of the asbestos used commercially in the world is crysotile, which is mined primarily in Canada and USSR. Crocidolite and amosite are mined in southern Africa, and anthophyllite in Finland.

Asbestos has many properties which has made it increasingly valuable industrially. Between 1877 and 1967 world production of asbestos has increased from 50 tons to 4 million tons per year. It is incombustible and resistant to high temperatures, and is therefore used as an insulation material. Its fibres are strong, and are used to strengthen and reinforce cement products and insulation boards. Asbestos can be woven into textiles, and is also used in the manufacture of friction materials such as brake linings.

Asbestos exposure may therefore occur in a wide variety of occupations: in miners and millers in those countries where it is mined, and in those transporting asbestos. In the United Kingdom the major risks of exposure have been to those engaged in the manufacture of asbestos textiles and asbestos-containing products, and to those working in the insulation industry. Insulation workers are exposed when lagging and stripping asbestos containing insulating materials, such as in power stations and in boiler rooms. In the past, naval vessel construction workers were particularly heavily exposed when lagging in confined spaces, and when spraying asbestos fibre, usually crocidolite, onto the bulkheads of naval vessels.

Three patterns of *benign pleural reaction* to inhaled asbestos can be distinguished: discrete pleural plaques, diffuse pleural thickening and pleural effusions. *Pleural plaques* are localized thickenings of the parital pleura and have been distinguished from *diffuse thickening* of the visceral pleura by occupying less than four interspaces, and not involving the costophrenic angles. Diffuse pleural thickening, although not always visible on the chest radiograph, invariably accompanies asbestosis, but can also occur in its absence. Pleural plaques are discrete areas of hyaline fibrosis. They are seen on the chest radiograph when of sufficient thickness or when sufficiently calcified (Fig. 17.4). They are rarely seen until twenty or more years after the onset of exposure. They are almost invariably bilateral and are asymmetrical. They are most commonly seen along the lateral chest wall, in the middle

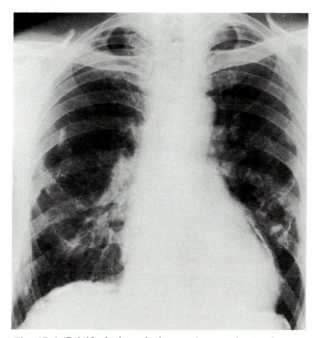

Fig. 17.4 Calcified pleural plaques in an asbestos lagger.

and lower lung zones, and along the line of the diaphragm. *En face*, calcified pleural plaques are irregular in outline and peripherally calcified.

The risk of developing a mesothelioma in those who have been exposed to asbestos is unrelated to the presence or absence of these pleural diseases. Pleural plaques do not interfere with lung function, but diffuse pleural thickening may on occasions be of sufficient severity to do so by compression of the underlying lung. The presence of pleural plaques is very suggestive of previous asbestos exposure, but other causes of pleural thickening and calcification, such as a previous empyema (particularly tuberculous) or haemothorax should be excluded. These are frequently unilateral, often involve the costophrenic angles, and are not typically calcified peripherally.

The relationship between benign *pleural effusions* and asbestos exposure is much less well documented than the other forms of benign pleural disease. However, otherwise unexplained pleural effusions, both unilateral and bilateral, have been reported in those with occupational asbestos exposure. The effusions may be an incidental finding on a chest radiograph, or may present with pleuritic chest pain, or with breathlessness if sufficient fluid has accumulated. Spontaneous resolution usually occurs, but the effusions may recur. The fluid is a sterile serous or serosanguinous exudate, with a preponderance of either neutrophils of lymphocytes. Other causes of similar but otherwise unexplained pleural effusion, particularly a tuberculous effusion, should be excluded before accepting asbestos exposure as the cause of the effusion. Pleural effusion as the presenting feature of either a malignant mesothelioma or a lung cancer should be particularly remembered in those who have had asbestos exposure.

Asbestosis is diffuse pulmonary fibrosis caused by inhalation of asbestos fibres. Its frequency in those occupationally exposed is related to both the degree and duration of exposure. When exposure was heavy, as before the 1931 regulations and during World War II, asbestosis developed in some individuals with exposures of less than one year usually after an interval of ten or more years from the onset of exposure. With improved dust control, few working with asbestos in the 1960s have developed asbestosis who have been exposed for less than 10 or 15 years. With increased recognition of the disease, and the appearance of disease attributable to exposures during the period of inadequate dust control, the number of individuals who have been awarded industrial compensation for asbestosis has been rising: 192 persons were compensated between 1957 and 1961, 398 between 1962 and 1966 and 730 between 1967 and 1971.

Asbestos fibres are ingested by alveolar macrophages and transported centrally to the alveoli within the walls of the first and second order respiratory bronchioles, where they provoke a local fibrotic reaction. This spreads peripherally to involve the whole acinus producing a diffuse, interstitial fibrosis. The fibrosis commences subpleurally in the lower lobes and spreads both within the lobes and to involve the middle lobe and lingula, the lower lobes tending to remain the most severely affected.

Asbestosis causes breathlessness on exertion, slowly increasing in severity with progression of the disease. Clubbing of finger and toe nails is frequently present; dependant end inspiratory crackles, not altered by coughing, are usually audible at the bases of the lungs.

The characteristic abnormalities seen on the chest radiograph are of small irregular opacities predominantly in the lower zones (Fig. 17.5). These changes may be classified according to their profusion and size by the ILO/UC classification. With progression of the disease these small irregular opacities become more profuse, together with a gradual reduction in lung volume, and may be accompanied by localized pleural plaques or by diffuse pleural thickening. Irregular opacities on the chest radiograph which predominantly affect the middle and upper zones of the lungs are rarely due to asbestosis.

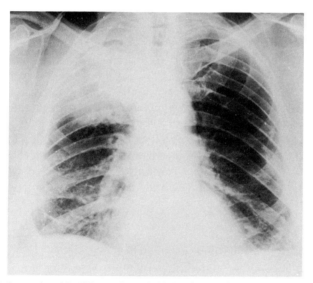

Fig. 17.5 Asbestosis with diffuse pleural thickening and lung cancer in an asbestos lagger.

Asbestosis causes a restrictive ventilatory defect, with a reduction in FEV_1 proportionate to the reduction in FVC, as well as a reduction in total lung capacity (TLC) and residual volume (RV), and a decrease in the carbon monoxide gas transfer test ($DLCO$) and in the gas transfer coefficient (KCO). However, because of the frequency of chronic airway disease evidence of a coexisting obstructive ventilatory defect is often found in those with asbestosis.

The diagnosis of asbestosis is made on finding the appropriate clinical, physiological and radiographic features of the disease in a person who has had substantial occupational asbestos exposure.

Discrete pleural plaques or diffuse pleural thickening when present with the typical basal small irregular opacities on the chest radiograph is virtually diagnostic of asbestosis. In the absence of such pleural abnormalities, asbestosis is indistinguishable from cryptogenic fibrosing alveolitis, and from fibrosing alveolitis associated with rheumatoid disease, SLE and scleroderma, except that progression of the pulmonary disease may be more rapid in these other conditions than in asbestosis. In general, where features suggestive of one of these other diseases are absent, a patient who has basal end inspiratory crackles heard on examination of the chest with irregular opacities predominantly affecting the lower zones of the lungs on the chest radiograph, who has had sufficient asbestos exposure, with an adequate interval between the onset of exposure and the development of the disease (generally in excess of ten years), should be diagnosed as having asbestosis.

Where the diagnosis remains in doubt, lung biopsy is justifiable to exclude fibrosing alveolitis, of which some forms are responsive to treatment. Lung biopsy performed solely in support of a claim for compensation is not justifiable.

Asbestosis causes both respiratory disability and a decreased expectation of life. Those diagnosed by the pneumoconiosis medical panel as having asbestosis have a death rate about 2.5 times that of the average death rate from all causes of men of the same age in England and Wales, and about 8.5 times the average death rate for lung cancer. Of those dying, about 35% die of lung cancer, 20% from other respiratory disease (including asbestosis), and 10% from mesothelioma (pleural and peritoneal).

(b) Talc pneumoconiosis

Talc is a hydrated magnesium silicate, which microscopically appears as flat polygonal plates. Other minerals, particularly tremolite and anthophyllite asbestos, and quartz are found in the rock from which it is mined, and commercial talc contains variable amounts of these other minerals.

Talc is used industrially as a paint filler, as a constituent of ceramics and roofing materials, in the rubber industry to prevent adhesion of rubber in moulds and to aid extrusion, and also in cosmetic powders. Talc pneumoconiosis has been described in talc miners and millers, and in some commercial users, such as the rubber industry.

Exposure to commercial talc may involve exposure not only to talc but also to tremolite and anthophyllite asbestos and to quartz. Three separate types of histological reaction may occur in the lungs, the dominant pattern depending on the composition of the inhaled talc: ill defined nodular lesions, which may show incomplete whorling due to quartz with talc; diffuse interstitial fibrosis produced by the asbestos, spreading peripherally from the respiratory bronchioles, resembling asbestosis; foreign body granulomata probably due to the talc alone. Birefringent needle-shaped particles may be demonstrated with polarized light in close association with these lesions. Massive lesions can develop with the nodular pattern of reaction.

Breathlessness on exertion is generally associated with either the diffuse fibrotic pattern of disease or in the nodular form when massive lesions have developed. Finger clubbing and basal end inspiratory crackles can be found in the diffuse fibrotic type of disease. Talc pneumoconiosis generally progresses slowly and rarely shortens life, although premature death may occur with widespread massive lesions and diffuse pulmonary fibrosis.

Three different patters of abnormality may be seen on the chest radiograph:

1. Small rounded opacities particularly in the mid zones resembling the changes of silicosis. Massive lesions can also develop in association with this type of disease.
2. Small irregular opacities predominantly in the lower zones resembling the changes seen in asbestosis.
3. Mixed pattern.

Little abnormality occurs in the early stages of the nodular disease, but a restrictive ventilatory defect with impaired gas transfer can occur later. The changes in the diffuse fibrotic disease are the same as those of asbestosis.

Massive lesions can develop in the nodular form of the disease. There is little evidence of an increased risk of tuberculosis, lung cancer or malignant mesothelioma.

The diagnosis is made on the radiographic appearances, together with the clinical and functional findings, in the presence of an appropriate occupational history. Lung biopsy is justifiable in a patient in whom the diagnosis is in doubt, to exclude other treatable causes of similar radiographic abnormalities.

17.1.6 Dusts which cause small rounded opacities on the chest radiograph which may progress to upper lobe fibrosis – extrinsic allergic alveolitis and chronic beryllium disease

Widespread small rounded opacities are seen on the chest radiograph in the acute stages of both beryllium disease and extrinsic allergic alveolitis. Both are diseases characterized by granulomatous inflammation in the lungs, and in both, fibrosis can develop which predominantly involves the upper lobes.

Upper lobe fibrosis is of course also characteristic of mixed dust fibrosis, with or without complicating tuberculosis, and of silicosis complicated by tuberculosis.

(a) Extrinsic allergic alveolitis

Extrinsic allergic alveolitis describes a group of diseases characterized by a granulomatous inflammatory reaction, which may progress to fibrosis, in alveolar walls and respiratory bronchioles. It is caused by a local hypersensitivity reaction to inhaled organic dusts. A large number of agents have been identified as causes of extrinsic allergic alveolitis of which some of the more important are given in Table 17.4. Of these, the two diseases seen most commonly in the United Kingdom are farmer's lung and bird fancier's lung (pigeon fancier's and budgerigar fancier's lung). Contaminants of humidifier systems, both in the home and at work have also recently been recognized as causes of extrinsic allergic alveolitis.

Table 17.4   Some causes of extrinsic allergic alveolitis

Disease	Antigen source	Causal antigen
Farmer's lung	Mouldy hay, straw, grain etc.	*Micropolyspora faeni*
Bagassosis	Mouldy bagasse	*Thermoactinomycetes sacchari*
Pigeon fancier's lung Budgerigar fancier's lung } Bird droppings		Avian serum proteins
Mushroom worker's lung		
Malt worker's lung	Mouldy maltings	*Aspergillus clavatus*
'Ventilation pneumonitis'	Contaminated humidifier water	Thermophilic actinomycetes
'Humidifier fever'	Contaminated humidifier water	? Amoebae

The disease has three distinguishable modes of presentation which are related primarily to the pattern and intensity of exposure to the causal antigen: acute, subacute and chronic. Acute allergic alveolitis follows intermittent heavy exposures. Recurrent episodes of breathlessness with fever and 'flu-like symptoms, such as headache, shivering and myalgia often with associated weight loss, develop some four to eight hours after exposure and persist, in the absence of further exposure, for some seven to ten days. Scattered end inspiratory crackles may be heard on examination of the chest. Small ill-defined rounded opacities are seen on the chest radiograph, often in all three lung zones. These usually resolve spontaneously in the absence of further exposure within about four to six weeks, but can persist. Continuous heavy exposure can cause subacute allergic alveolitis. Instead of recurrent episodes following intermittent exposure, the symptoms experienced are increasingly severe breathlessness, malaise and weight loss with persistent fever. The abnormalities on examination of the chest and of the chest radiograph are similar to the acute disease, although the shadows on the chest radiograph may be larger or become confluent. In both forms of the disease the changes in lung function test measurements are the same: a restrictive ventilatory defect with a decrease in the carbon monoxide gas transfer test. With avoidance of further exposure to the causal antigen both acute and subacute extrinsic allergic alveolitis are usually largely or completely reversible diseases.

With continued antigen exposure chronic irreversible changes in lung function occur, due to the development of pulmonary fibrosis. The disease may also present at this chronic stage in those with light exposure to the causal antigen of lung duration. Typically such patients complain of increasing limitation of activities from breathlessness, usually without associated constitutional symptoms, apart from weight loss. Scattered end inspiratory crackles may be heard on examination of the chest. Small rounded opacities on the chest radiograph are associated with contraction and destruction of the upper lobes, often with cyst formation. Lung function test measurements typically show a restrictive ventilatory defect with impairment of carbon monoxide gas transfer. Patients with the disease may also have evidence of coexisting airway narrowing, which may be a consequence of the disease or due to unrelated causes, such as cigarette smoking.

The diagnosis of extrinsic allergic alveolitis is based upon recognition of the appropriate clinical, radiographic and functional features of the disease, identification of a potential source of antigen in the patient's home or working environment, and the demonstration of precipitating antibodies in the serum to the causal antigen.

(i) *Farmer's lung*

The most important occupational cause of extrinsic allergic alveolitis is farmer's lung, which may present in any of the three ways described above. It is caused by an allergic reaction to *Micropolyspora faeni* which grows in mouldy hay, straw or cereal grain in which the water content exceeds 35% and the temperature is 50° C or more. These growth requirements are fulfilled when organic vegetable matter is harvested in poor conditions and stored damp, which allows moulding with self-heating to occur. Exposure to *M. faeni* occurs when bales of mouldy hay or straw are opened for animal feeding, and when mouldy grain is moved or threshed, particularly when such operations are carried out in poorly ventilated barns or sheds.

The diagnosis of acute and subacute farmer's lung is based upon recognition of the temporal relationship of the illness to the occupational exposure, the appearances of the chest radiograph and the finding of serum precipitins to mouldy hay and *M. faeni*. Almost all patients who have acute or subacute disease have serum precipitins, but these may also be found in up to 20% of healthy farmers. Acute and subacute allergic alveolitis has to be distinguished from influenza, viral pneumonia, miliary tuberculosis, sarcoidosis and silo filler's lung (which is also an occupational disease of farmers, see p. 492). Lung biopsy is usually not necessary, but should be performed where the diagnosis remains in doubt. Characteristically, 'sarcoid-like' non-caseating epithelioid and giant cell granulomata are seen in alveolar walls and respiratory bronchioles. These histological appearances may be distinguished from those of sarcoidosis by the presence of giant cells with characteristic clefts and by greater involvement of the alveolar walls in the inflammatory process in extrinsic allergic alveolitis.

The diagnosis of chronic farmer's lung can be more difficult, particularly in the absence of a previous history of intermittent episodes of acute disease. Furthermore serum precipitins are usually not found if exposure has not occurred for three years or more. Lung biopsy may not show granulomata after a year from the last exposure. Diagnosis has in these circumstances to be based on a history of occupational exposure and the exclusion of other diseases causing upper lobe fibrosis. The more important of these are pulmonary tuberculosis, sarcoidosis, allergic bronchopulmonary aspergillosis, mixed dust fibrosis and chronic beryllium disease.

Micro-organisms contaminating humidification systems have also been identified as causes of extrinsic allergic alveolitis. Two different clinical patterns of reaction occur. A disease very similar to farmer's lung which has been called 'ventilation pneumonitis' has been described from the United States. It occurs in those working in office blocks and in those living in blocks of flats in which the humidification system has become contaminated by thermophilic actinomycetes. Those affected have symptoms and functional abnormalities typical of extrinsic allergic alveolitis; ill defined small rounded opacities with fibrosis and contraction of the upper lobes develop on the chest radiograph. Precipitins to thermophilic actinomycetes are found in the serum of those affected. Humidification systems are an important potential allergenic source to remember in those with extrinsic allergic alveolitis, which can easily be overlooked.

(ii) *Humidifier fever*
A similar disease, which has been called 'humidifier fever', is due to a reaction to micro-organisms growing in water reservoir tanks. It occurs in those working in factories where water is recirculated for air humidification, or for pressure generation. Those affected have symptoms typical of recur-

rent attacks of acute allergic alveolitis. Breathlessness, associated with fever, shivering, myalgia, malaise, and headache develops about four hours after starting work. Usually symptoms occur on the first day back at work after an absence over a weekend or on holiday, and improve spontaneously over the following 12 to 36 h, despite continuing exposure at work during the remainder of the working week. Lung function measurements made before and after a working day in which symptoms occur, show the development of a restrictive ventilatory defect and of a decrease in the carbon monoxide gas transfer test. These abnormalities improve spontaneously during the working week, and recur, with the return of symptoms, on returning to work after an absence. The chest radiograph in those with 'humidifier fever' is normal during acute attacks. Furthermore, despite recurrent attacks, in some over periods of several years, measurements of lung function show no irreversible changes, and abnormalities do not develop on the chest radiograph. Lung biopsy findings have not been reported.

Those with the disease have serum precipitins to extracts made from the water or baffle plate jelly of the humidifier tank from their place of work, but not to extracts from these materials made from other factories where outbreaks of the disease have occurred. The causative agent has not yet been identified with certainty, but there is some evidence that it may be amoebae growing in the water tanks.

'Humidifier fever' should be remembered in the differential diagnosis of those with recurrent febrile illnesses of uncertain origin. It is diagnosed by obtaining a history of 'Monday symptoms', demonstrating the appropriate changes in lung function measurements which occur on the first day back at work after an absence, and by finding serum precipitins to an extract of humidifier water or jelly from the individuals place of work. Recognition of the disease can save those affected much unnecessary, often invasive, investigation.

(b) Beryllium disease

Exposure to beryllium fume and to the dust both of beryllium metal and several of its compounds causes two quite distinct diseases. Exposure to high concentrations of these materials can cause an acute inflammatory reaction which is confined to the respiratory tract, and which in those most severely affected causes acute pulmonary oedema. This is acute beryllium disease; where not fatal, it is usually followed by complete recovery, although chronic beryllium disease has been reported in a small proportion of those who recover. Acute beryllium disease is considered with the other causes of occupationally caused acute pulmonary oedema on p. 492. Chronic beryllium disease may follow acute beryllium disease, but more usually occurs without a preceding acute illness, in those exposed over a long period to relatively low concentrations of dust or fume. Chronic beryllium disease is very similar to sarcoidosis, with non-caseating epithelioid and giant cell granulomata occurring in the lungs as well as in several other affected organs.

Beryllium is extracted from the ore beryl, an aluminium beryllium silicate which is mined in South Africa, the United States, South America and India. Beryllium disease has not been reported in those mining and otherwise exposed to beryl, but both acute and chronic beryllium disease occurs in those extracting beryllium from the ore in which beryllium sulphate, beryllium fluoride and beryllium hydroxide are produced. Beryllium oxide is derived from the hydroxide by calcination.

Beryllium has several important industrial applications. Until about 1950 beryllium phosphors were used in fluorescent strip lighting tubes. The beryllium phosphors were contaminated by unreacted beryllium oxide, and exposure to the dusts of these compounds occurred in those preparing the phosphors, manufacturing the tubes, and those disposing of the tubes or accidentally breaking them. Up to 1966 about half the cases of chronic beryllium disease had occurred in those working in the fluorescent lighting industry; since about 1950 beryllium phosphors have been replaced in fluorescent lights by halophosphates.

The addition of small amounts of beryllium to other metals produces alloys of great tensile strength. Beryllium copper alloy is the most commonly used. In addition to its tensile strength it is also non-sparking and non-magnetic. It is used in integrated circuits in electrical and electronic equipment. Industrial beryllium copper alloys, which contain 2% and 0.5% beryllium, are prepared from a 4% master alloy. Exposure to beryllium fume can occur in those preparing the industrial and master alloys, as well as in any process involving heat treatment of the 2% industrial alloy or the welding of beryllium alloys. Drilling and machining beryllium metal or beryllium alloys can produce respirable beryllium dust, particularly where dry processes are used.

Respiratory disease is the most common mode of presentation of chronic beryllium disease. Symptoms may develop within months to several years of exposure, usually within five years of last exposure, but in some 10% of cases, symptoms have developed after an interval of more than ten years from last exposure. Patients usually present with increasing exertional dyspnoea, or with a dry unproductive cough. In the cases originally described in those working in the fluorescent lighting industry these symptoms were often accompanied by lethargy and considerable weight loss. With greatly improved industrial hygiene, exposures to beryllium in those with the disease have been less severe, and such features are now unusual. Furthermore, with regular screening of those working with beryllium, cases of the disease may be identified by finding abnormalities on a chest radiograph in those without respiratory symptoms. Scattered inspiratory crackles may be heard on examination of the chest, but frequently no abnormal physical signs are present.

The abnormal appearances of the chest radiograph and their progression are very similar those seen in sarcoidosis (Fig. 17.6). Widespread ill-defined small rounded opacities are seen predominantly in the upper and mid-zones which may be associated with bilateral hilar lymph node enlargement.

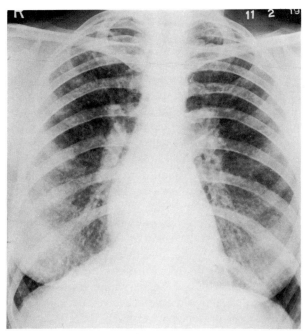

Fig. 17.6 Beryllium disease in a beryllium worker.

Unlike sarcoidosis, hilar lymph node enlargement does not occur in the absence of radiographic evidence of pulmonary involvement, and the hilar lymph nodes are not as enlarged as in sarcoidosis. As in sarcoidosis, linear opacities, due to fibrosis radiating from the hilum, with contraction of upper lobes may develop. Spontaneous resolution of the pulmonary shadows rarely occurs in beryllium disease. The shadows may remain unchanged for several years, but they tend to be progressive. Measurements of lung function show a restrictive ventilatory defect with an impaired carbon monoxide gas transfer test.

Spontaneous pneumothorax has been reported in about 15% of cases of beryllium disease. Hypercalcaemia can also occur, with nephrolithiasis in about 10% of cases. Hepatosplenomegaly has been reported in some 5% of cases.

The diagnosis of beryllium disease is based upon finding the appropriate clinical, radiographic and lung function abnormalities in a patient who has had exposure to beryllium dust or fume, which can have occurred ten or more years in the past. The most important differential diagnosis is from sarcoidosis, which although very similar to beryllium disease, does differ in several important respects. Manifestations of sarcoidosis which do not occur in beryllium disease include uveitis, erythema nodosum and lupus pernio, cystic changes in the bones of the hands and feet and involvement of the salivary and lachrymal glands. Bilateral hilar lymph node enlargement without pulmonary involvement does not occur in beryllium disease, and unlike sarcoidosis spontaneous resolution of radiographic abnormalities is unusual. The tuberculin test is positive in those with beryllium disease as frequently as in the population from which they have come, and the Kveim test is negative. Hyperglobulinaemia with a predominant increase in IgG can occur in both sarcoidosis and beryllium disease. The increased IgG is less likely to be associated with increases in IgA and IgM in beryllium disease than in sarcoidosis.

Beryllium can be estimated quantitatively both in urine and in other tissues, including the lung. Finding beryllium in the urine or in biopsy or postmortem specimens of lung tissue, however, is evidence only of past exposure to beryllium, and not of beryllium disease. Although it is usual to find beryllium in the lungs of those with beryllium disease, there is unfortunately no correlation between the concentration of beryllium in the lungs or urine and the severity of the disease. Furthermore, beryllium may be absent from the urine in those with chronic beryllium disease, and is irregularly distributed in the lungs, and will not necessarily be found in a lung biopsy specimen. However, the presence of beryllium in the lungs of a patient with widespread pulmonary granulomata makes the diagnosis of beryllium disease very likely.

The beryllium patch test, in which a 2% solution of beryllium sulphate or nitrate is applied to the skin of the forearm for 48 hours, should not be performed, as it may provoke an exacerbation of the disease. Other *in vitro* tests of lymphocyte sensitization to beryllium are at present being developed and assessed.

Beryllium disease also requires differentiation from those diseases other than sarcoidosis which produce small round opacities on the chest radiograph (Table 17.2) and from those causing upper lobe fibrosis, which include pulmonary tuberculosis, chronic extrinsic allergic alveolitis and chronic allergic bronchopulmonary aspergillosis.

17.2 Occupational asthma

Occupational asthma is variable airway narrowing causally related to agents inhaled in the working environment. It affects only a proportion (usually a minority) of those exposed to the agents causing the disease and usually develops only after an initial symptom-free period of exposure, which can vary between different individuals from weeks to years. Asthmatic reactions tend to recur on re-exposure to the causal agent at atmospheric concentrations which do not affect others similarly exposed. Although occupational exposures are a relatively infrequent cause of asthma, the recognition of occupational asthma is important. Avoidance of exposure to the causal agent can be followed by complete remission of symptoms and restoration of normal lung function.

A large number of agents to which exposure occurs at work have been reported as causing asthma. Those of most importance in the United Kingdom are listed in Table 17.5, with some of the more common circumstances in which exposure to them occurs. It is to be expected with increasing recognition of occupational asthma, and the continuous introduction of new materials into industrial processes that the number of agents which cause occupational asthma will increase.

Table 17.5   Some causes of occupational asthma

Causal agents	Circumstances of exposure
Biological causes	
B. subtilis enzymes (alcalase etc.)	Enzyme detergent industry
Small mammal urine proteins (rats, mice etc.)	Animal laboratory workers
Grain, flour and their contaminants	Food industry (millers, bakers etc.); farmers
Wood dusts (W. red cedar, Iroko, etc.)	Wood mills, carpenters
Colophony (as soft solder flux)	Electronics industry
Antibiotics (penicillins etc.)	Pharmaceutical industry
Chemical causes	
Di-isocyanates (toluene (TDI), diphenylmethane (MDI), hexamethylene (HDI and naphthalene (NDI))	Polyurethane foam manufacture Printing industry Synthetic paints and rubber adhesives
Epoxy resin curing agents (phthalic anhydride, trimellitic anhydride, triethylene tetramine etc.)	Surface coatings Adhesives
Complex salts of platinum (particularly ammonium hexachlorplatinate)	Platinum refining

The characteristic symptom of occupational asthma is episodic breathlessness, which may be associated with cough, wheezing and chest tightness, temporally related to occupational exposures. Those affected may themselves appreciate that their symptoms develop during the working week, often increasing as the week progresses, improve when away from work such as at weekends or on holidays, and recur on return to work. Symptoms may develop within minutes of exposure (immediate symptoms) or only after an interval of several hours from the onset of exposure (late symptoms). Late symptoms can commence during the latter part of the working day or in the evening after returning home. On occasions, however, symptoms may not be easily recognized as asthmatic and their relationship to occupational exposure is unclear. Breathlessness without wheezing or chest tightness, which varies little from day to day, may persist for several days, or even weeks, after exposure has ceased, and can easily be attributed to the effects of cigarette smoking or bronchial infection. Failure of symptoms to improve over a weekend does not exclude the diagnosis of occupational asthma. Failure to recognize some improvement in symptoms during a two- or three-week holiday, or to appreciate a deterioration on returning to work, is unusual. Patients with occupational asthma often find that in addition to occupational exposures, other stimuli, such as exercise, upper respiratory tract infections and emotional upset also provoke asthmatic reactions.

In general, any patient diagnosed as having occupational asthma should be advised to avoid further exposure to the causal agent. Relocation within the same organization is often possible, but avoiding exposure may mean the loss of current employment. Such advice can only be given where the physician is confident that the patient's symptoms are related to an occupational exposure. Where possible this requires some objective evidence of the relationship. Inhalation testing with the specific agent suspected of causing the disease was developed for this purpose. Such tests, particularly with occupational agents, are potentially hazardous, and should only be conducted by those experienced in their techniques. They are also very demanding on resources: individuals on whom such tests are performed must be admitted to hospital for observation by medical staff for at least 24 hours after testing. Other methods of investigation are increasingly employed: lung function measurements made in relation to periods of occupational exposure are used to demonstrate work-related airway narrowing, and skin tests, where appropriate, to provide evidence of a specific immunological reaction to the putative cause.

When seen away from their place of work, many patients with occupational asthma have either normal lung function or airway narrowing which fails to improve after bronchodilator inhalation. Single pre- and postshift measurements of lung-function may provide evidence of occupational asthma, but are often found to be unhelpful and may be misleading (Fig. 17.7). The most useful method of demonstrating work-related asthma has been shown to be the regular measurement of peak expiratory flow rates, made by the subject himself, over several weeks to include both periods at work and absences from work.

Printer with TDI exposure

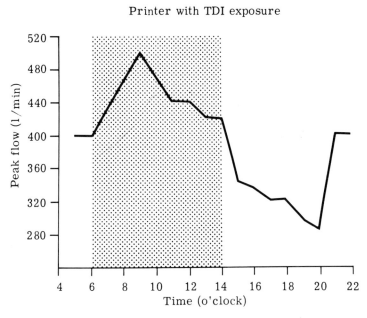

Fig. 17.7 Peak flow measurements recorded before, during and after a day at work in a printer sensitive to TDI. Although the record shows considerable variation in peak flow measurements, with diurnal variation and a late reaction, measurements before and after the working shift would not have shown a decrease in peak flow rates.

The patient is asked to measure his peak flow every two hours from waking to sleeping and record each time the best of three measurements. A minimum record requires two weeks at work with two two-day rest periods. An adequate record for demonstrating the absence of work-related asthma, requires in those with a normal peak flow a two-week period at work which shows a less than 15% diurnal variation. Those with a decreased peak flow require a period at work followed by at least ten days away from work, and a further two-week period at work, to allow identification of those whose recovery is delayed. Prophylactic drugs such as sodium cromoglycate and corticosteroids should not be taken during the period of the record, as these can mask significant changes. The frequency with which other forms of treatment, such as bronchodilators, should be recorded and, if possible, kept constant during days at work and days at home. The mean peak flow for each day should be plotted, together with the maximum and minimum values recorded for that day.

Three different patterns of asthmatic reactions have been described, which seem to depend primarily upon the time taken for recovery, and the cumulative effect of repeated exposures. Such patterns may not always be apparent, particularly where intermittent occupational exposure to the causal agent may be occurring.

1. Equivalent deterioration in peak flow measurements each day. This occurs in those who have a sufficiently rapid recovery after work that the patient returns to work each day with his normal peak flow (Fig. 17.8).

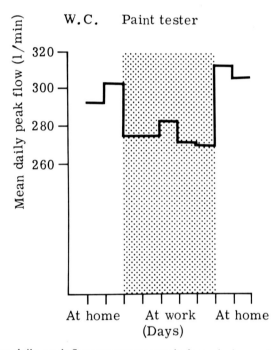

Fig. 17.8 Mean daily peak flow measurements before, during and after a working week in a paint spray tester sensitive to HDI. Record shows equivalent deterioration in mean peak flow rates during each day of the working week, with recovery on first day of weekend.

2. Progressive deterioration in peak flow measurements each day during the working week, with improvement which takes three days or less (Fig. 17.9). The combination of a three-day recovery period with a late reaction on the first day back at work produces a weekly pattern with the first working day as the best of the week ('Monday best' pattern).

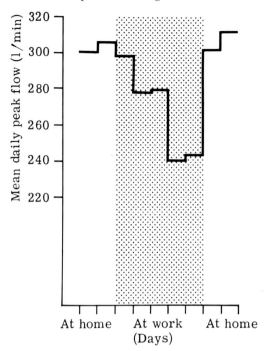

Fig. 17.9 Mean daily peak flow measurements before, during and after a working week in a scientist sensitive to the locusts with which he worked. Record shows progressive deterioration during the working week with return to normal peak flow on the first day of the weekend.

3. Progressive deterioration week by week. This occurs where the period of recovery is greater than three days, and patients return to work at the beginning of each working week without recovery of normal lung function (Fig. 17.10). Week-by-week deterioration in peak flow develops which progresses to a stage of 'fixed' airways obstruction, when the record plateaus. Recovery may not start for up to ten days after last exposure, and can continue for up to three months. This pattern appears to be particularly common in those with occupational asthma due to di-isocyanates and to wood dusts. Asthma may easily not be recognized in patients with this pattern of reaction, which requires an adequate period of recovery to allow symptomatic and functional improvement to occur.

Immediate skin prick test reactions can be elicited in those with occupational asthma due to soluble allergens which provoke an IgE mediated reaction. Such allergens include the *B. subtilis* enzyme, alcalase, the complex platinum salt, ammonium hexachlorplatinate, wheat and rye flour and rat and mouse urine. Unfortunately, the relationship of a positive skin test reaction to disease in those exposed to these agents has with several agents not been investigated. With two allergens, however, rat urine proteins and ammonium hexachlorplatinate, a positive skin prick test reaction to the causal allergen has been found to be a sensitive (few false negatives) and specific (few false positives) index of asthma in those exposed. However, further assessment of the relationship of skin test reactions to disease in those exposed to these and other agents causing occupational asthma will be required before physicians can judge their diagnostic value in individual patients.

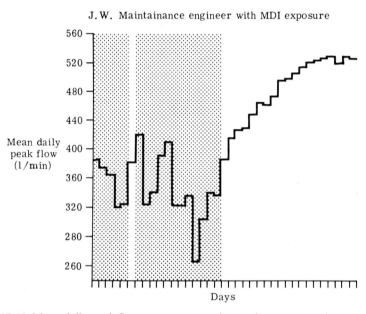

Fig. 17.10 Mean daily peak flow measurements in a maintenance engineer sensitive to MDI. Record shows measurements over 2 periods of 5 and 12 consecutive days at work with 1 day off work between these two periods, followed by a 19-day period away from work. Measurements during working weeks are variable, reflecting intermittent exposures to MDI. Full recovery only reached after 16 days away from work.

Serological tests are at present being developed for identifying specific antibodies to agents which cause occupational asthma. In the past two to three years, methods for demonstrating IgE or IgG antibody or both to TDI, MDI, trimellitic anhydride, phthalic anhydride and ammonium hexachlorplatinate have been reported. If these methods are validated, and the tests can be introduced into clinical practice, the diagnosis of occupational asthma due to these agents may be greatly simplified.

There remain four important indications for inhalation testing: where an individual is suspected of reacting to an agent not as yet recognized as being a cause of occupational asthma; where, as may occur, an individual with work-related asthma is exposed to several well recognized causes of occupational asthma; where genuine doubt remains about the diagnosis of occupational asthma after all other appropriate investigations (including work records of peak flow measurements) have been completed; and where the symptoms experienced at work are of such severity that it is not thought justifiable for the patient to be further exposed to the working environment. Inhalation testing whose sole purpose is in support of a legal claim is, we believe, unjustifiable.

The aim in an inhalation test is to expose the affected individual to a single agent only, in circumstances which resemble as closely as possible the conditions of exposure at work. Unlike exposures at work, exposures of short duration to individual agents in carefully controlled conditions can be carried out in inhalation tests. The exposure concentrations in inhalation tests should be related to the exposures experienced at work, and the physical conditions of exposure, such as the temperature to which materials are heated and the size of dust particles, should be repeated.

Several different methods for inhalation testing with occupational agents have been developed, which depend primarily on the physical state of the different materials. Inhalation of nebulized extracts is used for exposure to extracts of soluble allergens, such as urine and serum proteins. This traditional method of inhalation testing is not applicable to the majority of occupational agents. Liquids, such as TDI and formaldehyde, which are volatile at room temperature, can be painted onto a flat surface in an enclosed space. The atmospheric concentration achieved can be varied by using different concentrations of the material in solution, and measured with an appropriate monitor. Exposure to dusts, such as wood dust, pharmaceutical agents (for example antibiotics) and complex platinum salts can be achieved by asking the patient to tip the material between two trays in an enclosed chamber. Wood dusts can be used without dilution, but antibiotics and complex platinum salts require dilution in dried lactose powder to avoid exposure to excessive atmospheric concentrations. Materials which are heated at work, such as the soft solder flux, colophony, should generally be heated to the same temperatures during the inhalation test, so that exposure will be to similar degradation products.

At least four patterns of asthmatic reaction provoked by inhalation testing may be distinguished. Immediate reactions develop within minutes and improve spontaneously over one to one and a half hours (Fig. 17.11). Late reactions develop an hour or more after exposure, most commonly after an interval of three to four hours, persist for up to 24 to 36 hours before resolving spontaneously. A dual reaction is a late reaction preceded by an

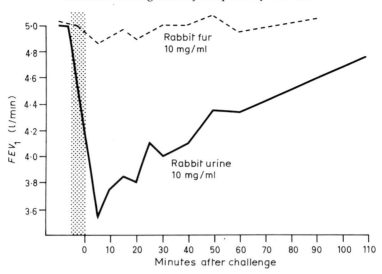

Fig. 17.11 Inhalation test with extracts of rabbit fur and rabbit urine in a laboratory animal worker. Record shows immediate asthmatic reaction provoked by rabbit urine extract.

immediate reaction (Fig. 17.12). Recurrent nocturnal reactions may follow a single exposure of short duration: asthmatic reactions occur during the night waking the patient from sleep, with complete or partial improvement in lung function occurring during the intervening daytimes. Because of these recurrent reactions it is essential that an adequate interval is left between exposures to different agents. This will ensure that any reaction provoked by one agent is not incorrectly attributed to the subsequent exposure to a different agent.

17.3 Byssinosis

Byssinosis is an occupational disease of textile workers, caused by inhalation of the dust emitted during the preparation and cleaning of cotton, flax, and soft hemp fibres, before spinning. It occurs principally in the cotton industry, in the opening and blowing room, cardroom and winding room workers, in those preparing flax in factories manufacturing linen, and in those making ropes and twines from soft hemp. Byssinosis usually only develops after several years of exposure to these dusts, and is more prevalent among cigarette smokers than among non-smokers.

In the early stages of the disease, those affected complain of chest tightness and breathlessness, which develops towards the end of a working shift on the first day back at work after a weekend or holiday absence (often a

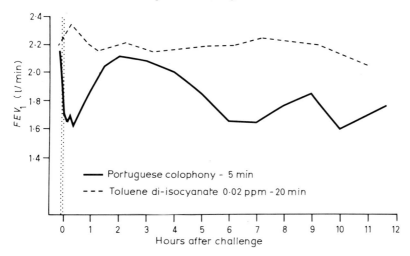

Fig. 17.12 Inhalation testing of an electronics factory employee exposed at work to both TDI and colophony. Record shows no reaction provoked by 20 min exposure to TDI at atmospheric concentrations of 0.02 ppm (threshold limit value), but dual (immediate and late) reaction provoked by exposure to heated Portuguese colophony for 5 min.

Monday). These symptoms resolve spontaneously within a short period of leaving work. No symptoms occur on the Tuesday or subsequent days of the working week, but will recur on returning to work after an absence. With progression of the disease, symptoms increase in severity, and extend into Tuesday and subsequent days of the working week. Eventually, usually after several years, effort dyspnoea develops, with airway narrowing, which persists throughout the working week, and over weekends and holidays. At this stage the disease is indistinguishable from chronic obstructive bronchitis.

Byssinosis does not produce any abnormalities on the chest radiograph and does not cause any specific pathological changes in the lungs. It has therefore to be diagnosed primarily on the characteristic history of respiratory symptoms which in the early stages of the disease are worst at the beginning of the working week. At this early stage, measurements of lung function on the first day back at work after absence will show a fall in FEV_1 across the working shift, of between about 200 and 400 ml. In the later stages of byssinosis, when irreversible airway narrowing has developed, such acute changes do not occur, and the disease can only be distinguished from non-occupational causes of chronic airway narrowing by obtaining a past history of symptoms typical of the disease in its initial stages.

Transient airway narrowing is characteristic of byssinosis in the early stages of the disease, but conventionally byssinosis is distinguished from occupational asthma. Although this distinction may be artificial, byssinosis does differ from other forms of occupational asthma in at least two important respects. Unlike the characteristic 'Monday symptoms' of byssinosis, symptoms and lung function in occupational asthma tend to deteriorate progressively during the working week (*vide supra*). Furthermore, although asthma in those with occupational asthma may persist, despite avoidance of exposure to the causal agent, patients with occupational asthma do not tend to develop the irreversible airway narrowing which is characteristic of the later stages of byssinosis.

17.4 Irritant respiratory reactions

Several gases and fumes, if inhaled in sufficient concentration, can provoke an acute irritant reaction in the airways or alveoli or both. The site of reaction within the respiratory tree is related to the solubility of the gas, and to the dose inhaled. Highly soluble gases such as ammonia dissolve in the upper respiratory tree and are rarely inhaled in sufficient concentration to penetrate into the alveoli. They cause immediate irritation to the eyes, nose, throat and upper airways, and those affected remove themselves rapidly from exposure, thereby minimizing the dose inhaled. Poorly soluble gases such as the oxides of nitrogen (NO_2 and N_2O_4) and phosgene, and fumes such as cadmium and beryllium do not dissolve in the upper respiratory tract, and can penetrate into the alveoli. Immediate irritant symptoms of the eyes, nose, throat and upper airways do not occur and exposure may continue for prolonged periods. With sufficient exposure, pulmonary oedema develops after an interval of up to twelve hours. Chlorine gas is of intermediate solubility. It affects the upper respiratory tract alone after a short-lived exposure to small concentrations of the gas, but pulmonary oedema occurs rapidly after heavier or more prolonged exposures. Exposures to irritant gases or fumes in enclosed or poorly ventilated areas are particularly hazardous.

Hazardous exposures to chlorine gas can occur after an accidental damage to containers in which chlorine is being stored or transported. Exposure to oxides of nitrogen can occur in several different circumstances. Farmers may be affected by the gas generated in silos by the anaerobic fermentation of plant nitrates. These are converted into nitrites, which combine with organic acids to form nitrous acid, which decomposes into nitrogen dioxide. The gas begins to form a few hours after filling the silo, peaks between one and five days, and may persist in toxic concentrations for up to two weeks. Inhalation results in silo fillers' disease. The combination of atmospheric oxygen and nitrogen produced at the high temperatures of electric arc and oxyacetylene welding and oxyacetylene cutting, any operation where nitric acid acts upon a metal, and the detonation of explosives in mines, can also all produce oxides of nitrogen.

Recovery from acute pulmonary oedema after nitrogen dioxide exposure can be followed by a further similar episode, which occurs after an interval of two to six weeks in the absence of any further exposure. The cause of this second reaction is unclear, but may be the result of a secondary infection in previously damaged lungs. In addition to pulmonary oedema, exposure to oxides of nitrogen can cause an obliterative bronchiolitis which may or may not be preceded by attacks of pulmonary oedema. Welders and metal cutters in addition to oxides of nitrogen are particularly at risk from exposure to several other irritant gases and fumes, including cadmium fume when welding or cutting cadmium plated or alloyed metals, and phosgene gas, when welding or cutting metals which have been incompletely dried after degreasing with carbon tetrachloride or trichloroethylene, which decompose to produce phosgene at high temperatures.

Pulmonary oedema, caused by the inhalation of irritant gases and fumes, produces blotchy, homogeneous, often widespread, opacities on the chest radiograph. The normal sized heart, the absence of upper lobe venous distension, and the peripheral rather than perihilar distribution of the shadowing, suggest pulmonary oedema caused by an inhaled irritant rather than by cardiac disease.

Exposure to an irritant gas or fume should be considered particularly as a potential cause of pulmonary oedema in those without evidence of cardiac disease, when a history of exposure to one of the recognized causal agents should be sought.

17.5 Occupational cancer of the lungs and pleura

The risk of developing lung cancer is increased in those occupationally exposed to a number of different materials. Lung cancers caused by occupational exposures have no specific features which allow them to be distinguished from lung cancers not so caused. Attributing lung cancer in an individual to a specific occupational exposure has therefore to be a judgement of reasonable probability, which is based on a knowledge of the patient's occupational history. The latent interval between the onset of exposure and the development of lung cancer is usually in excess of twenty years. A history of all employments since leaving school, and, where possible, of the materials to which exposure occurred during each employment, has to be obtained if any potential occupational cause of a lung cancer is to be identified.

The more commonly recognized occupational causes of lung cancer are listed in Table 17.6 with some of the circumstances in which exposure to them can occur. Of these the most important contemporary cause is asbestos, which in addition to causing lung cancer can also cause pleural and peritoneal, mesothelioma. Although asbestosis and lung cancer are independent risks of asbestos exposure, they are caused by similar levels of asbestos exposure. They therefore frequently coexist, and where this occurs it is reasonable to attribute the lung cancer, in addition to the pulmonary fibreosis, to the asbestos exposure. Lung cancer which may be attributable to asbestos exposure also occurs in those without asbestosis, but asbestos exposure cannot be identified as the cause of the lung cancer in this situation with as much confidence as in those with coexisting asbestosis. Asbestos exposure is associated with an increased risk of developing lung cancer in non-smokers, but the risk of developing lung cancer in those exposed to asbestos is greatly increased in cigarette smokers.

Table 17.6 Some causes of occupational lung cancer

Cause	Circumstances of exposure
Asbestos (all fibre types)	Asbestos miners and millers
	Asbestos textile and product manufacturers
	Asbestos insulation workers (laggers, strippers and sprayers)
Irradiation	Uranium miners
	Cumberland haematite miners
Coal tar (benzpyrene)	Coke oven workers
Nickel (? nickel subsulphide)	Nickel refiners
Arsenic	Arsenical sheep dip manufacturers
	Copper smelters
	(arsenic contaminates copper ore)
Chromates	Manufacture of bichromates from chromite ore
Bischloromethyl ether	Ion exchange resin manufacturers

Whereas the risk of developing lung cancer is increased in those exposed to all types of asbestos fibre, the risk of developing a mesothelioma is a particular hazard of exposure to the amphiboles, crocidolite and amosite. Exposure to asbestos sufficient to cause a mesothelioma is usually substantial but is generally of shorter duration than that necessary to cause lung cancer and asbestosis. Furthermore, the latent interval from initial asbestos exposure to the development of a mesothelioma is between twenty and fifty years. Many of those who are now developing mesotheliomas were exposed to asbestos in World War II in the naval dockyards or in the manufacture of gas masks. Exposures which can be of relatively short duration and latent intervals of up to fifty years can on occasions make it difficult to identify an asbestos exposure responsible for a mesothelioma. Mesotheliomas present with breathlessness, due to the accumulation of effusion in the pleural space, or with chest pain from invasion by the tumour of the chest wall. Evidence of pleural effusion, irregular nodular protuberances of the pleura, and ipsilateral contraction of the hemithorax may be seen on the chest radiograph. The diagnosis is made histologically. Two histological patterns can be distinguished: tumours with spindle-shaped cells, and tumours with glandular-like structures. The glandular pattern has to be differentiated from an adenocarcinoma involving the pleura. Adenocarcinomas may secrete a PAS positive glycoprotein. Mesotheliomas can secrete hyaluronic acid which is stained with Alcan Blue (prior incubation with hyaluronidase eliminates this reaction). Unfortunately the majority of both of these tumours secrete neither.

17.6 Summary

Exposure to agents in the working environment can cause a wide spectrum of lung diseases, which include asthma, alveolitis, fibrosis and cancer. Where there are no manifestations of the disease which are specific to an occupational cause, the diagnosis can only be a judgement based on reasonable probability. This demands a knowledge of the different manifestations of occupational lung diseases, the degree and circumstances of exposure which are sufficient to cause the diseases, and the non-occupational diseases from which they must be distinguished. Diagnosis can only be more certain if specific features of a disease can be identified, or where the relationship between the disease and occupational exposure can be validated in the individual.

Further reading

Advisory Committee on Asbestos, (1979), *Asbestos*, Final report, Vols 1 and 2, HMSO.
Becklake, M. R. (1976), Asbestos related diseases of the lung and other organs: their epidemiology and implications for clinical practice. *Am. Rev. resp. Dis.,* **114**, 187.
Burge, P. S., O'Brien, I. M. and Harries, M. G. (1979), Peak flow records in the diagnosis of occupational asthma due to colophony. *Thorax*, **34**, 308.
Burge, P. S., O'Brien, I. M. and Harries, M. G. (1979), Peak flow records in the diagnosis of occupational asthma due to isocyanates. *Thorax*, **34**, 317.
Davies, R. S. and Pepys, J. (1977), Occupational asthma, In: *Asthma*, (eds T. J. H. Clark and S. C. Godfrey, Chapman and Hall, London.
Morgan, W. K. C. and Lapp, N. L. (1976), Respiratory disease in coal miners. *Am. Rev. resp. Dis.*, **113**, 531.
Muir, D. C. F. (ed.), *Clinical Aspects Of Inhaled Particles* William Heinemann, London.

Pepys, J. and Hutchcroft, B. S. (1975), Bronchial provocation tests in etiologic diagnosis and analysis of asthma. *Am. Rev. resp. Dis.* **112**, 829.
Pneumoconiosis and related occupational diseases. Notes on diagnosis and claims for industrial injuries scheme benefits (1979), HMSO
Rogan, J. M. (ed), (1972), *Medicine In The Mining Industries* William Heinemann, London.
Ziskind, M., Jones, R. J. and Weill, H. (1976), Silicosis. *Am. Rev. resp. Dis.*, **113**, 643.

References

1. Parkes, W. R. (1974), *Occupational Lung Disorders*, Butterworths, London.
2. Cochrane, A. C. (1962), The attack rate of progressive massive fibrosis. *Br. J. indust. Med.*, **19**, 52.
3. Caplan, A. (1953) Certain unusual radiological appearances in the chest of coal miners suffering from rheumatoid arthritis. *Thorax*, **8**, 29.

Nomenclature

Spirometric units

BLI	bronchial lability index
epp	equal pressure point
f_c	cardiac frequency
f_r	breathing frequency
FET	forced expired time
FEV_1, FEV_2 . . .	forced expired volume in one second, in two seconds, etc.
FIV_1, FIV_2 . . .	forced inspired volume in one second, in two seconds, etc.
FRC	functional residual capacity
FVC	forced vital capacity
MVV	maximum voluntary ventilation
PEF	peak expiratory flow
R_{AW}	airway resistance
RV	residual volume
SG_{AW}	specific airway conductance
TLC	total lung capacity
V_s	stroke volume
VC	vital capacity

Gas-exchange units

(See Piiper, J., Dejours, P., Haab, P. and Rahn, H. (1971) Concepts and basic quantities in gas exchange physiology. *Respir. Physiol.*, **13**, 292–300.)

C	mass concentration of gas in liquid
D	diffusion factor
$\dot{D}$	diffusion in unit time
$DLCO$	mass transfer of CO per unit of pressure gradient per unit time for the lung as a whole (sometimes written $D_L CO$)
FX	fractional concentration of gas X

F_EX	fractional concentration of gas X in expired air
F_IX	fractional concentration of gas X in inspired air
G	conductance of a route for a substance ($d\dot{M}/dP$)
KCO	mass transfer of CO per unit time per unit of pressure gradient per litre of accessible gas in the lung
M	mass of a gas (mol)
$\dot{M}$	mass flow of a gas (mol/min)
P	pressure
PX	partial pressure of gas X
Q	quantity of blood
$\dot{Q}$	blood flow
$\dot{Q}_s$	anatomical shunt blood flow
R	respiratory exchange ratio at lips
RQ	true metabolic respiratory quotient in the tissues
V	volume of gas
$\dot{V}$	volume flow of a gas
	expressed STPD it is a mass flow ($\dot{M}$)
	expressed BTPS it is a volume flow
β	capacitance of compartment for a substance (dM/dP)

Subscripts

(Capitals refer to the gas phase, lower case to the blood or tissue phases. A bar over any subscript denotes a mixture.)

a	arterial
A	alveolar
b	blood
c	capillary, or cardiac
c$'$	end capillary
D	dead space
E	expired air
Ē	mixed expired air
i	inorganic
I	inspired air
Ī	mixed inspired air
L	whole lung
m	mouth
p	pleural, or pulmonary
r	recoil
t	tissue, or total
T	tidal, or total
v	venous
v̄	mixed venous

Index